Third Edition

Platinum Notes

Surgical Sciences (2012–13)

Volume–3

- Surgery
- Orthopedics
- ENT
- Obstetrics & Gynecology
- Ophthalmology
- Anesthesiology

Ashfaq Ul Hassan MBBS MS
Lecturer Anatomy
SKIMS Medical College Bemina,
Srinagar, Jammu and Kashmir
India

JAYPEE BROTHERS MEDICAL PUBLISHERS (P) LTD
New Delhi • Panama City • London

Published by
Jaypee Brothers Medical Publishers (P) Ltd

Corporate Office
4838/24 Ansari Road, Daryaganj, **New Delhi** - 110002, India
Phone: +91-11-43574357, Fax: +91-11-43574314

Offices in India
- **Ahmedabad**, e-mail: ahmedabad@jaypeebrothers.com
- **Bengaluru**, e-mail: bangalore@jaypeebrothers.com
- **Chennai**, e-mail: chennai@jaypeebrothers.com
- **Delhi**, e-mail: jaypee@jaypeebrothers.com
- **Hyderabad**, e-mail: hyderabad@jaypeebrothers.com
- **Kochi**, e-mail: kochi@jaypeebrothers.com
- **Kolkata**, e-mail: kolkata@jaypeebrothers.com
- **Lucknow**, e-mail: lucknow@jaypeebrothers.com
- **Mumbai**, e-mail: mumbai@jaypeebrothers.com
- **Nagpur**, e-mail: nagpur@jaypeebrothers.com

Overseas Offices
- **Central America Office, Panama City, Panama,** Ph: 001-507-317-0160
  e-mail: cservice@jphmedical.com, Website: www.jphmedical.com
- **Europe Office, UK,** Ph: +44 (0) 2031708910, e-mail: info@jpmedpub.com

Platinum Notes: Surgical Sciences (2012-13) (Volume–3)

First Edition: **2010**
Second Edition: **2011**
Third Edition: **2012**

ISBN : 978-93-5025-918-4

Typeset at JPBMP typesetting unit

Printed in India by Gopsons Papers Ltd.

Contributors

Ghulam Hassan MBBS MS
Ex-Prof and Head
Anatomy, GMC, Srinagar

Zahida Rasool MBBS
Medical Consultant
IUST Awantipora, Kashmir

Muneeb Ul Hassan MBBS
Assistant Surgeon
Directorate of Health Services Kashmir

Shabinul Hassan BDS
Resident SKIMS Soura

Life so short, the art so long...-Hippocrates

Preface

The news of **NEET** and changing pattern of the Examinations of **AIPG, AIIMS, DNB** and state level exams prompt me to introduce new changes with new ideas and new topics for the third edition of Platinum notes.

I am hence once again pleased to present a newer, more simplified, interesting, easy, palatable, lucid and High yield book for the Medical students.

After an excellent positive feedback and unexpected success of the First Edition and Second Edition of Platinum Notes, I am pleased to again update Platinum notes and present the Third Edition of Platinum Notes.

It gave me immense pleasure and satisfaction to read the comments for my book from students all over the country.

The book because of its contents and the amount of concentrated knowledge contained in it has been not only been able to compete but also surpass its counterparts. This gives me immense satisfaction taking into account that Platinum has been able to achieve a great place during its first edition only and I would provide my little amount of wisdom hopefully annually updating Platinum on yearly basis to tailor the book to the needs of Medical students.

A Substantial feedback from students especially preparing for AIPGE Examinations has prompted me to bring this third edition best suited for this examination and I would thank the appreciators of my book for all their comments. But at the same time I would be more thankful to the critics who pointed out certain deficiencies in my first edition and due to their healthy criticism I have been able to add what was deficient.

I thank medical students from all over India especially the students of Maharashtra, Rajasthan, Delhi, Karnataka, Tamil Nadu, Uttar Pradesh, Bihar, Kerala, Kolkata and Jharkhand for their feedback. In the first instance I would not have expected the response but thanks to Almighty for everything.

I would like to express great satisfaction at my personal level as to the feedback of students appearing for AIIMS, PGI, DNB, UPSC for their continuous feedback via emails.

I would like to express my apology to all those students to whose queries I could not respond via email. I hope you will continue guiding me similarly in future as well.

Wishing you a good academic career.

Ashfaq Ul Hassan

Acknowledgments

No word would be sufficient to thank the **Almighty** for all the necessary guidance and courage he provided me throughout my life and especially for preparation of this project and blessings to **Prophet Muhammad** (PBUH).

I would firstly like to express my special gratitude to my parents particularly my father **Prof Ghulam Hassan,** Ex-Prof and Head, Anatomy, GMC Srinagar who has been a role academic model to me and provided me guidance, necessary facilities and most of all good wishes. Without his guidance and support I would not have been able to accomplish this task. As a consequence of constant interaction with him, I have learnt the maximum in my life.

I would like to take this as an opportunity to thank my academically brilliant and favorite teachers from whom I have imbibed a lot. I would wholeheartedly like to express my thanks to my seniors, academically brilliant colleagues who have laid a major emphasis on my life. I personally and whole heartedly acknowledge the following:

- Prof Ghulam Hassan MS Ex-Prof and Head, Department of Anatomy, GMC Srinagar
- Prof Showqat Zargar Prof and Head Gastroenterology Department/Director SKIMS, Soura
- Prof AR Trag Vice Chancellor, IUST, Awantipora
- Prof GQ Allaqaband MD Ex-Principal, Ex Head Deptt of Medicine, GMC/SMHS Srinagar
- Prof Nelofer Geelani, Vice Principal SKIMS Medical College SKIMS Bemina
- Dr Sheikh Aijaz Additional Professor Surgery, SKIMS Soura
- Prof Mehraj Din Ex Director SKIMS Soura
- Prof Saleh Al Damegh, Director Al Raji Group of Colleges, KSA
- Prof Abdullah Al Gasham Dean Al Qasim University, KSA
- Prof Khursheed Iqbal Dean DM Cardiology, SKIMS Soura
- Prof AH Ahanger HOD CVTS SKIMS, Soura
- Prof Syed Amin Tabish, Head Hospital Adminstration, SKIMS Soura
- Prof AH Zargar Prof and Head Endocrinology, Ex-Director SKIMS, Soura
- Prof Pervez Shah DM Neurology, SMHS Hospital Srinagar
- Dr Tanveer Masood MD Professor, Medicine, SMHS Srinagar
- Prof Riyaz Unthoo MBBS MS, Head of The Department Opthomology, SKIMS Bemina
- Dr Arshad Farooq MBBS MD Paediatrics, SKIMS Bemina
- Dr Masood Kirmani MBBS MS Head of The Department, ENT, SKIMS, Bemina
- Dr Khursheed MBBS MD Head Microbiology, SKIMS Bemina
- Dr Rashid MBBS MD Head Pathology, SKIMS, Bemina
- Dr Manzoor, Consultant Dermatology, SKIMS Bemina
- Dr Rifat MBBS MD, Head Obstetrics/Gynaecology, SKIMS Bemina
- Prof Anil Bhan MS Mch CVTS Surgeon, Med City, Gurgaon, Delhi
- Prof Sameer Kaul Consultant Oncologist, New Delhi
- Dr Sajjad Reshi MRCP Interventional, Cardiologist, Cardiff, UK
- Dr Sunil Munshi MRCP Consultant Leicster General Hospital, Leicester, UK
- Dr AY Izideen MRCS Consultant Surgeon, Prince Charles Hospital, UK
- Dr Manzoor Dar MS MRCS, UK
- Dr Maki Alvi Ashraf, MRCOG Consultant Gynaecologist, UK
- Prof Altaf MS MRCS, Prince Charles Hospital, UK
- Prof RN Bargotra, Ex-Prof and Head, GMC, Jammu
- Dr RD Mehra Prof, Department of Anatomy, AIIMS, New Delhi

- Prof Showqat Jeelani Head Surgery Department, SMHS, Srinagar
- Dr Asif MBBS MS, Consultant ENT, SKIMS Bemina
- Dr Riyaz Malik MBBS MD, Lecturer, Paediatrics, SKIMS Bemina
- Dr Farhana Ahad Pukhta, Lecturer Physiology, SKIMS Medical College Bemina
- Dr Nusrat MBBS MS Lecturer, Opthomology, SKIMS Bemina
- Dr Ashfaq Bhat MBBS MD Lecturer SPM, SKIMS, Bemina
- Dr Afiya MBBS MD Pathology, Lecturer SKIMS Bemina
- Dr Sajid Wani MBBS Tutor Demonstrator, Microbiology, SKIMS Bemina
- Dr Talib Khan Lecturer Anesthesiology, SMHS Srinagar

Special Mention of My Favorite, Academically Brilliant Teachers

- Prof Ghulam Hassan Ex-Prof and Head Anatomy GMC Srinagar
- Prof Pervez Shah MD DM Neurology, SMHS Srinagar
- Dr Tanveer Masood MD Associate Prof, Medicine, SMHS Srinagar
- Dr Rouf Ahamed MS Prof ENT Department SMHS Srinagar
- (Late) Dr Tajamul Assistant Surgeon Medicine, SMHS Srinagar
- Mr TN Kaul Teacher CMS, Tyndale Biscoe School, Srinagar

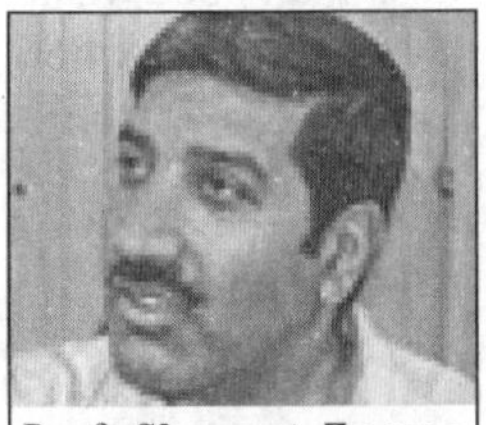
Prof. **Showqat Zargar**

"I am extremely obliged to Prof Showqat Zargar *MBBS MD DM* ***Director and Head Department of Gastroenterology SKIMS, Soura for his help, support and moral boosting approach, guidance for this project and allowing me to be a Member and a part of SKIMS fraternity."***

No words to express my gratitude to **Dr Zahida Rasool**, Medical Consultant for her help in contributing their academic skills and all needed support help for every part during the preparation of this book. Her idea and effort at adding vital information and latest topics has been a real help.

The acceptance of my work by **Shri Jitendar P Vij** (Chairman and Managing Director) and overall incharge of Jaypee Brothers Medical Publishers (P) Ltd. and his interest and overall supervision of the whole project deserves special thanks.

I would specially like to express my renewed gratitude and thanks to **Mr Bhupesh Arora** (General Manager) Jaypee Brothers Medical Publishers (P) Ltd. for his improved suggestions for third edition. His constant help, guidance and exhaustive interaction throughout the course of preparation of this book has been of immense help. It has taken long, interactive and detailed sessions between both of us which have helped in making the project a success. I admire the working ability and highly professional attitude of this gentle man.

I would like to thank **Manas Yadav & Tahira Parveen** for all expertise at printing and giving the final look of the book and working really hard on the project. His effort at final formatting of the book has been commendable.

Author /Editor in Chief:

Ashfaq Ul Hassan

I would like suggestions from the readers of this book, not only for improving the quality of the book but also for aiding all future candidates in their career.

Contact: *ashhassan@rediffmail.com*

From the Publisher's Desk

We request all the readers to provide us their valuable suggestions/errors (if any) at: jaypeemcqproduction@gmail.com

so as to help us in further improvement of this book in the subsequent edition.

Abbreviations

1°	Primary
2°	Secondary
#	Fracture
ACE	Angiotensin converting enzyme
ACE-I	Angiotensin converting enzyme inhibitor
ACTH	Adrenocorticotropic hormone
ACh	Acetylcholine
Adr	Adrenaline
AD	Autosomal dominant
ADH	Anti-diuretic hormone
AF	Atrial fibrillation
AFB	Acid-fast bacilli
AFP	Alpha-fetoprotein
A.k.a	Also known as
ALL	Acute lymphocytic leukemia
AML	Acute myelogenous leukemia
ANA	Antinuclear antibody
ANS	Autonomic nervous system
AP	Anteroposterior
AR	Autosomal recessive
ARDS	Acute respiratory distress syndrome
ARF	Acute renal failure
AS	Aortic stenosis
ATP	Adenosine triphosphate
ASD	Atrial septal defect
AV	Atrioventricular
A/E	All except
Acc/ to	According to
Ad/E, ad/e	Adverse effects
A/W or a/w	Associated with
BBB	Bundle branch block
bid	Twice a day
BMR	Basal metabolic rate
BP	Blood pressure
BPH	Benign prostatic hypertrophy
BUN	Blood urea nitrogen
B/L	Bilateral
BM	Bone marrow, basement membrane
b/n or b/w	Between
C/S	Culture and sensitivity
Ca2+	Calcium
CABG	Coronary artery bypass graft
CAD	Coronary artery disease
CCF	Congestive cardiac failure
CT	Computerized tomography
CHF	Congestive heart failure
CHO	Carbohydrate
CML	Chronic myelogenous leukemia
CMV	Cytomegalovirus
CN	Cranial nerves
CNS	Central nervous system
CO	Cardiac output
C/O	Complaining of
COLD	Chronic obstructive lung disease
COPD	Chronic obstructive pulmonary disease
CPK	Creatine phosphokinase
CRF	Chronic renal failure
CRP	C-reactive protein

CSF	Cerebrospinal fluid	**EUA**	Examination under anesthesia.
CVA	Cerebrovascular accident	**FBS**	Fasting blood sugar
CVP	Central venous pressure	**FEV**	Forced expiratory volume
CVS	Cardiovascular system	**FFP**	Fresh frozen plasma
CXR	Chest X-ray	**FRC**	Functional residual capacity
Ca	Carcinoma/Cancer	**FTT**	Failure to thrive
C/c	Complication	**FVC**	Forced vital capacity
C_T	Chemotherapy	**FA**	Fatty acid
C/I	Contraindication	**FFA**	Free fatty acid
Cl/f	Clinical features	**GFR**	Glomerular filtration rate
CTD	Connective tissue disease	**GH**	Growth hormone
Cont./L	Contralateral	**GIT**	Gastrointestinal tract
Cx	Cervix	**GTT**	Glucose tolerance test
D and C	Dilation and curettage	**GU**	Genitourinary
DI	Diabetes insipidus	**HAV**	Hepatitis A virus
DIC	Disseminated intravascular coagulopathy	**HCG**	Human chorionic gonadotropin
DIP	Distal interphalangeal joint	**HDL**	High density lipoprotein
DKA	Diabetic ketoacidosis	**Hb**	Hemoglobin
dL	Deciliter	**HIV**	Human immunodeficiency virus
DM	Diabetes mellitus	**HLA**	Histocompatibility locus antigen
DTR	Deep tendon reflexes	**H/O**	History of
DVT	Deep venous thrombosis	**HR**	Heart rate
d/to	Due to	**HSV**	Herpes simplex virus
D/g	Diagnosis	**HTN**	Hypertension
DOC	Drug of choice	**HS**	Hereditary cpherocytosis
Ds, d/s	Disease, disease	**HCC**	Hepato cellular carcinoma
DM	Diabeties mellitus	**HD**	Hodgkin's cisease
ECG	Electrocardiogram	**I and D**	Incision and drainage
ECT	Electroconvulsive therapy	**IDDM**	Insulin dependent diabetes mellitus
ECHO	Echocardiography	**Ig**	Immunoglobulin
EMG	Electromyogram	**IM**	Intramuscular
EOM	Extraocular muscles	**INR**	International normalized ratio
ESR	Erythrocyte sedimentation rate	**ITP**	Idiopathic thrombocytopenic purpura
ERCP	Endoscopic retrograde cholangio-pancreatography	**IV**	Intravenous
		IVP	Intravenous pyelogram

IVU	Intravenous urogram
ICT	Intracranial tension
IOC	Investigation of choice
ILD	Interstitial lung disease
IOT	Intraocular tension
Ipsi/L	Ipsilateral
JVP	Jugular venous pressure
K+	Potassium
K/as	Known as
LAE	Left atrial enlargement
LBBB	Left bundle branch block
LDH	Lactate dehydrogenase
LMN	Lower motor neuron
LE	Lupus erythematosus
LP	Lumbar puncture
LV	Left ventricle
LVH	Left ventricular hypertrophy
LN	Lymph node
MAO	Monoamine oxidase
MEN	Multiple endocrine neoplasia
MI	Myocardial infarction or mitral insufficiency
mL	Milliliter
MMR	Measles, mumps, rubella
MRI	Magnetic resonance imaging
MRSA	Methicillin resistant staph aureus
MG	Myasthenia gravis
Mc or MC	Most common
MN	Malnutrition
M/m	Management
Ms, m/s	Muscle
Na	Sodium
NIDDM	Non-insulin dependent diabetes mellitus
NSAID	Non-steroidal anti-inflammatory drugs
n.or nv	Nerve
NHL	Non-Hodgkin's lymphoma
OCG	Oral cholecystogram
PA	Posteroanterior
PDA	Patent ductus arteriosus
PMN	Polymorphonuclear leukocyte (neutrophil)
PP	Patient profile
PT	Prothrombin time, or physical therapy
PTCA	Percutaenous transluminal coronary angioplasty
PTH	Parathyroid hormone
PTT	Partial thromboplastin time
P/g	Prognosis
P_x	Prophylaxis
PBC	Primary bilary cirrhosis
RA	Rheumatoid arthritis
RBBB	Right bundle branch block
RBC	Red blood cell
RIA	Radioimmunoassay
RNA	Ribonucleic acid
RTA	Renal tubular acidosis
RVH	Right ventricular hypertrophy
Rx	Treatment
R, or T/t	Treatment
R_T	Radiotherapy
SBE	Subacute bacterial endocarditis
SGOT	Serum glutamic-oxaloacetic transaminase
SGPT	Serum glutamic-pyruvic transaminase
SIADH	Syndrome of inappropriate antidiuretic hormone
SLE	Systemic lupus erythematous
SCLC	Small cell lung carcinoma
SM	Smooth muscle
Supf.	Superficial
SqCC	Squamous cell carcinoma
TIBC	Total iron binding capacity
tid	Three times a day
TSH	Thyroid stimulating hormone
TT	Thrombin time

TTP	Thrombotic thrombocytopenic purpura
TURP	Transurethral resection of prostate
TOC	Treatment of choice
UC	Ulcerative colitis
UMN	Upper motor neuron
URI	Upper respiratory infection
US, U/S	Ultrasound
UTI	Urinary tract infection
UVA	Ultraviolet A light
U/L	Unilateral
VF	Ventricular fibrillation
VDRL	Venereal disease research laboratory (test for syphilis)
V/Q	Ventrilation-perfusion
VT	Ventricular tachycardia
vWD	von Willebrand's virus
VZV	Varicella zoster virus
V/s	Vessel
Vs	Versus (= against)
WBC	White blood cell
WPW	Wolff-Parkinson-White
WG	Wegner's granulomatosis
WT	Wilm's tumor
XLR	X linked recessive
Yr	Year
Zn	Zinc
ZES	Zollinger Ellison Syndrome
——	Reaction block by, inhibited by
~	Denotes heading
!	Increase

Contents

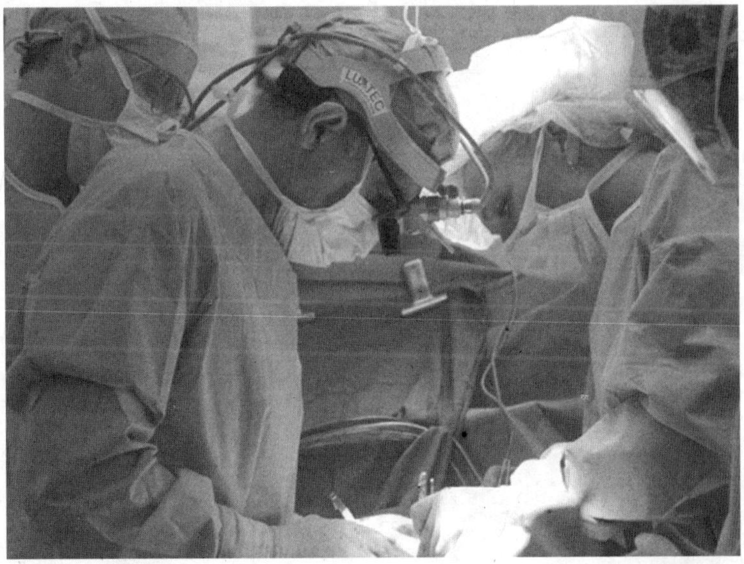

SURGERY

➲ Vascular Surgery

⇨ Hemorrhage

Primary Hemorrhage

Primary Hemorrhage occurs at the time of injury or operation.

Reactionary Hemorrhage

Reactionary hemorrhage may follow primary hemorrhage within 24 hours (usually 4–6 hours) and is mainly due to

- **Rolling ('slipping') of a ligature,**
- Dislodgement of a clot or cessation of reflex vasospasm.

The precipitating circumstances are: (1) the rise in blood pressure and the refilling of the venous system on recovery from shock; and (2) restlessness, coughing and vomiting which raise the venous pressure (e.g. reactionary venous Hemorrhage within a few hours of thyroidectomy).

Secondary Hemorrhage

Secondary hemorrhage occurs after 7–14 days, and is due to infection and sloughing of part of the wall of an artery.

Predisposing factors are:

- Pressure of a drainage tube,
- A fragment of bone,
- A ligature in an infected area or cancer.

Secondary hemorrhage is prone to occur with anorectal wounds, for example after hemorrhoidectomy.

- <u>**Hypovolemic Shock:**</u> Hypovolemic shock occurs from **hemorrhagic losses, such as with trauma, gastrointestinal bleeding, or ruptured aneurysms, or from plasma volume losses.** Shock arising from plasma volume losses may be due to extravascular fluid sequestration, as might occur in **pancreatitis, burns, and bowel obstruction, or it may arise from excessive gastrointestinal, renal, or insensible fluid losses and multiple organ dysfunction.** **DNB 2011**
- Multiple organ failure is the most common cause of death in intensive care units. More recently, it has become increasingly clear that noninfectious insults, such **as trauma, pancreatitis, burns, and massive transfusions, may produce a syndrome of multiple organ dysfunctions.**
- **The concept of shock has evolved over the centuries from the earliest descriptions in antiquity of traumatic wounds and hemorrhage. Hippocrates (460-380 B.C.) recognized certain principles of wound care, such as elevating a wounded extremity and applying various extracts to a bleeding wound to effect coagulation, but the correlation between blood loss and death had not yet been made. The appearance of a patient in shock or other preterminal conditions was described and has been referred to as Hippocratic facies, the presence of which signaled imminent death.** **KCET 2012**

➲ Vascular Malformations: High Yield for AIPGMEE, AIIMS, PGI 2012/2013

- **Hemangioma:** Are malformations of developing blood vessels. They commonly appear in the skin but may develop in any organ.

- **Strawberry Naevus:**
  - ✓ Usually appear at about a week of age and may rapidly enlarge in the first few months of life.
  - ✓ Usually **resolve spontaneously** by intravascular thrombosis. **JK BOPEE**
  - ✓ This process is normally complete by 5-7 years of age leaving only a minor blemish or none at all.
- **Stork Mark:** Is a superficial capillary hemangioma which may be seen on the forehead, bridge of the nose and upper eyelids. The lesion is often v-shaped pointing down to the nose and there is a corresponding mark on the nape of the neck.
- **Port-wine Stain (Naevus Flammeus):**
  - ✓ Unlike a strawberry naevus this is present at birth and may be very disfiguring, as it becomes darker and increasingly nodular with age.
  - ✓ **Persists (P for P)** **DNB 2003**
- **Sturge-Weber Syndrome**
  - ✓ Is a severe form of port wine stain on the scalp and face, in the distribution of one of the branches of the **trigeminal nerve**, associated with an underlying vascular anomaly of the arachnoid covering the cerebral hemisphere.
  - ✓ This leads to **epilepsy, hemiplegia and mental retardation.** **AIIMS 2004**
- **Cavernous Hemangioma:**

These may occur alone or in association with a capillary lesion in the overlying skin. They increase in size after birth but usually in proportion to the growth of the infant. Most resolve spontaneously but some persist requiring excision.

Vascular Ectasias

— **Vascular ectasias are common lesions characterized by local dilation of preexisting vessels; they are not true neoplasms.**

Spider Telangiectasia

— This **non-neoplastic vascular lesion grossly resembles a spider**; there is a radial, often pulsatile array of dilated subcutaneous arteries or arterioles (resembling legs) about a central core (resembling a body) that blanches when pressure is applied to its center.

— It is commonly seen on the face, neck, or upper chest and is most frequently associated with **hyperestrogenic states such as pregnancy or cirrhosis**

Hereditary Hemorrhagic Telangiectasia (Osler-Weber-Rendu Disease)

— In this autosomal dominant disorder, the telangiectasias are malformations composed of dilated capillaries and veins.

— Present from birth, they are widely distributed over the skin and oral mucous membranes, as well as in the respiratory, GI, and urinary tracts. Occasionally, these lesions rupture, causing serious epistaxis (nosebleeds), GI bleeding, or hematuria.

Hemangiopericytomas:

- Are rare tumors derived from pericytes-myofibroblast-like cells that are normally arranged around capillaries and venules.
- Hemangiopericytomas can occur as slowly enlarging, painless masses at any anatomic site, but they are most common on the lower extremities (especially the thigh) and in the retroperitoneum.
- They consist of numerous branching capillary channels and gaping sinusoidal spaces enclosed within nests of spindle-shaped to round cells. The tumors may recur after excision, and roughly half metastasize, usually hematogenously to lungs, bone, or liver.

⇨ Kasabach-Merritt Syndrome

Hemangiomas **associated with a generalized bleeding disorder caused by the trapping of platelets within them which produces a profound** thrombocytopenia. COMED 2007

Several **Types of vascular tumors** have been associated with this syndrome such as.

- **Capillary/cavernous hemangiomas**
- **Infantile hemangioendothelioma**
- **Kaposiform hemangioendothelioma**
- **Lymphangioma,**
- **Tufted angioma**

Patients are at risk of bleeding complications including intracranial hemorrhage. PGI 2009

Certain medications used include

- Corticosteroids
- Alpha-interferon
- Chemotherapy (e.g. vincristine)
- Radiation therapy

⇨ Lymphangioma

- ✓ Are similar to hemangiomas but involve lymphatics. They may also occur anywhere in the body but in particular they may present as a cystic hygroma
- ✓ Most commonly arising in the cervical region

⇨ Cystic Hygroma

This developmental lymphangioma is derived from the primitive embryonic jugular venolymphatic sacs complete excision is the therapy of choice; however, this is not always possible, as the mass may be more solid in nature and infiltrate structures such as the tongue or pharynx. The cystic form is frequently intimately adherent to vital structures (e.g., vagus nerve, phrenic nerve) that should not be sacrificed.

- ✓ **Sclerosing agents,** PGI 2011
- ✓ **Ateroid injection,**
- ✓ **Irradiation**
- ✓ **Injection of a bleomycin-fat emulsion or**
- ✓ **Intralesional streptococcal lysin**
- ✓ **Excision** PGI 2011

⇨ Klippel Trenauny Syndrome:

- Congenital AV fistulas
- Hemangiomas
- Varicose veins
- Hypertrophy of limbs

Aneurysms: Important Points for 2011/2012

The most common type of "**true aneurysm**" is fusiform type.	
The most common site of **arterial aneurysm** is Infra renal part of Abdominal Aorta.	
Popliteal Aneurysms are the **most common Peripheral** aneurysms.	
The most common site for **dissecting aneurysms** is Ascending Aorta.	
MC Causeof AAA IS A: Abdominal Aortic Aneurysm is Atherosclerosis.	**AI 1996**
"**Cirsoid aneurysms**" are common in superficial temporal artery.	**PGI 1988**

Types of Aneurysms

- **Berry aneurysm:** occurs in circle of willis
- **Micro aneurysms:** seen in Diabetes and Hypertension
- **Mycotic aneurysms:** are seen in **bacterial** infections.
- **Aortic dissecting Aneurysms:** Due to degeneration of tunica media. Occur in Marfans Syndrome and Hypertension.
- **Syphilitic aneurysms or Luetic aneurysms:** involve ascending Aorta
- **Pseudoaneurysm follow trauma usually.** **JIPMER 1993**

Abdominal Aortic Aneurysm: Important Points for 2011/2012

- AAAs, are the **most common type of aortic aneurysm.**
- Most are **true aneurysms** that involve all three layers
- AAAs are mostly due to **atherosclerosis**
- May present as a **large, pulsatile mass above the umbilicus.** A bruit may be heard from the turbulent flow in a severe atherosclerotic aneurysm or if thrombosis occurs.
- Once an aneurysm has ruptured, it presents with a classic "**pain-hypotension-mass**" **triad**. The pain is classically reported in the abdomen, back or flank. It is usually acute, severe and constant, and may radiate through the abdomen to the back.
- ❐ **Medical therapy** of aortic aneurysms involves strict blood pressure control. This does not treat the aortic aneurysm per se, but control the rate of expansion of the aneurysm.
- ❐ **Surgical Treatment** The definitive treatment for an aortic aneurysm is surgical repair of the aorta.
- ❐ A Rapidly expanding **aneurysm** should be operated on as soon as feasible, since it has a greater chance of rupture.
- ❐ A Slowly expanding **aortic aneurysms** may be followed by routine diagnostic testing (i.e. CT scan or ultrasound imaging).

➲ Sinus of Valsalva Aneurysm: High Yield for 2011/2012

- ❒ Is a **dilatation of the aortic sinus** that eventually ruptures into **cardiac chamber, the pulmonary artery, or the pericardium.**
- ❒ The cause may be either **congenital or acquired**, and the most common cause of an acquired sinus of Valsalva aneurysm is bacterial endocarditis.
- ❒ The vast majority of sinuses of Valsalva aneurysms are asymptomatic before they rupture, but if symptomatic they present as obstruction to either the left or right outflow tract, heart block, or embolization.
- ❒ When sinus of Valsalva aneurysms rupture, they present with symptoms of an **acute left-to-right shunt and these include dyspnea, palpitations, and chest pain.**
- ❒ Finally, associated defects occur commonly with congenital sinus of Valsalva aneurysms, the most common being ventricular septal defect followed by aortic insufficiency.

➲ The Subclavian Steal Syndrome: High Yield for AIPGMEE, AIIMS, PGI 2012/2013

- ❒ Occurs when there is **reversal of flow in the ipsilateral vertebral artery** distal to a stenosis or occlusion of the proximal subclavian. The neurologic symptoms reported in these patients most commonly include vertigo, limb paresis, and paresthesias. Bilateral cortical visual disturbances, ataxia, syncope, and dysarthria
- ❒ Because of the reduction of pressure in the subclavian artery distal to the obstruction, blood flows antegrade up the contralateral vertebral artery, into the basilar artery, and retrograde down the ipsilateral vertebral artery to supply collateral circulation to the upper extremity.
- ❒ Thus, blood supply is presumably "stolen" from the basilar system and may compromise regional or total cerebral blood flow.

➲ Trimodal Pattern of Mortality

- **Most trauma deaths** occur within the first hour of injury, often before the victim arrives at hospital. It accounts for 50% of deaths after trauma and the cause of death is usually severe brain or cardiovascular injury. Such deaths can only be reduced by preventive strategies in the community.
- **A second peak** occurs between 1 and 4 hours after injury, and accounts for 30% of deaths. These are preventable with appropriate early diagnosis and treatment of severe life threatening injuries, such as pneumothorax, flail chest, abdominal hemorrhage, pelvic and long bone injuries. This period during which lives can be saved by prompt and efficient treatment has been called the golden hour.
- **A third peak** occurs days or weeks after the initial trauma and due to multiple organ failure (MODS) and overwhelming infection. It accounts for 20% of trauma deaths. Appropriate initial care can prevent late complications and death.

⇨ Arterial Diseases

Burgers Disease (Thromoangitis Obliterans)☛

Affects **small and medium sized** arteries.	PGI 2004
Affects young	PGI 1988
Affects **smokers**☛☛	PGI 1988

- Ankle pressure index is low here.
- Coldness and numbness of toes is the first sign.
- **Xanithol nicotinate is used for treatment** MAHE 2005
- **Lumbar sympathetectomy is done.** TN 1990

Peripheral or sympathetic nerve blocks may provide temporary pain relief, especially when the disease is accompanied by severe vasospasm. PGI 2011

When nerve blocks prove beneficial, dorsal or lumbar sympathectomy may provide more lasting benefit. PGI 2011

Anticoagulants, dextran, phenylbutazone, inositol niacinate, and corticosteroids have all been recommended. Other therapies used are

- **Prostaglandin therapy**
- **Pentoxifylline**
- **Intra-arterial infusion of urokinase, followed by small-vessel balloon catheter angioplasty and anticoagulation**
- **"Martorells sign"** is positive.

Remember:

Raynauds disease: Affects arterioles. Features are: Blanching, Dusky cyanosis, Red engorgement
Raynauds phenomenon is vasospastic condition of diverse etiology
Lerieches syndrome Is due to aortoiliac occlusion
Butchers thigh is due to injury to Femoral Artery in Femoral Triangle.

⇨ Leriche's Syndrome

Chronic occlusion of the aortic bifurcation by thrombosis

Characteristic symptoms of thrombotic occlusion of the terminal aorta include

- **Extreme liability to fatigue of both lower limbs, described as a weariness rather than the typical intermittent claudication;** JKBOPEE 2012
- **Symmetrical atrophy of both lower limbs without trophic changes in the skin or nails;**
- **Pallor of the legs and feet; and**
- **Inability to maintain a stable erection due to inadequate arterial flow to the penis from hypogastric arterial obstruction, thus reducing the blood flow through the internal pudendal artery and its blood flow to the corpora cavernosa.**

The physical findings include absence of pulses in the abdominal aorta and in the arteries distally. **JKBOPEE 2012**

The 5 Ps characteristic of peripheral arterial occlusion. DNB 2011

Pain

Pallor

Paralysis

Pulselessness

Paresthesia

Deep Venous Thrombosis: High Yield for AIPGMEE, AIIMS, PGI 2012/2013

- Most important consequences of this disorder are "**pulmonary embolism**" and the "**syndrome of chronic venous insufficiency.**"
- Deep venous thrombosis of the iliac, femoral, or popliteal veins is suggested by **unilateral leg swelling, warmth, and erythema, Pain** **AI 1990, CMC 2001**
- **Earliest sign is rise in temperature.**
- **occurs less frequently in the upper extremity** than in the lower extremity,
- The noninvasive test used most often to diagnose deep venous thrombosis is **duplex venous ultrasonography** **PGI 1997**
- Impedance plethysmography measures changes in venous capacitance during physiologic maneuvers.
- It is much less sensitive for diagnosing deep venous thrombosis of the calves.
- Heparin is used for DVT Prophylaxis **PGI 1997**
- **Thrombolytic therapy, bandaging arre effective.** **MAHE 2007**
- **Magnetic resonance imaging (MRI)** is another noninvasive means to detect deep vein thrombosis. Its diagnostic accuracy for assessing proximal deep vein thrombosis is similar to that of duplex ultrasonography. It is useful in patients with suspected thrombosis of the superior and inferior venae cavae or pelvic veins.

Signs of DVT

Holmans sign:	Forced dorsiflexion of ankle causes pain in calf. ☛ **COMED 2000**
Mosses sign:	Pain in calf on squeezing calf muscles
Pratts sign:	Lateral squeezing of calf muscles causes pain
Phlergma alba dolens:	Swollen leg (whitish) with edema and blanching☛
Phlegm cerulae dolens:	Painful (blue) leg☛

Varicose Veins

- Are **dilated, tortuous superficial veins** that result from defective structure and function of the valves of the saphenous veins, from intrinsic weakness of the vein wall, from high intraluminal pressure, or, rarely, from arteriovenous fistulas.
- **Primary varicose veins** originate in the superficial system and occur two to three times as frequently in women as in men. Approximately half of patients have a family history of varicose veins. ☛
- **Secondary varicose veins** result from deep venous insufficiency and incompetent perforating veins or from deep venous occlusion causing enlargement of superficial veins that are serving as collaterals.
- **Duplex imaging is gold standard.** **JIPMER 2003**

► **Management:**

- Varicose veins can **usually be treated with conservative measures**
- **External compression stockings** provide a counterbalance to the hydrostatic pressure in the veins.
- **Small symptomatic varicose veins can be treated with sclerotherapy,** in which a sclerosing solution is injected into the involved varicose vein and a compression bandage is applied.
- **Ethanolamine oleate is used as sclerosant** **PGI 1988**
- **Surgical therapy usually involves extensive ligation and stripping of the greater and lesser saphenous veins**
- **Broide Tredlenburg test demonstrates sapheno femoral incompetence** **ORISSA 1998**
- **Ecchymosis is the commonest complication of stripping.** **AIIMS 1992**
- **Cocket and Dodds operation is subfascial ligation operation.** **AP 1996**

Arteriovenous Fistula (AVF): High Yield for AIPGMEE, AIIMS, PGI 2012/2013

AVF may be congenital or acquired (by trauma of a penetrating wound, or surgically created for renal dialysis)

Physiological Effects of Fistula:

- ✓ Increased pulse pressure (Increased systolic and decreased diastolic)
- ✓ Enhanced venous return result in increased HR and increased CO
- ✓ Left ventricular enlargement and later cardiac failure may occur
- ✓ A congenital fistula in the young may cause overgrowth of limb
- ✓ In the leg, indolent ulcers may result from relative ischemia below the short circuit.

Clinical Signs

- **A pulsatile swelling**
- **A thrill on palpation**
- **Continuous bruit on auscultation**

"Nicoladoni Sign or Branham Sign":

Pressure on the artery **proximal to fistula** causes the swelling to diminish in size, a thrill or bruit to cease, the pulse rate to fall and the pulse pressure return to normal. **AIIMS 2009**

"In patients with arteriovenous fistulas, the cardiac output may be increased, and compression of the fistula, which diminishes the flow, is followed by a slower heart rate (Branham's or Nicoladoni's sign) and a lower cardiac output. Nicoladoni described a patient with an arteriovenous fistula in whom compression of the fistula (with cessation of flow through it) caused a decrease in the pulse This bradycardic reaction was later described by Branham and also bears his name." **DNB 2011**

⇨ Trophic Ulcers

Are included in neurogenic ulcers which are caused by various factors such as impairment of nutrition of the tissues, inadequate blood supply and neurological deficit e.g., a bedsore.

The neurological conditions which predispose to formation of trophic ulcers include:

- Diabetes
- Tabes dorsalis
- Alcoholic peripheral neuritis
- Spina bifida
- Meningomyelocele
- Leprosy
- peripheral nerve injury
- paraplegia
- Syringomyelia
- Transverse myelitis

Lymphatic Diseases

Lymphoedema Congenita	Present at birth
Lymphoedema Praecox	Starts at puberty
Lymphoedema Tarda	Starts at adulthood
Milroys Disease	Congenital lymphedema of familial type AMU 1985

Cellulitis in Lymphedema DNB 2011

- The eczema and ulceration seen in venous disease are not characteristic of swelling due to lymphedema. Approximately half of patients with lymphedema experience recurrent spontaneous attacks of bacterial cellulitis most often caused by staphylococcus. These episodes are characterized by increased swelling due to local inflammation, pain, and high fever. This increased susceptibility to bacterial infection is believed to be related to loss of local immune defenses because of diminished lymphatic function. If cellulitis occurs, it should be treated promptly with effective antibiotics and bedrest with elevation of the involved extremity.
- Cellulitis is most frequently caused by gram-positive organisms, and antibiotics effective against these organisms should be given empirically and adjusted if necessary after the bacterial culture is known.

Virchows triad: endothelial injury +hypercoagubility+stasis	DNB 2008
Cocket and Dodd surgery: subfascial ligation	UPSC 2008
Broide Tredlenburg test demonstrates: saphenofemoral incompetence	Orrisa 98
Tredlenbergs test denotes: perforator incompetence	JIPMER 2K
Investigation of choice for peripheral aneurysm: Ultrasound	UP 2008
Most common cause of mycotic aneurysm: Staph	DNB 2008
Fogarty catheter is used for: removal of clots from vessels	UPSC 2009

Total Parentral Nutrition: High Yield for AIPGMEE, AIIMS, PGI 2012/2013

Infusion Technique and Patient Monitoring

- Partial and short-term total parenteral nutrition can be provided via a peripheral vein if the majority of the energy is supplied by isotonic fat solutions;
- Long-term total parenteral nutrition using glucose as the chief energy source requires administration via a central vein catheter so the hypertonic solution can be rapidly diluted in a high-flow system.
- The preferred site for central vein infusion is the superior vena cava.
- Tunneled catheters and implanted subcutaneous ports require operating room insertion and are more stable for long-term use.
- Central catheters should be changed when clinically indicated; routine changes are costly and hazardous.

As Primary Therapy		As Supportive Therapy
Indications:		Indications:
▶ GIT fistulas		➡ Acute radiation enteritis
▶ Renal failure		➡ Acute chemotherapy toxicity
▶ Esophageal cancer		➡ Ileus
▶ Gastric cancer		➡ After Major surgery
▶ Short bowel syndrome	PGI 05	
▶ Severe burns	PGI 05	
▶ Hepatic failure		
▶ Crohns disease		

Complications:

- Air embolism
- Hydrothorax, pneumothorax, hemothorax
- Catheter embolism
- Injury to thoracic duct,brachial plexus
- Catheter sepsis
- Weight losss in 7 days. ORISSA 1999

Metabolic:

- Hyper, hypo (sodium, potassium, magnesium, calcium, phosphate) AIIMS 2003
- Zinc and vitamin deficiency
- Azotemia
- Metabolic bone disease
- Essential fatty acid deficiency AIIMS 2003

1

SURGERY

⇨ Complications of Parenteral Nutrition (Detailed) Important Topic

Mechanical Complications

These Include

- **Pneumothorax,**
- **Brachial plexus injury,**
- **Subclavian or carotid artery puncture,**
- **Hemothorax,**
- **Chylothorax,**
- **Thrombosis or pulmonary embolism** may occur secondary to central venous catheter use.

Infectious complications

Sepsis occurs secondary to contamination of the central venous catheter.

Mc Complication **AIPGME 2012**

Metabolic complications

Metabolic complications can be divided into Early or nutrient relatej and **Late or related to long term administration.** Early complicatio include, among others, hyperglycemia, refeeding syndrome, and lipid metabolism abnormalities. Complications associated with long-term PN infusion include steatosis, cholestasis, and metabolic bone disease.

- **Hyperglycemia**-is the most common metabolic complication associated with PN administration.
- **Hypoglycemia**- Abrupt discontinuation of TPN can produce rebound hypoglycemia in patients with limited oral intake.
- **Hyperlipidemia**
- **Refeeding syndrome-** is defined as severe electrolyte and fluid shifts that may result from refeeding after severe weight loss (protein- calorie malnutrition).

Hepatobiliary complications

Hepatic dysfunction is a common manifestation of long-term parenteral nutrition support. It includes **elevated serum transaminases and alkaline phosphatase. Steatosis, steatohepatitis, lipidosis, chloestasis, fibrosis and cirrhosis** can occur.

Biliary complications include **acalculous cholecystitis, gallbladder sludge, and cholelithiasis.**

Metabolic Bone disease- including **osteomalacia or osteopenia** may be seen with long-term TPN.

⇨ Refeeding Syndrome

- Is defined as **severe electrolyte and fluid shifts that may result from refeeding after severe weight loss (protein- calorie malnutrition).**
- In starvation, energy is derived principally from fat metabolism. **TPN results in a shift from fat to glucose as the predominant fuel and rapid anabolism** increases the production of phosphorylated intermediates of glycolysis. These intermediates trap phosphate, producing profound hypophosphatemia. Hypophosphatemia is the hallmark of the refeeding syndrome and has been reported in patients being repleted both parenterally and enterally.

- Hypokalemia and hypomagnesemia also occur.
- The lack of phosphate and potassium lead to a relative ATP deficiency, resulting in the insidious onset of respiratory failure and reduced cardiac stroke volume.The refeeding syndrome can be life threatenting if not promptly treated.
- Because of these risks, the rate of TPN administration in a severly malnourished patient should be slowly increased over several days.

➲ Wounds and Tissue Repair: High Yield for AIPGMEE, AIIMS, PGI 2012/2013

The types of healing are customarily divided into repair by first, second, or third intention.

Primary or first intention healing ☛occurs in closed wounds in **which the edges are approximated**, such as a **clean skin incision** closed with sutures. The incisional defect re-epithelializes rapidly, and matrix deposition seals the defect. **DELHI 1992**

Second intention healing occurs when the **wound edges are not apposed,**☛ such as an open punch skin biopsy wound, a deep burn, and an infected wound left open to granulate. Granulation tissue fills the wound, and the wound contracts and re-epithelializes.

Delayed primary or third intention healing occurs when an **open wound is secondarily closed several days after injury.** Such a wound is initially left open because of gross contamination. A classic example is wound management after removal of a ruptured appendix. After the peritoneum and fascia are closed to prevent evisceration, the skin and subcutaneous tissue are left open and the wound is packed loosely with sterile moist gauze. The wound is closed several days later after wound contamination has markedly diminished.

A scar is loosely defined as an abnormal, disorganized collection of collagen following wound repair. The collagens are a large group of triple-helix structural matrix proteins.

Types of Collagen:

- **Type I collagen** is the major structural component of bones, skin, and tendons.
- **Type II** is found predominantly in cartilage.
- **Type III** is found in association with Type I, although the ratio varies in different tissues.
- **Type IV** collagen is found in **basement membranes** in association with mucopolysaccharides and laminin **JK BOPEE**
- **Type V** is found in the cornea in association with Type III and is important in maintaining transparency.

➲ Clinical Factors that affect Wound Healing

- **Nutrition**
  - Protein depletion impairs wound healing
  - Vitamin C (ascorbic acid) deficiency causes scurvy. In patients with this deficiency, wound healing is arrested during fibroplasia. ☛ **AI 1993**
  - Vitamin A (retinoic acid) requirements increase during injury. Severely injured patients require supplemental vitamin A to maintain normal serum levels. Vitamin A also partially reverses the impaired healing in chronically steroid-treated patients.

- Vitamin B 6 (pyridoxine) deficiency impairs collagen cross-linking.
- Vitamin B1 (thiamine) and vitamin B2 (riboflavin) deficiencies cause syndromes associated with poor wound repair.
- VITAMIN E has **inhibitory role in wound healing** ☛ MAHE 05
- Deficiencies of trace metals such as **zinc and copper**, **Oxygen** AI 1993
- Anemia, and↓ Perfusion
  - **Oxygen** is required for successful inflammation, angiogenesis, epithelialization, and matrix deposition.
  - **Anemia** ☛
  - **Diabetes Mellitus and Obesity**☛
  - **Corticosteroids, Chemotherapy, and Radiation Therapy**☛
  - **Infection** MP 2008

- **Best method of skin disinfection is: tincture iodine.** TN 1990
- **Bacterial spores get destroyed by: autoclaving.**
- **Sharp instruments are sterilized by hot air oven.** UP 2001
- **Disposable items are best sterilized by ethylene oxide.** KAR 2002

⇨ Keloids

- Keloids are made of dense **connective tissue.**
- Keloids are best treated by **intrakeloidal injection of triamiclonolone**

Feature	**Hypertrophic scar**☛	**Keloid**☛
Hereditary	Not Familial	May be familial AI 1998
Race	No predilection	Common in blacks
Sex	No Predilection	Common in females
Borders	Confined to wound☛☛	Outgrow wound☛
Course	Subsides	Rarely subsides PGI 2006
	➡ Does not extend beyond wound margin. ➡ Red, raised, tender. ➡ Remodelling phase↑☛ ➡ Where tension of skin is more☛ AI 2001 ➡ Best scars seen in old people. PGI 1989	May turn malignant. PGI 2006 Recurrence common. PGI 2007 **Sternum mc site.** PGI 1996 **Appears after surgery in few days.** JIPMER 1995 **Best treated by intralesional steroidal application.** UPSC 1995 **Excision and repair are even better** UPSC 2001

1

SURGERY

⇨ Wounds

Clean Wound	✓ No violation of Mucosa ✓ No inflammation ✓ No drains ✓ No need of any prophylactic antibiotic Eg: varicose Vein Surgery Elective Herniotomy
Clean Contaminated wound	✓ Violation of mucosa but no spillage ✓ Need of Prophylactic antibiotic Eg: **Elective Cholecystectomy** **KCET 2012, APPG 2006**
Contaminated wound	✓ Preexisting infection ✓ Spillage of visccus contents ✓ Need of Prophylactic Antibiotic Eg: Appendicectomy

⇨ Sutures

Absorbable:	
✓ **PDS**	**KCET 2012**
✓ **Vicryl (Poly glactin)☛**	
✓ **Dexon (Poly glycolic acid)☛**	**PGI 1997**
✓ **Catgut**	
Non Absorbable:	
✓ **Nylon☛**	
✓ **Prolene**	**PGI 1997**
✓ **PTFE**	
✓ **Silk☛**	
✓ **Thread**	

⇨ Catgut **DNB 2011**

- ❒ The origin of the name catgut or **kittegut** is from a very delicate musical instrument called a kitte—a type of fiddle that required fine gut for its strings.
- ❒ **Catgut** is made from the **intestines of cattle or sheep.**
- ❒ Chromic catgut has been treated with a chromium salt to retard its absorption by conditioning the surgical gut to resist digestion by the body; its absorption is delayed up to 20 days.
- ❒ Catgut acts as an active foreign body in the tissue and may interfere with wound healing. Plain catgut usually evokes a greater inflammatory reaction than chromic catgut. Repair with plain catgut is extremely helpful in children for whom the prospect of suture removal is frightening and often equated with the discomfort of suture placement. This repair is also helpful for patients who have to travel soon after the operative procedure

➲ Sutures and Preservatives

Sutures	Preservatives
➠ Catgut	Isopropyl alcohol☛ AIIMS 1996
➠ Proline	Isopropyl alcohol☛
➠ Vicryl	None
➠ Silk	None

⇨ Grafting Related Terms

- **Imbibition:** Refers to absorption of nutrients into the graft. ☛
- **Inosculation:** donor and recipient capillaries become aligned. ☛
- **Revasculaization:** is completed by connecting vessels into arterioles and venules.

Skin grafts Skin grafts are harvested from a donor site and transferred to a recipient site on which they must survive, a process known as take.

- All skin grafts initially adhere to the recipient bed by the formation of fibrin. Oxygen and nutrients diffuse through by a process known as plasmatic imbibition to keep the graft alive.
- New blood vessels then grow from the recipient site and link up with dermal capillaries to re-establish a blood supply, a process known as inosculation.
- Thin skin grafts are more likely to survive by imbibition and will revascularise readily and are therefore more likely to take than thicker grafts.

Partial-thickness skin grafts☛ (Theirsch graft) PGI 2004

- Consist of **epidermis and a variable thickness of dermis.**☛
- Partial-thickness grafts are used to resurface relatively large areas of skin defect and are particularly useful in burns.

Full-thickness grafts (Wolfes Graft)☛ AIIMS 2002

- Consist of **epidermis and all of the dermis;**☛
- The donor site will not epithelialise and must be closed, usually directly. Full-thickness grafts are most commonly used in repairing defects on the face.

Composite grafts

- **Consist of skin and some underlying tissue** such as fat and cartilage.☛ COMED 01
- Again, donor sites must be closed directly. Composite grafts carry the highest risk of failure.

➲ Biologic Dressings: High Yield for AIPGMEE, AIIMS, PGI 2012/2013

Viable cutaneous allograft is the **biologic dressing of choice**, against which all other available materials must be evaluated. In the operating room using sterile technique, allograft skin is harvested from cadavers free of jaundice, cutaneous malignancy or infection, and viral disease. The harvested grafts are spread on fine-mesh gauze that is thinly impregnated with petrolatum, placed in sterile containers, and then refrigerated for up to 2 weeks. Alternatively, the tissue can be frozen using cryoprotective techniques. If refrigerated, such tissue performs better as a biologic dressing the sooner after harvest it is used.

1

SURGERY

⇨ Cutaneous Allograft

- Prevents wound desiccation;
- Promotes maturation of granulation tissue;
- Limits bacterial proliferation in the burn wound;
- Prevents exudative protein and red blood cell loss;
- Decreases wound pain, thereby facilitating movement of involved joints;
- Diminishes evaporative water loss from the burn wound surface, thus decreasing heat loss; and serves to protect tendons, vessels, and nerves.

⇨ Lyophilized Allograft Skin

- Has an indefinite shelf life
- Is easily reconstituted;
- Shows less adherence to the wound than viable allograft skin, and
- If harvested at too great a thickness, undergoes dermal-epidermal separation after application to the wound with subsequent desiccation of the exposed dermis.

⇨ Cutaneous Xenografts

- Are less effective as physiologic dressings and allow survival of greater numbers of subgraft bacteria, presumably because such tissue is not vascularized by the host.
- Such tissues are not rejected in the true sense of the word but slough following necrosis.

⇨ Amnion

- Is physiologic dressing that is **readily available and inexpensive.** ☚
- Since the amniotic tissue will desiccate and spontaneously separate from the wound bed if left exposed, it must be covered with occlusive dressings that preclude continuous observation of the dressing and underlying wound bed.
- Amnion, like cutaneous xenografts, is **not vascularized by the host**, and biologic union occurs by ingrowth of granulation tissue.

➲ Swellings of Skin: High Yield for AIPGMEE, AIIMS, PGI 2012/2013

❐ **Lipoma**	➨ Universal tumor
❐ **Adiposis dolorosa (Dercums disease)**	➨ Multiple lipomata
❐ **Cavernous hemangioma**	➨ Arises from **veins**☚
❐ **Plexiform hemangioma**	➨ Arises from **Arteries**☚
❐ **Warts**	➨ Human pappiloma Virus

❐ Rhinophyma (Potato Nose)	➨ Acne Rosacea
❐ Cavernous Lymphangioma	➨ Cystic Hygroma
❐ Sebaceous cyst	➨ Wen
❐ Buschke lownstein tumor	➨ Massive veneral wart
❐ Marjolins growth	➨ Squamous cell carcinoma
❐ Bedsore	➨ Trophic ulcer
❐ Pilomatrixoma	➨ Calcifying epithelioma
❐ Potts puffy tumor	➨ Skull osteomyelitis
❐ Rasp berry tumor	➨ Umblical adenoma MP 2003

⇨ Sebaceous Cyst DNB 2011

- Is also called as Wen.
- It usually lies in dermis.
- It is a retention cyst. DNB 01
- Its contents are **sebum and keratin.**
- Common sites are face and scalp.
- They **don't occur on** palm and scalp.
- **Cocks peculiar tumor is a complication.** AIIMS 2001

⇨ Lipoma

- ✓ Most common site: trunk
- ✓ "Slipping margin "sign positive.
- ✓ Pedunculated lipoma is called: lipoma arborscens

➲ Lipomatosis

Multiple symmetric lipomatosis (Madelung disease) High yield for 2011-2012 AIPGME

- ▶ It is characterized by a symmetric, progressive growth of nonencapsulated subcutaneous adipose tissue, primarily in the neck (bull neck with buffalo hump and double chin) and supraclavicular and shoulder regions.
- ▶ Fat may also accumulate in the trunk and proximal limbs, though the distal arms and legs are spared. Rarely, laryngeal, tracheal, or vena caval compression may occur from deep lipomatous infiltration in the neck and mediastinum.
- ▶ Many patients also have peripheral neuropathy; hypertriglyceridemia and hyperuricemia are uncommon. Serum HDL cholesterol levels are usually elevated, and diabetes mellitus has not been reported.

Forms of lipomatosis

- **Mediastinal lipomatosis** is characterized by local overgrowth of adipose tissue in the mediastinum. It occurs in patients with Cushing's syndrome and can occasionally cause tracheal compression.
- **Pelvic lipomatosis** is characterized by overgrowth of pelvic fat, causing bladder dysfunction (frequency, dysuria, and nocturia), constipation, and lower abdominal pain. Bilateral ureteral obstruction may also occur.
- **Epidural lipomatosis** occurs in obese patients or in those receiving exogenous steroid therapy. Fat deposition most often occurs in the thoracic or lumbar spine, causing back pain, radicular pain, or spinal cord compression. Laminectomy may be indicated for cord compression.

Adiposis dolorosa (Dercum disease) High yield for 2011-2012 Aipgme

- This is a rare disease of unknown etiology that mainly affects obese postmenopausal women
- It is characterized by the presence of multiple circumscribed or diffuse painful subcutaneous fat deposits on the trunk and limbs, particularly near the knees.
- Patients also report weakness, fatigue, and emotional lability.

- **Mc type: subcutaneous**
- **Painful: neurofibroma**
- **Vascular: naevolipoma**

Dercums disease:

- ✓ **Adiposis dolorosa**
- ✓ **Fatty deposits on limbs/trunk with facial sparing**
- ✓ **Rare disease**
- ✓ **Multiple painful lipomas in adult life.**

⇨ Ulcers of Skin

- **Rodent ulcer:** Basal Cell Carcinoma **JKBOPEE**
- **Martorells ulcer:** Hypertensive/Atherosclerotic ulcer
- **Bazins ulcer:** Erythrocyanoid ulcer
- **Snail track ulcer:** Syphilitic ulcer

⇨ Premalignant Skin Lesions

- **Bowens disease**
- **Solar keratoses**
- **Radiodermatitis**
- **Marjolins ulcer**

⇨ Tumors Affecting Skin: DNB 2011

Desmoid tumors of the abdominal wall are benign fibrous tumors that arise from the musculoaponeurotic abdominal wall. These tumors are **histologically benign** but frequently are **locally invasive and are prone torecurrence after local excision.** They **present as firm, subcutaneous masses that grow slowly. They should be widely excised to prevent local recurrence. They do not have a propensity toward metastasis.**

Primary malignancies of the abdominal wall are uncommon. Any of the cutaneous neoplasms may affect the abdominal wall and are treated like skin cancers elsewhere. Sarcomas arising from the abdominal wall are uncommon and are best treated by surgical excision.

The abdominal wall is occasionally the **site of metastasis from primary malignancies located elsewhere.** In particular, tumors of the ovary and prostate may metastasize to the lower abdominal wall. Tumors of the stomach, uterus, lung, kidney, breast, and colon occasionally give rise to metastases located within the abdominal wall.

➲ Basal Cell Carcinoma: High Yield for AIPGMEE, AIIMS, PGI 2012/2013

- **Basal Cell Carcinoma BCC** is a malignancy arising from epidermal basal cells.
- **Also called as rodent ulcer.**
- Commonest site face. AI 1995
- The **most common type** is **noduloulcerative** BCC, which begins as a small, **pearly nodule**, often with small telangiectatic vessels on its surface. COMED 2008
- The nodule grows slowly and may undergo central ulceration.
- Direct spread seen. MAHE 2007
- Lymphatic spread does not occur. AI 89
- **Mohs micrographic excision procedure is used for BCC.** KAR 2006

⇨ Squamous Cell Carcinoma

Squamous Cell Carcinoma : Primary cutaneous SCC is a malignant neoplasm of **keratinizing epidermal cells.**

Unlike BCC, which has a very low metastatic potential, SCC can **metastasize and grow rapidly**. The clinical features of SCC vary widely.

- **Actinic keratosis predisposes to SCC.** AIIMS 2002
- **Bowens disease**
- **Lichen planus**
- **DLE** PGI 1997

➲ Marjolin's Ulcer: High Yield AIPGME 2011/2012

- Refers to an **aggressive ulcerating squamous cell carcinoma** presenting in an area of previously **traumatized, chronically inflamed, or scarred skin.**

- They are commonly present in the context of chronic wounds including
  - **Burn injuries,**
  - **Venous ulcers,**
  - **Ulcers from osteomyelitis, and**
  - **Post radiotherapy scars.**
- Slow growth, painlessness (as the ulcer is usually not associated with nerve tissue), and absence of lymphatic spread due to local destruction of lymphatic channels.
- Histologically, the tumour is a well-differentiated squamous cell carcinoma. This carcinoma is aggressive in nature, spreads locally and is associated with a poor prognosis. 40% occur on the lower limb and the malignant change is usually painless.

The Glomus Tumor: High Yield for AIPGMEE, AIIMS, PGI 2012/2013

- Is a rare and **benign vascular** neoplasm
- Arises from the **neuroarterial structure** called a **glomus body**
- The most common site of glomus tumors is **subungual** and in the hand (Digits) **AIIMS 2008**
- Affect **women** three times more commonly than men.
- The lesions are usually solitary but multifocal tumors are also seen.
- Clinically, glomus tumors are characterized by a triad of
  - **Sensitivity to cold,**
  - **Localized tenderness and**
  - **Severe intermittent pain.**

Treatment of glomus tumors consists of **surgical excision.**

Keratoacanthoma

Keratoacanthoma, typically appears as a dome-shaped papule with a central keratotic crater, expands rapidly, and commonly regresses without therapy.

This lesion can be difficult to differentiate from SCC.

Benign. **PGI 2000**

Self limiting corse.

Affects elderly men usually.

Melanoma: High Yield for AIPGMEE, AIIMS, PGI 2012/2013

Melanomas originate from melanocytes, pigment cells normally present in the epidermis and sometimes in the dermis.

An alternative prognostic scheme for clinical stages I and II melanoma, proposed by **Clark**, is based on the anatomic level of invasion in the skin. **(Clark's Level)**

- Melanomas may spread by the **lymphatic channels or the bloodstream.** PGI 2008
- The earliest metastases are often to regional lymph nodes.
- Most common site for Malignant melanoma is **skin** (90%).
- Cutaneous melanoma arises from **epidermal melanocytes.** AIIMS 2001
- **Junctional melanoma** predisposes to MM.
- May be **familial.** AIIMS 1987

Early detection of melanoma may be facilitated by applying the **"ABCD rules"**:

- A asymmetry, benign lesions are usually symmetric;
- B border irregularity, most nevi have clear-cut borders;
- C color variegation, benign lesions usually have uniform light or dark pigment;
- D diameter >6 mm (the size of a pencil eraser).

- **Lentigo maligna** is the least common type
- It is also known as Hutchinsons freckle.
- Face is the most common site involved by it AIIMS 2001

- **Superficial spreading is the most common type** AIIMS 2001
- It may occur at any site on body

- **Nodular Melanoma** is the most malignant type PGI 1999
- It is common in younger age group.
- **Acral lentigous** occurs on palms and soles especially
- **Amelanotic** has the worst prognosis

- **"Clarks level"is classification based on level of "invasion into skin."**
- **"Breslows staging"** is based on **thickness of invasion.**
- **No's of MM (Malignant Melanoma)**
- No incisional biopsy
- No induration
- No role of radiotherapy
- Not known usually before puberty

⇨ Soft Tissue Tumors: DNB 2011

- **Mc soft tissue tumor in a child is Rhabdomyosarcoma.**
- **Mc type: embryonal rhabdomyosarcoma.**
- **Resection is the treatment of choice.** PGI 2000
- **Soft toissue sarcomas mostly spread hematogeneously.**

1

SURGERY

- **But lymphatic metastasis is seen in enbryonal rhabdomyosarcoma.** **AI 2005**
- **Lower extremity is the commonest site.** **AIIMS 2002**
- **Grade of tumor detects prognosis.** **AIIMS 1996**
- **Liposarcoma is the mc retroperitoneal tumor.**
- **Lymphoma and retroperitoneal sarcoma are mc retroperitoneal malignant lesions.**

Genetic syndromes such as neurofibromatosis, familial adenomatous polyposis, and the Li-Fraumeni syndrome have all been shown to be associated with the development of soft tissue sarcoma. Ionizing radiation and lymphedema are **well-established antecedents to the development of soft tissue sarcoma.**

Retroperitoneal Fibrosis

- Retroperitoneal fibrosis characterized by **extensive fibrotic encasement of the retroperitoneal tissues**
- Most common in men over age 50 who have renal failure secondary to obstructive uropathy
- Diffuse desmoplastic involvement of the retroperitoneum may alternatively give rise to obstructive jaundice or small or large bowel obstruction
- Classic diagnostic triad includes:
  - **Bilateral hydronephrosis/hydroureter**
  - **Medial deviation of the ureters**
  - **Extrinsic ureteric compression at the L4-5 level**

Over 67% of cases are idiopathic

Known etiologies include:

- ✓ **Drugs**
- ✓ **Inflammatory disorders**
- ✓ **Retroperitoneal hemorrhage**
- ✓ **Peri-aneurysmal (abdominal aortic aneurysm [AAA]) inflammation**
- ✓ **Irradiation**
- ✓ **Urinary extravasation**
- ✓ **Cancer**

- Most common drugs associated with retroperitoneal fibrosis are methsergide and b-blockers

Retroperitoneal Sarcoma: High Yield for AIPGMEE, AIIMS, PGI 2012/2013

- **Mesenchymal-derived soft-tissue neoplasms**
- **Metastasize via the hematogenous route with the majority of metastases to the liver or lung**
- **Behavior tends to be dictated by tumor grade rather than cell type of origin**
- **Rarely cause symptoms until they grow to a large size**
- **Vague abdominal symptoms are the most common presenting complaint**
  - ✓ Account for 15% of all sarcomas and 55% of all retroperitoneal tumors
  - ✓ Most common variant is a liposarcoma

Symptoms and signs

Nonspecific vague abdominal symptoms most common complaint

- ✓ Abdominal discomfort
- ✓ Early satiety
- ✓ Nausea and vomiting
- ✓ Weight loss
- ✓ Palpable abdominal mass

Chest film or thoracic CT scan: May demonstrate pulmonary metastases

Abdominal CT scan or MRI

- — Demonstrates the soft-tissue neoplasm and its relationship to adjacent retroperitoneal structures.
- — MRI is typically more accurate than CT scan in defining the extent of tumor and invasion of surrounding structures.

➲ Paragangliomas High Yield for 2011-2012

- ► **Are generally benign, slow growing tumors** arising from widely distributed.
- ► Paraganglionic tissue thought to originate from the **neural crest.**
- ► **Paraganglia are distributed throughout the head and neck and superior mediastinum along the course of the major vasculature.**
- ➦ **Paraganglia are also found in the orbit, the larynx, and along the course of the vagus nerve.**
- ➦ **All paragangliomas are closely related to one another and to pheochromocytomas of the adrenal gland.**
- ➦ **Their histiologic appearance is similar to the normal histology of the paraganglia.**
- ➦ They consist of clusters of **Type I or chief cells** which are members of the amine precursor and uptake decarboxylase (APUD) family and **Type II or sustentacular cells (modified Schwann cells).**
- ➦ **These two cell types are arranged into clusters with a core of chief cells surrounded by the sustentacular cells embedded in a fibrous stroma.**
- ➦ **The** clusters of cells make up the histologic structure termed **Zellballen.** **JK 2010**
- ➦ **Nuclear pleomorphism and cellular hyperchromatism are common in paragangliomas and should not be considered evidence of malignancy.**
- ➦ **Malignancy can not be determined histologically but is reserved for the presence of local, regional or distant metastasis.**
- ➦ **Additional studies using immunohistochemical techniques revealed that malignant glomus tumors are characterized by the presence of MIB-1, p53, Bcl-2 and CD34.**
- ➠ **A Glomus <u>jugulare</u> tumor** grows in the temporal bone of the skull, in an area called the jugular foramen near jugular bulb. (IX, X, XI) nerves are at risk). The jugular foramen is also where the jugular vein and several important nerves exit the skull. **This area contains glomus bodies, which are nerve fibers that normally respond to changes in body temperature or blood pressure.**
- ➠ **A Glomus <u>tympanicum</u> tumor** are located in the middle ear on promontory of cochlea. Usually present with pulsatile tinnitus, conductive hearing loss, blue mass behind tympanic membrane.

► Intravagal **Paragangliomas:** Arise most commonly at the level of the nodose ganglion but may occur at any point along the course of the vagus nerve in the neck. The mean age at presentation is about 50 years of age. Intravagal paragangliomas are more common in females than males. Intravagal paragangliomas usually present as a painless neck mass located behind the angle of the mandible. Vagal paragangliomas can bulge into the pharynx and cause dysphagia.

Salivary Glands: High Yield for AIPGMEE, AIIMS, PGI 2012/2013

Pleomorphic Adenoma

✓ **Mc benign salivary gland tumor.** ☛	AI 2002
✓ **Most common site is superficial lobe.**	
✓ **Malignant transformation is uncommon**	
✓ **Treatment is by superficial parotidectomy (Pateys operation)** ☛	PGI 2000

Warthin's Tumor:

✓ **Second Most common** benign tumor of parotid gland.	
✓ Consists of **epithelial + lymphoid elements** (Adenolymphoma) ☛	AIIMS 2005
✓ Common **in males** in 5th - 7th decade.	
✓ Bilateral in about 10% cases. ☛	
✓ Encapsulated.	
✓ Shows **Hot Spot** in Tc-Pertechnate scan.	
✓ Superficial parotidectomy is the treatment.	AIIMS 2001

Adenoid Cystic Carcinoma

❑ Also called as **cylindroma/ treacherous tumor**	
❑ Mc cancer of minor salivary glands. ☛	
❑ Invades **Perineural space and lymphatics** ☛	AIPGME 2012, KCET 2012
❑ Treatment is radical parotidectomy	

Mucoepidermoid Cancer

❑ Mc malignant salivary gland tumor. ☛	
❑ **Arises from mucin secreting cells and epidermal cells**	PGI 1999
❑ Mc malignant tumor of parotid	
❑ Mc radiation induced salivary tumor	

Remember:

► Most tumors of major salivary glands are **benign.** ☛	
► Pleomorphic adenoma is the **most common benign salivary gland tumor.** ☛	JK BOPEE 2011
► Most of the **minor** salivary gland tumors are **malignant**	PGI 2006

- Most common site of minor salivary gland tumor is **oral cavity**
- Most of salivary gland tumors are **radioresistant**
- **Godwins Tumor** is Benign Lymphoepithelial tumor of parotid
- **Calculi** are commonest in **submandibular duct** AIIMS 1999
- **Most common organism as a cause of acute parotitis is staph aureus**
- Most common cause of acute parotitis is mumps
- Most of submandibular calculi are **radiopaque**
- **Sialolithiasis is stones in salivary ducts**
- **Sialadenosis is non inflammatory swelling affecting salivary glands**
- **Freys syndrome** (gustatory sweating) occurs after parotid surgery due to involvement of auriculotemporal nerve
- **Sialography is not done in acute infection of salivary glands** AI 2005

Chest Wall:

Poland's Syndrome

- Hypoplasia of the skin and subcutaneous tissue of the anterior chest;
- Absence or hypoplasia and upward displacement of the nipple and breast;
- Pectoral and axillary hypotrichosis;
- Absence of the sternocostal portion of the pectoralis major muscle;
- Absence of the **pectoralis minor** muscle;
- Absence of portions of costal cartilages two to four or three to five;
- Ipsilateral hand anomalies (mitten hand, or brachysyndactyly);
- Absence of latissimus dorsi and serratus anterior muscles; and
- Scoliosis

Breast

- **Modified sweat gland**
- **"Axillary tail of Spence" is prolongation of breast tissue into axilla**
- **"Foramen of langer" is the space through which axillary tail passes.**
- **"Ligaments of cooper " attach breast to superficial fascia**
- **"Mammary ridge" is the embryonic precursor.**
- **"Subareolar plexus of Sappy" is a lymphatic plexus**
- **Peau d orange is lymphatic permeation.** PGI 1988
- **Blood supply: internal mammary artery, lateral thoracic, superior thoracic and acromiothoracic arteriers**

➲ Gynecomastia: High Yield for AIPGMEE, AIIMS, PGI 2012/2013

Can be Physiologic or Pathologic:

- **Physiologic gynecomastia** is seen in newborn infants, pubescent adolescents and elderly individuals.
- **Pathologic gynecomastia** can be caused by a decrease in the production and/or action of testosterone, by an increase in the production and/or action of estrogen, or by drug use; however, gynecomastia can also be idiopathic. Conditions that result in primary or secondary hypogonadism and cause decreased testosterone production and/or action include the following:
  - Klinefelter syndrome
  - Congenital anorchia
  - Testicular trauma
  - Testicular torsion
  - Viral orchitis
  - Kallmann syndrome
  - Pituitary tumors
  - Malignancies that increase the serum human chorionic gonadotropin (hCG) (e.g., large cell lung cancer, gastric carcinoma, renal cell carcinoma, hepatoma)
  - Renal failure
  - Hyperthyroidism
  - Malnutrition
  - Androgen insensitivity syndrome

⇨ Risk Factors for Breast Cancer

► Race: White females☚	
► Age: elderly☚	
► Family history +☚	PGI 2001
► Relatives (true)	PGI 2002
► Non breastfeeding mothers	
► ↑Fatty food intake	PGI 2002
► Nulliparity	PGI 2001
► BRCA 1 and BRCA2 mutations☚☚☚	
► Cancer in other breast☚	
► Mammary dysplasia/ Atypical hyperplasia / Sclerosing adenosis	PGI 2005
► Early menarche☚☚	
► Late menopause☚	
► Late first pregnancy	
► Atypical Hyperplasia is a major factor from pathological view point for breast cancer.	DNB 2011

High Yield Points

- MC disorder of breast:Fibroadenosis
- MC tumor of breast: Fibroadenoma
- MC carcinoma of breast: Ductal/Schirrous carcinoma
- Mc bilateral tumor: Lobular carcinoma of breast
- Mc inviolved: Lymph nodes are Axillary group
- MC cause of breast discharge: Duct ectasia
- Mc cause of bloody discharge: Duct pappiloma
- Mc site of metastasis of breast ca: Bone
- Mc site of breast ca: Upper outer quadrant
- FIRST INVESTIGATION FOR BREAST LUMP: FNAC
- BEST INVESTIGATION FOR BREAST LUMP: BIOPSY

Invasive Ductal Carcinoma

- Is by far the most common variant, accounting for approximately 75% to 80% of all invasive breast.
- Invasive ductal carcinoma develops from **epithelial cells of the terminal duct.**
- Histologically, it is composed of **small, glandular, duct like structures**, lined by variably.
- Anaplastic cells. The most common mode of presentation is a palpable mass in the breast.
- **PET scan** is sensitive for diagnosis. **AIPGME 2012**

The Colloid (Mucinous) Variant

- **Is relatively rare** (about 1% to 2%) and occurs
- More frequently in older women. Histologically, this carcinoma is characterized by
- Abundant mucin secretion.
- It is associated with a better prognosis than the ductal type.

Invasive Lobular Carcinoma

- Is the second most frequent histologic type of breast adenocarcinoma, accounting for approximately 10% of all cases.
- Its presumed cellof origin is the lobular cell.
- The most typical histologic characteristic is the presence ofcancer cells lined up in orderly rows **("single-file").**

Inflammatory Breast Cancer

- Is a pattern of invasive breast cancer in which the neoplastic cells infiltrate widely through the breast tissue.
- The cancer involves dermal lymphatics and therefore has a high incidence of systemic metastasis and a poor prognosis. If the lymphatics become blocked, then the area of skin may develop **lymphedema and "peau d'orange," or orange peel appearance**. The overlying skin in inflammatory breast cancer is usually **swollen, red, and tender.**

❐ A 16 year old female has firm, rubbery mass in right breast moving with palpation	Fibroadenoma	Most common benign tumor Pop corn calcification
❐ A 16 year old female has firm, rubbery mass in right breast is 8 cms in diameter	Giant Fibroadenoma	
❐ A 30 year old female has history of bilateral breast tenderness related to menstrual cycle with lumps coming and going.	Fibrocystic disease	
❐ A 30 year old female has bloody discharge from nipple. No other palpable masses are seen.	Intraductal Pappiloma	
❐ A 30 year old lactating mother has red, hot, tender mass with fever and leucocytosis	Breast abscess	
❐ A 55 year old woman has 3.5 cms hard mass in her left breast with ill defined borders and not mobile. The skin overlying has orange peel appearance	Breast ca	Adenocarcinoma MC Arises from terminal duct.
❐ A 60 year old has headaches not responding to medications. She had undergone Modified radical Mastectomy 1 year back	Brain metastasis from Breast ca	

Van Nuys Prognostic Classification for Breast Cancer	MAH 2012
❐ Group 1 Non-high nuclear grade without necrosis	
❐ Group 2 Non-high nuclear grade with necrosis	
❐ Group 3 High nuclear grade with or without necrosis	

➲ Galactocele: High Yield for AIPGMEE, AIIMS, PGI 2012/2013

❐ Is a milk-filled cyst☚
❐ **Round, well circumscribed**, and **easily movable** within the breast.
❐ Usually occurs **after the cessation of lactation** or when feeding frequency has been curtailed significantly.
❐ **Inspissated milk** within a large lactiferous duct is responsible.
❐ The tumor is usually located in the **central portion of the breast or under the nipple.**
❐ Needle aspiration produces **thick, creamy material** that may be tinged dark-green or brown. Although it appears purulent, the fluid is sterile.
❐ The treatment is needle aspiration. Withdrawal of thick milky secretion confirms the diagnosis,
❐ Operation is reserved for those cysts that cannot be aspirated or that become super infected.

➲ Phyllodes Tumor: High Yield for AIPGMEE, AIIMS, PGI 2012/2013

✓ Serocystic disease of Broide or Cystosarcoma Phyllodes ☚	JK 2007
✓ Name is **misnomer** as it is rarely cystic or rarely develops into sarcoma.	
✓ **Phyllodes: Leaf.** It is a **benign** breast tumor. It is a **stromal** breast tumor.	

✓	They presents as a **large, massive tumor with uneven bosselated** surface. ☛
✓	They are however mobile and resemble fibroadenoma
✓	They account for **less than 1%** of all breast neoplasms.
✓	This is predominantly a tumor of **adult women,** with very few examples reported in adolescents.
✓	Patients typically present with **a firm, palpable mass.** ☛
✓	These tumors are **very fast growing,** and can increase in size in just a few weeks.
✓	Occurrence is most common **between the ages of 40 and 50,** prior to the menopause.
✓	The common treatment for phyllodes is **wide local excision.** Other than surgery, there is no cure for phyllodes, as chemotherapy and radiation therapy are not effective. ☛☛

⇨ Indicators of Poor Prognosis in Breast Cancer

►	↑PCNA, Ki67 expression☛☛
►	↑bcl2 expression☛
►	↓bax expression
►	↑HER 2 expression☛☛☛
►	↑EGFR expression
►	↑p53 expression

⇨ Characteristics of Advanced Breast Carcinoma

❒	Edema.
❒	Redness.
❒	Nodularity or ulceration of the Skin.
❒	Presence of large primary tumor.
❒	Fixation to chest wall.
❒	Enlargement, shrinkage.
❒	Retraction of breast.
❒	Marked axillary lymphadenopathy.
❒	Supra clavicular LAP.
❒	Oedema of ipsilateral arm.
❒	Distant metastasis.

✓	Angiosarcoma and lymphangiosarcoma develop as a complication of lymphedema in patients of breast cancer. ☛☛☛
✓	A greenish discharge is usually due to duct ectasia
✓	Mondors disease is thrombophelibitis of breast (superficial veins) ☛ PGI 2006

⇨ Treatment of Breast Cancer

PGI 2002

Stage I, II:

- ✓ Breast Conserving Therapy ☛☛
- ✓ MRM + Systemic Therapy

Stage III (operable)

- ✓ MRM + Chemotherapy + Radiotherapy☛☛☛

Stage IV

- ✓ Palliative

⇨ Surgeries Commonly Asked

- ► QUART: (Quadrenectomy) +axillary block dissection+ radiotherapy
- ► Lumpectomy: Removal of tumor +2cm rim of normal breast atleast☛
- ► Simple Mastectomy: Removal of breast +skin
- ► MRM (Pateys): Removal of breast+axillary block dissection☛
- ► Radical Mastectomy: MRM + removal of pectoral muscles+thoracodorsal nerve+artery to latissmus dorsi
- ► Extended Radical Mastectomy: Radical mastectomy+removal of internal mammary lymph nodes
- ► Had field operation cone excision of major duct ☛

Stage I: BREAST CCONSERVATIVE THERAPY/LUMPECTOMY + AXILLARY CLEARANCE + RADIOTHERAPY. PGI 2002

Stage II: BREAST CCONSERVATIVE THERAPY/LUMPECTOMY+AXILLARY CLEARANCE+ RADIOTHERAPY. PGI 2002

Stage III: NEO ADJUVANT CHEMO+ MRM+ RADIOTHERAPY (OPERABLE)

Stage III inoperable/IV: PALLIATIVE (RADIOTHERAPY)/HORMONAL ABLATION/CHEMOTHERAPY

Breast Reconstruction:

May be performed at the time of mastectomy for breast cancer or later.

First, the existing skin can be stretched by placing a tissue expander underneath it and gradually inflating the expander until the skin has stretched to the required amount. The expander then acts as an implant.

Second, the skin and volume component of the breast can be replaced by **the latissimus dorsi musculocutaneous flap with or without an underlying silicone breast implant.**

Third, the skin and volume component of the breast can be replaced by a **transverse rectus abdominis musculocutaneous flap (TRAM flap).**

⇨ Paget Disease of Breast

- ➠ Infiltrating ductal carcinoma involving the nipple epithelium
- ➠ 1% of all breast cancers
- ➠ No age group predilection
- ➠ Changes may be limited to the nipple, extend to the areola, or to the skin around the areola
- ➠ 50-60% have a palpable tumor

- If lesion is confined to nipple only, axillary metastases present in only 5% of patients
- Paget disease of the breast has been associated with **breast carcinoma developing in males who had Klinefelter syndrome.**

SYMPTOMS AND SIGNS

- Burning and pruritus of the nipple
- Superficial erosion or ulceration of the nipple
- Serous or bloody nipple discharge
- Nipple retraction

IMAGING FINDINGS

- Mammography may show thickening of the nipple, calcifications, or lesion anywhere in the breast

Male Breast Cancer: High Yield for AIPGMEE, AIIMS, PGI 2012/2013

- Breast cancer occurring in the mammary gland of males is **infrequent**, accounting for no more than 1% of the incidence in women.
- It generally occurs at an **older age.**
- The average age at diagnosis is **10 years older in men** than in women.
- Probably because the breast tissue is scant in men, breast tumors in males **involve the pectoralis major muscle more commonly.**
- Delay in diagnosis also must play a role in the more advanced presentation of male breast cancer.
- Histologically, tumors of the male breast are most commonly **infiltrating ductal carcinomas** that are similar in appearance to their counterparts in females.
- Male breast cancer very often contains **steroid hormone receptors.**
- The treatment of carcinoma in the male breast depends on the stage and local extent of the tumor. If the underlying pectoral muscle is involved, radical mastectomy is the procedure of choice. Alternatively, modified radical mastectomy with excision of the involved portion of muscle is adequate treatment.
- **For smaller tumors**, which are movable across the chest wall, modified radical mastectomy appears to be the procedure of choice. Because of the local aggressiveness of these tumors, some authors have advocated the use of postoperative radiation therapy.
- The presence of nodal metastases appears to have at least the same prognostic power in men as in women.

Risk Factors are

- Conditions with **Hyperestrogenic** and **Hypoandrogenic** states.
- **Cirrhosis of liver**
- **Undescended testis**
- **Mumps orchitis**
- **Klienfilters syndrome**
- **May accompany gynecomastia**

- Most common variety is **infiltrating ductal cancer.**
- Presents with **unilateral lump** with majority being **Estrogen receptor positive.**

1

⇨ Mondor Disease (Thrombophlebitis of the Thoracoepigastric Vein)

Essential Features

- **Thrombophlebitis of the thoracoepigastric vein over breast or upper abdomen**
- **More common in women**
- **Self-limited, often within 3 wks**
- **Little to no risk of thromboembolism**
- Occasionally follows radical mastectomy

Symptoms and Signs

- Breast pain
- Superficial abdominal pain
- Localized tender, cord-like structure in subcutaneous tissue of abdomen thorax or axilla

⇨ Remember to Differentiate it From Menetrier'e Disease Which is:

- **Gastric pits are elongated and tortuous** with replacement of parietal & chief cells, so mucosal folds of body and fundus are greatly enlarged.
- Most patients are **hypochlorhydic**
- Majority of patients in middle or old age have **protein losing enteropathy** due to protein leakage from gastric mucosa.
- Barium meal shows enlarged nodular and course folds
- Treatment with antisecretory drugs may reduce protein loss but unresponsive patients require partial gastrectomy

⇨ Tietze Syndrome

- **Painful, nonsuppurative inflammation of costochondral cartilage**
- **Unknown cause**
- **May represent seronegative rheumatic disease**
- **Often self-limited**
- **Unilateral or bilateral**
- **Involves second-fourth costal cartilages**

SYMPTOMS AND SIGNS

- Local swelling, tenderness in parasternal area

SURGERY

1

SURGERY

➲ Aorta:

⇨ Aortic Injury

- Widening of superior mediastinum> 8 cms is considered a reliable sign of Aortic injury.
- "PA view" is better than AP view in this type of injury
- X ray is used as a "screening tool "here.
- "Acceleration or deceleration" injuries are associated with aortic rupture.

⇨ Other Signs are

- ✓ Obscured aortic knob
- ✓ Widened mediastinum
- ✓ Deviation of left main stem bronchus
- ✓ Obliteration of aorticopulmonary window
- ✓ Deviation of nasogastric tube
- ✓ Left apical cap
- ✓ Opacification of aortopulmonary window.
- ✓ Left pulmonary Hilar hematoma

⇨ Zones in Neck Injury

- Zone I : Sternal notch to cricoid cartilage
- Zone II : Cricoid cartilage to angle of mandible
- Zone III : angle of mandible to base of skull

Remember:

- **Whiplash injury** is acute hyperflexion of spine. Especially cervical spine.
- **Coup and contre coup injuries** are a feature of brain.
- **Blast injuries** cause damage to lungs and intestines

⇨ Blast Injury

- Rupture of Tympanic membrane, dislocation of ear ossicles
- Injury to lungs
- Perforation of stomach, gut.
- Conjuctival hemorrhage in eyes.

➲ Thoracic Outlet Syndrome: High Yield for AIPGMEE, AIIMS, PGI 2012/2013

- ❐ Thoracic outlet syndrome,
- ❐ Scalenus anticus syndrome,
- ❐ Cervical rib syndrome,
- ❐ Paget Schroetter syndrome,
- ❐ Costoclavicular syndrome, Cervical band syndrome,
- ❐ Cervicobrachial myofascial pain syndrome, Brachial plexopathy

1

SURGERY

- Thoracic outlet syndrome (TOS) is due to compression/irritation of brachial plexus elements **("Neurogenic TOS")** and/or subclavian vessels **("Vascular TOS")** in their passage from the cervical area toward the axilla. The usual site of entrapment is the **interscalenic triangle.**
- Provocation tests that can suggest the presence of thoracic outlet syndrome include:
  - **Adson's maneuver.**
  - **Wright test**
  - **Roos stress test**

A female with **recent tooth extraction** has huge hot, red, tender mass in left lower side of face **pushing up the floor of mouth**	**Ludwings Angina**
A 50 year old notices **coldness and tingling in his left hand and forearm** pain while doing **heavy work** along with **vertigo, blurred vision**	**Subclavian steal syndrome**
A 50 year old has **a 6 cms pulsatile mass deep in abdomen**	**AAA (Abdominal Aortic Aneurysm)**
A 65 year old has **sudden onset, tearing chest pain radiating to back** with BP 220/120 with **unequal arm pressures** and normal cardiac enzynes	**Dissecting aneurysm of Thoraxic Aorta**
A 20 year old with **BP 195/120 in upper limb** with **normal BP in lower limbs and rib notching**	**Coarctation of Aorta**

Neck

Dermoid Cysts

- These usually occur at sites of **embryological fusion.**
- These may be in the midline.
- A dermoid cyst in the neck may be mistaken for a thyroglossal cyst although **it will not move on swallowing or protrusion of the tongue.**
- A common site is the **external angular dermoid cyst in the eyebrow** area at the outer angle of the eye. Occasionally there may be a dumbbell extension intracranially.
- They occur if **ectodermal cells** become buried beneath the skin surface during development.
- An **inclusion dermoid cyst** may similarly arise secondary to trauma.

Cystic Hygroma

- Commonly arising in the neck, these **fluid filled lesions of lymphatic origin, (Lymphangioma)** PGI 1999
- **MC site: Posterior triangle of neck**
- Seen in **Turners syndrome, trisomies, fetal alcohol syndrome, multiple pterygium syndrome.** PGI 2000
- **Brilliantly translucent , positive cough impulse** AI 1991
- They are either present at birth, sometimes being diagnosed on antenatal ultrasonography, or may appear within the first 2 years or sometimes later.

- **Infection** leads to difficulty with subsequent surgery, which is thus best performed soon after diagnosis.
- **Excision is treatment of choice.** AI 2003
- Aspiration of the cysts and injection of a **streptococcal derivative 'OK432', bleomycin, picibanil** is a treatment that is proving to be an effective alternative to surgery.

⇨ Sternomastoid Tumor

- **Is due to infarction of sternomastoid muscle**☚
- Usually **during delivery**
- Infarcted muscle replaced by fibrosis
- Present **immediately after birth as a "swelling"** with the **new born keeping his/her neck to one side.**

⇨ Branchial Cyst

- Remanant of **Second branchial cleft**☚
- Mc site is **upper part of neck** at junction of upper **anterior border** of sternomastoid.☚☚ PGI 2006
- **Wallis made of lymphoid tissue.** PGI 2007
- **"NON" translucent**☚
- **Complete excision** is treatment of choice.

⇨ Ranula (Latin Rana = Frog)

- This is a **sublingual cyst** which may be small or may fill the **floor of the mouth.** ☚
- Extravasation cyst of sublingual glands TN 1991
- It may be related to a salivary or mucus gland.
- It is thin walled and contains **clear viscid fluid.** ↑☚
- Care is required **not to damage the submandibular duct** during its excision and marsupialization is often safer.

⇨ Chemodectoma

- **"Potato tumor"** or carotid body tumor.☚
- **"Benign tumor" but rarely metastasizes (unusual combination)**
- **Arises from "chemoreceptor zone".**☚
- <u>Non</u> chromaffin para ganglioma AIIMS 1997
- <u>Origin from Schwann cells</u> PGI 2005
- **Association with high altitude. Family history and Pheochromocytoma.**☚
- **Bipopsy is contraindicated.**☚
- **Usually unilateral**
- **Firm, rubbery, mobile from side to side, slow growing.**☚
- **Bruit** may be present
- **Angiogram** is diagnostic.
- **Good prognosis, rarely metastasizes.** PGI 2002
- **Surgical excision** is **"treatment of choice"**☚☚ AIIMS 2004

Branchial Cyst
➡ Arises from 2 nd Branchial cleft
➡ Located usually at anterior border of upper 1/3 of Sternomastoid
➡ Contains cholesterol crystals
Branchial Fistula
➡ Represents persists 2 nd Branchial Cleft
➡ Located usually at anterior border of lower 1/3 of Sternomastoid
Cystic Hygroma
➡ Represents lymphatic venous anastamotic failure
➡ Located usually in the neck at lower in posterior triangle
➡ Brilliantly translucent
Cervical Rib
➡ Mostly unilateral
➡ Mostly on right side

⇨ Surgically Important Thyroid Conditions

Ectopic Thyroid and Anomalies of the Thyroglossal tract
➡ Some **residual thyroid tissue** along the course of the thyroglossal tract is not uncommon, and may be lingual, cervical or intrathoracic. ➡ Very rarely the whole gland is ectopic.
Lingual thyroid
➡ This forms a rounded swelling at the **back of the tongue** at the **foramen cecum** (and it may represent the only thyroid tissue present. ☛ ➡ It may cause dysphagia, impairment of speech, respiratory obstruction or hemorrhage. ➡ It is best treated by full replacement with thyroxine when it should get smaller, but excision or ablation with radioiodine is sometimes necessary.
Median (thyroglossal) ectopic thyroid
➡ This forms a swelling in the **upper part of the neck** and is usually mistaken for a thyroglossal cyst.
Lateral aberrant thyroid
➡ There is no evidence that aberrant thyroid tissue ever occurs ➡ 'Normal thyroid tissue' found laterally, separate from the thyroid gland, **must be considered and treated as a metastasis** in a cervical lymph node from an occult thyroid carcinoma, almost **invariably of papillary type.** ☛☛
Struma ovarii
➡ Is not ectopic thyroid tissue, but **part of an ovarian teratoma.** ➡ Very rarely, neoplastic change occurs or hyperthyroidism develops.

➲ Struma Ovarii: High Yield for AIPGMEE, AIIMS, PGI 2012/2013

- Is a **rare ovarian tumor** defined by the presence of thyroid tissue
- Most commonly, they occur as part of a teratoma, but may occasionally be encountered with **serous or mucinous cystadenomas**
- Several variants of the tumor exist.
- Benign strumosis is a rare version of mature thyroid tissue implants throughout the peritoneal cavity.
- Strumal carcinoid is defined by the presence of carcinoid tissue within a struma and is exceptionally rare.
- The vast majority of struma ovarii are benign; however, malignant disease is found in a small percentage of cases.
- The symptoms of struma ovarii are similar to other ovarian tumors and are nonspecific in nature.
- The tumor can be characterized by radiological imaging; however, the final diagnosis is made upon **pathological and histological** examination of the tissue itself.

Surgical resection remains the definitive treatment for benign disease, and surgery with adjuvant radioiodine therapy has been shown to be successful in treating metastatic and recurrent disease

➲ Thyroglossal Cyst: High Yield for AIPGMEE, AIIMS, PGI 2012/2013

- This may be present in any part of the **thyroglossal tract**
- MC site is **beneath the hyoid**, in the region of the thyroid cartilage, and above the hyoid bone. **AI 1998**
- **Occupies the midline**, except in the region of the thyroid cartilage, where the thyroglossal tract is pushed to one side, usually to the left. **AI 2006**
- The **swelling moves upwards on protrusion of the tongue as well as on swallowing** because of the attachment of the tract to the foramen cecum. **AI 2006**

Never to be forgotten:

- ✓ **Subhyoid,** **AIIMS 1997**
- ✓ **Painless,** **AIIMS 1997**
- ✓ **Midline,**
- ✓ **Non transluminant but fluctuant swelling**

A thyroglossal cyst **should be excised (Sistrunks operation)** because infection is inevitable, owing to the fact that the wall contains nodules of lymphatic tissue which communicate by lymphatics with the lymph nodes of the neck. **DNB 2011**

Thyroglossal fistula

- Thyroglossal flstula is **never congenital.**
- It follows **infection or inadequate removal** of a thyroglossal cyst.
- The cutaneous opening of such a fistula is **drawn upwards on protrusion of the tongue.**
- A thyroglossal fistula is **lined by columnar epithelium**, discharges mucus, and is the seat of recurrent attacks of inflammation.

1

SURGERY

➲ Sistrunk's Operation

Because the thyroglossal tract is so closely related to the body of the hyoid bone, this central part must be excised, together with the cyst or fistula, or recurrence is certain. When the thyroglossal tract can be traced upwards towards the foramen cecum, it must be excised with the central section of the body of the hyoid bone, and a central core of lingual muscle.

▶ A 10 year old girl with round 1 cm mass in **midline of neck** moving with **movement of tongue**	**Throglossal duct Cyst**
▶ A 15 year old girl with round 1 cm on side of **neck beneath and in front of sternocleidomastoid.**	**Branchial cyst**
▶ A 6 year old with **fluid filled translucent mass** in supraclavicular area	**Cystic hygroma**
▶ A 35 year old with **enlarged lymph nodes in cervical region** with **night sweats and pruritis plus axillary lymphadenopathy**	**Lymphoma**

➲ De Quervain's Thyroiditis

Granulomatous thyroiditis - Subacute thyroiditis – De Quervain's thyroiditis

- This is due to a **virus infection.** **AI 2002**
- There is **pain in the neck, fever, malaise and a firm, irregular enlargement** of one or both thyroid lobes.
- There is a **raised erythrocyte sedimentation rate** and **AI 2002**
- **Absent thyroid antibodies, uptake of Iodine in the gland is low**
- The condition is **self limiting** - subsequent hypothyroidism is rare. **AI 2002**
- In 10 percent of cases the onset is acute, the goiter very painful and tender, and there may be symptoms of hyperthyroidism.
- **The specific treatment for the acute case with severe pain is to give prednisone.**

➲ Riedel's Thyroiditis

Riedel's thyroiditis

- Thyroid tissue is **replaced by cellular fibrous tissue** which infiltrates through the capsule into adjacent muscles, paratracheal connective tissue and the carotid sheaths.
- It may occur in association with **Retroperitoneal and Mediastinal fibrosis**
- The goiter may be unilateral or bilateral and is **very hard and fixed.**
- The **differential diagnosis from anaplastic carcinoma** can only be made with certainty by biopsy, when a wedge of the isthmus should also be removed to free the trachea.
- If unilateral, the other lobe is usually involved later and subsequent **hypothyroidism** is common.

⇨ Solitary Thyroid Nodules

- More common in females. **PGI 2006**
- Nodules classified as cold, warm or hot
- **Most solitary thyroid nodules are cold**

▶ MALT Lymphomas present at extra nodal sites.	PGI 05
▶ MALT Lymphomas are predisposed by H. pylori.	
▶ MALT Lymphomas are sensitive to chemotherapy.	

⇨ Pseudolymphoma

- Represents 10% of all gastric lymphomas.
- Pseudolymphoma is **benign gastric lymphomatosis**, characterized by lymphoid infiltration of the gastric wall, predominantly in the mucosa, without evidence of nodal disease.
- **Ulceration and extensive fibrosis** are present, commonly with chronic peptic ulcer disease.
- Pseudolymphoma may represent a **premalignant lesion** that can convert to malignant lymphoma

⇨ Mucosa-associated Lymphoid Tissue (MALT) Tumors

- Are **low-grade B-cell tumors** that demonstrate mucosally based lymphoid tissue.
- They have growth characteristics that are **less malignant** than those of lymphomas.
- MALT tumors are associated with **Helicobacter pylori**, and recent reports suggest that eradication of the H. pylori leads to regression of the tumor.
- MALT tumors can progress to high-grade lymphomas, since they frequently coexist.

⇨ Gastric Antral Vascular Ectasia (Gave)

- Is an **uncommon cause of chronic gastrointestinal bleeding or iron deficiency anemia.**
- The condition is assoicated with **dilated small blood vessels in the antrum, or the last part of the stomach.**
- It is also called **"watermelon stomach"** because streaky long red areas that are present in the stomach may resemble the markings on watermelon.
- GAVE is **associated with a number of conditions, including**
  - ✓ **Portal hypertension,**
  - ✓ **Chronic renal failure,**
  - ✓ **Collagen vascular diseases, particularly sclerodema.**
- Pathology: The endoscopic appearance of GAVE is similar to portal hypertensive gastropathy. Typical histologic changes include superficial hyperplestic antral mucosa, dilated capillaries containing fibrin thrombi and fibromuscular hypertrophy of the lamina propia.
- Clinical features; acute severe Hemorrhage is rare. Most patients presents with persistent inron deficiency anemia from continued occult blood loss.
- GAVE is treated with treatment through the **endoscope, including argon plasma coagulation and electrocautery.**
- Other medical treatments have been tried and include estrogen and progesterone therapy and anti-fibrinolytic drugs such as tranexamic acid.

➲ Other Conditions Seen:

⇨ GIST

- Originate from the **interstitial cell of cajal (intestinal pacemaker).**
- Common in stomach AIPGME 2011
- **Tyrosine kinase** activity is high in these Tumors.
- 70% spindle cells and 30% epithelial cells.
- Benign GIST are 2-3 times more frequent than malignant.
- Lymph node metastasis is rare.
- Liver is involved in metastasis.
- Manifest in fourth decade.
- Bleeding is the main presentation in gastric GIST, bleeding and obstruction in small intestinal.
- **Expresses CD117 and CD34.**
- Treatment margin negative resection and adjuvant therapy with **Imatinib**
- Follow up treatment is done with PET

Acute Gastric Dilatation:

- This condition usually occurs in association with some form of ileus which is not treated by nasogastric suction.
- The **stomach, which may also be atonic, dilates enormously.**
- Often the patient Vomits, is also dehydrated and has electrolyte disturbances. **PGI 2006**
- Failure to treat this condition can result in a sudden massive vomit with aspiration into the lungs. **PGI 2005**
- The **treatment is nasogastric suction, fluid replacement** and treatment of the underlying condition.
- Surgery is not advocated. **AIIMS 1997**

Trichobezoar and phytobezoar

Trichobezoar (Hair Balls) ☚

- Are unusual and are virtually exclusively found in **female psychiatric patients**, often young.
- It is caused by the pathological **ingestion of hair which remains undigested** in the stomach.
- The hair ball can **lead to ulceration and gastrointestinal bleeding, perforation or obstruction.**
- The diagnosis is made easily at **endoscopy** or, indeed, from a plain radiograph.
- Treatment consists of **removal of the bezoar** which may require open surgical treatment.

Phytobezoars ☚

- **Are made of the "vegetable matter"** and found principally in patients who have gastric stasis. **MANIPAL 2006**

Volvulus of the Stomach:

- **Rotation of the stomach** usually occurs around the axis and between its two fixed points, i.e., the cardia and the pylorus. ☚

- Rotation can occur in the **horizontal (organoaxial) "most common"** or vertical (mesenterioaxial) direction
- This condition is usually associated with **(paraoesophageal herniation)**
- The transverse **colon moves upwards to lie under the left diaphragm**, thus taking the stomach with it, and the stomach and colon may both enter the chest through the eventration of the diaphragm.
- The condition is **commonly chronic**, the patient presenting with difficulty in eating. An acute presentation with ischaemia may occur.

Ulcers

Are defined as a break in the mucosal surface >5 mm in size, with depth to the submucosa.

Duodenal ulcer	Gastric ulcer
More common	
More associated with **H. pylori**	Less common
Early age of onset	Associated with H. pylori
Occur most often in the **first portion of duodenum**), with ~90% located within 3 cm of the pylorus.	Later age of onset
	Occur most often in the lesser curvature
Less chances of malignancy	More chances of malignancy
No loss of weight	Loss of weight
Tenderness usually **in R. Hypochondrium**	Tenderness usually midline
Night pain **common**	Night pain uncommon

Curlings ulcer: GI ulcers in severe burns	UPSC
Cushings ulcer: GI ulcers in head Injury	

Giant Duodenal Ulcers (GDUs)

Are a subset of duodenal ulcers that have historically tesulted in greater morbidity than usual duocenal ulcers.

Criteria for definition:

- **Ulcer crater greater than 2 cm,**
- **Performance of the roentgen examination before surgical or pathological demonstration of ulcer.**
- **Proof that the lesion was benign and confirmation at surgery or post-mortem examintion**

Aetiology: GDUs have been most commonly associated with recent NSAID use and H pylori infection.

Clinical features: The most common of these symptoms is abdominal pain. The majority of GDUs also present with hemorrhage.

Most Common

MC Site of gastric ulcer	Lesser Curvature	
MC Site of duodenal ulcer	Duodenal Cap	COMED 2000
MC Site of carcinoma stomach	Antrum	
MC Site Zollinger-Ellison Syndrome	Pancreas	

1

SURGERY

Malignant Gastric Ulcer

- Ulcer≥2.5 cm
- Ulcer within a mass
- Folds that don't radiate from ulcer margin

⇨ Perforated Peptic Ulcer

- Is the **second most common complication** of peptic ulcer.
- Usually located anteriorly
- **Duodenal ulcer perforation is more common in younger.**
- **Gastric ulcer perforation is more common in older.**
- **Gastroduodenal artery bleeds in duodenal ulcer.** PGI 2000
- Free gas under diaphragm is indicative.
- Treatment is by: Nasogastric suction, acid suppression, broad spectrum antibiotics are used PGI 2001
- Exploratory laprotomy PGI 2001

Surgical Treatment of Duodenal Ulcers:

- **Highly selective vagotomy (Least chance of diahorrea/dumping syndrome)** AIIMS 2001
- **Selective vagotomy and drainage**
- **Truncal vagotomy and drainage**
- **Truncal vagotomy and anterectomy (Lowest chance of recurrence)** AI 2002

Surgical Treatment of Gastric Ulcers:

- **Distal gastrectomy**
- **Vagotomy, pyloroplasty and ulcer excision**

➲ GI Bleeding: Causes

⇨ ABCDEFGHI:

- **Angiodysplasia**
- **Bowel cancer**
- **Colitis**
- **Diverticulitis/Duodenal ulcer**
- **Epitaxis/ Esophageal (cancer, esophagitis, varices)**
- **Fistula (anal, aortaenteric)**
- **Gastric (cancer, ulcer, gastritis)**
- **Hemorrhoids**
- **Infectious diarrhea/IBD/Ischemic bowel**

- **Hematemesis indicates an upper GI source of bleeding** (above the ligament of Treitz). Melena indicates that blood has been present in the GI tract for at least 14 h. Thus, the more proximal the bleeding site, the more likely melena will occur.
- **Hematochezia usually represents a lower GI source of bleeding**, although an upper GI lesion may **bleed** so rapidly that blood does not remain in the bowel long enough for melena to develop.
- **GIB of obscure origin** Obscure GIB is defined as recurrent acute or chronic bleeding for which no source has been identified by routine endoscopic and contrast studies. Push enteroscopy, with a specially designed enteroscope or a pediatric colonoscope to inspect the entire duodenum and part of the jejunum, is generally the next step. Push enteroscopy may identify probable bleeding sites in 20 to 40% of patients with obscure GIB. If enteroscopy is negative or unavailable, a specialized radiographic examination of the small bowel (e.g., Enteroclysis) should be performed.
- **Occult GIB** is manifested by either a **positive test for fecal occult blood or iron deficiency anemia.**
- **Peptic ulcers are the most common cause of** <u>**UGIB**</u>, accounting for about 50% of cases. **Mallory-Weiss tears** account for 5 to 15% of cases. **Hemorrhagic or erosive gastropathy** [e.g., due to nonsteroidal anti-inflammatory drugs (NSAIDs) or alcohol] and erosive esophagitis often cause mild UGIB, but major bleeding is rare.

Dumping Syndrome

Dumping syndrome consists of a series of **vasomotor and gastrointestinal signs and symptoms and occurs in patients who have undergone vagotomy and drainage (especially Billroth procedures).**

Early Dumping

- Takes place **15 to 30 min** after meals
- Consists of crampy abdominal discomfort, nausea, diarrhea, belching, tachycardia, palpitations, diaphoresis, light-headedness, and, rarely, syncope.
- Cause: **rapid emptying of hyperosmolar gastric contents** into the small intestine, **AI 1999**
- Fluid shift into the gut lumen with plasma volume contraction and acute intestinal distention.
- Release of vasoactive gastrointestinal hormones (vasoactive intestinal polypeptide, neurotensin, motilin)

Late Dumping

- Typically occurs **90 min to 3 h** after meals.
- **Vasomotor symptoms** (light-headedness, diaphoresis, palpitations, tachycardia, and syncope) predominate during this phase.
- This component of **dumping** is thought to be **secondary to hypoglycemia** from excessive insulin release.

- Dumping **syndrome** is most noticeable after **meals rich in simple carbohydrates** (especially sucrose) and **high osmolarity.**
- Ingestion of **large amounts of fluids** may also contribute.
- Up to **50% of postvagotomy and drainage patients** will experience **dumping syndrome** to some degree.
- Signs and symptoms **often improve with time**
- **Dietary modification** is the cornerstone of therapy for patients with **dumping syndrome.**

- **Small, multiple (six) meals devoid of simple carbohydrates** coupled with elimination of liquids during meals is important.
- **Antidiarrheals and anticholinergic agents** are complimentary to diet.
- The somatostatin analogue **octreotide** has been successful in diet refractory cases.

Short Bowel Syndrome

Clinical problems that often occur following resection of varying lengths of small intestine

Features:

- **Diarrhea and/or steatorrhea,** **AIIMS 1996**
- **Increase in renal calcium oxalate calculi** is observed in patients with a small-intestinal resection with an intact colon and is due to an increase in oxalate absorption by the large intestine, with subsequent hyperoxaluria.
- **Gastric hypersecretion** of acid **AI 1998**

Treatment:

- Diet should be **low-fat, high-carbohydrate** to minimize the diarrhea proton pump inhibitor may be helpful.
- **Fat-soluble vitamins**, folate, cobalamin, calcium, iron, magnesium, and zinc are the most critical factors to monitor on a regular basis.
- If these approaches are not successful, **TPN** represents an established therapy that can be maintained for many years.
- **Intestinal transplantation** is beginning to become established as a possible approach for individuals with extensive intestinal resection who cannot be maintained without **TPN**.

Bacterial Overgrowth Syndrome or Stagnant Bowel Syndrome

- **Diarrhea, steatorrhea, and macrocytic anemia** whose common feature is the proliferation of colon-type bacteria within the small intestine.
- Due to **stasis caused by**
  - ✓ **Impaired peristalsis (i.e. functional stasis),**
  - ✓ **Changes in intestinal anatomy (i.e. anatomic stasis),**
  - ✓ **Direct communication between the small and large intestine.**
- Presence of increased amounts of a colonic-type bacterial flora, such **as E. coli or Bacteroides**, in the small intestine.
- **Macrocytic anemia** is due to cobalamin, not folate, deficiency.
- **Steatorrhea** is due to impaired micelle formation as a consequence of a reduced intraduodenal concentration of bile acids and the presence of unconjugated bile acids.
- Best established by a **Schilling test** which should be abnormal following the administration of ^{58}Co-labeled cobalamin, with or without the administration of intrinsic factor.
- Following the administration of tetracycline for 5 days, the Schilling test will become normal, confirming the diagnosis of bacterial overgrowth.

Ulcerative Colitis	Crohn's Disease
❒ Involves rectum always☛☛	❒ Involves ileum mostly
❒ May cause "**pancolitis**"	❒ Non diffuse involvement
❒ **Diffuse involvement**	❒ Called "**regional enteritis**"☛
❒ Retrograde spread to ileum is **backwash ileitis**	
❒ Disease of continuity	❒ Skip lesions☛☛ AI 96
❒ Pseudopolyps present☛ AI 94	❒ Pseudopolyps absent☛
❒ Limited to mucosa and submucosa	❒ Transmural inflammation
❒ Non caseasting granulomas not seen☛☛	❒ Non caseasting granulomas seen☛☛☛
❒ Creeping fat not seen	❒ Creeping fat seen☛☛ JK BOPEE
❒ Crypt abscess. PGI 2006	❒ Crypt abcess also seen. PGI 2006
❒ Strictures, ulcerations, fistula less frequent	❒ Strictures,ulcerations, fistula frequent
❒ Toxic megacolon occurs AI 96	❒ Rare
❒ Malignant transformation +++☛☛	❒ Malignant transformation +
❒ Malignant transformation +	
❒ Malignant transformation from dysplastic sites. PGI 98	
❒ **Takes 10 years to develop.** PGI 1999	
❒ **Common in younger patients**	
❒ **Associations of UC:**	
➨ **pyoderma gangreonosum** PGI 1999	
➨ **Erythema nodosum**	

⇨ Surgery in UC

There are several well-identified complications that require urgent **operation for survival**. These include

- ❒ **Massive, unrelenting hemorrhage;** ☛☛
- ❒ **Toxic megacolon with impending or frank perforation;** ☛
- ❒ **Fulminating acute ulcerative colitis that is unresponsive to steroid therapy;**
- ❒ **Obstruction from stricture;**
- ❒ **Suspicion or demonstration of colonic cancer.**

- ❒ The largest numbers of colectomies for ulcerative colitis are performed for less dramatic indications, as the disease enters an intractable chronic phase and becomes both a physical and a social burden to the patient.
- ❒ **For Hemorrhage/Bleeding**: Prompt surgical intervention is indicated after hemodynamic stabilization. More than 50% of patients with acute colonic bleeding have toxic megacolon, so one should be suspicious of the coexistence of the two complications. Uncontrollable hemorrhage from the entire colorectal mucosa may be the one clear indication for emergency proctocolectomy. If possible, the rectum should be spared for later mucosal proctectomy with ileoanal anastomosis.

1

SURGERY

⇨ Acute Toxic Megacolon

- ❐ Can occur in both ulcerative colitis and Crohn's disease.
- ❐ Its incidence is higher in ulcerative colitis. ☛☛
- ❐ Patients usually present clinically with the **onset of abdominal pain and severe diarrhea (greater than 10 stools per day), followed by abdominal distention and generalized tenderness.** ☛☛
- ❐ Once megacolon and toxicity develop, fever, leukocytosis, tachycardia, pallor, lethargy, and shock ensue. It is important to note that any of these manifestations can **be masked** by chronic steroid use and the generally poor nutritional condition of the patient.
- ❐ An abdominal radiograph usually shows dilation of the transverse and occasionally the sigmoid colon that is greater than 5 cm. and averages 9.2 cm. Thickening and nodularity of the bowel wall due to mucosal inflammation are also noted.
- ❐ **Initial treatment for toxic megacolon includes intravenous fluid and electrolyte resuscitation, nasogastric suction, broad-spectrum antibiotics to include anaerobic and aerobic gram-negative coverage, and total parenteral nutrition to improve nutritional status.** Proctoscopy may be helpful in determining the etiology of the attack, as may culture of the stool.

⇨ Adipose Tissue Changes of Crohns Disease

- ✓ **Fat Hypertrophy**
- ✓ **Fat Wrapping (Creeping fat)** — **JK BOPEE**
- ✓ More than **50%** of intestinal surface may be covered by fat especially along the **antimesentric border** and sometimes leading to the **obliteration of bowel mesentry angle.**
- ✓ Creeping fat is well demonstrated by **CT scan.**

⇨ Ulcers in GIT

- ➨ Transverse Ulcers: TB☛☛
- ➨ Longitudnal Ulcer: Crohns Disease☛
- ➨ "Flask" shaped Ulcer: Amebic ulcer☛ — COMED 2002

⇨ Ileal Resection: DNB 2011

Early Complications

The main complications of ileal resection operation in the early postoperative period are **intestinal obstruction from adhesions, intra-abdominal abscess, wound infection, anastomotic leaks, bleeding from areas of operation, phlebothrombosis and pulmonary embolism, atelectasis and pulmonary infections, urinary retention, and enterocutaneous fistulas.**

Late Complications

- Resection of the ileum can result in **malabsorption of vitamin B 12.** The ileum is the sole site of absorption of this vitamin.
- The ileum is also the area of intestine where bile salts are actively absorbed. Extensive ileal resections can result in **depletion of the bile salt pool, resulting in steatorrhea** from lack of sufficient bile salts in the enteric lumen for the formation of bile salt micelles. Micelles are needed for solubilization of fatty acids and their subsequent absorption. Steatorrhea may cause binding of calcium ion by fatty acids, making calcium unavailable in the enteric lumen for binding to oxalates. The unbound oxalate then passes into the large intestine, where it is absorbed. The absorbed oxalate is excreted in the urine, where it may precipitate to form **oxalate urinary stones.** Uric acid stones may also form in subjects with postresection diarrhea, with its resultant sodium, potassium, and water loss. The urine output decreases, the urine becomes more acidic, and uric acid urinary stones can form.
- Extensive resections may leave insufficient small intestinal mucosa for the digestion and absorption of foodstuffs, vitamins, water, and electrolytes. **The short bowel syndrome** then develops. This condition is characterized by **crampy abdominal pain, diarrhea, borborygmi, abdominal distention, and weight loss.**

⇨ Tumors of Small Bowel

Benign:

- Adenoma
- Lipoma
- Angioma
- Hamartoma

Malignant:

- Adenocarcinoma
- Carcinoid
- Lymphoma
- Sarcoma

⇨ Small Intestine

- Blood Supply. The small intestine receives its blood supply from the **superior mesenteric artery,** the second large branch of the abdominal aorta.
- **Peyer's patches** are lymph nodules aggregated in the submucosa of the small intestine. These lymphatic nodules are most abundant in the ileum, but the jejunum also contains them.
- Mucosa. The mucosal surface of the small intestine contains numerous circular mucosal folds called the **plicae circulares (valvulae conniventes, or valves of Kerckring).** These folds are 3 to 10 mm. in height; they are taller and more numerous in the distal duodenum and proximal jejunum, becoming shorter and fewer distally.
- **Intestinal villi** barely visible to the naked eye resemble tiny finger-like processes projecting into the intestinal lumen.

1

SURGERY

⇨ Acute Mesenteric Ischemia and Infarction

Classified as occlusive or nonocclusive.

Occlusion accounts for about 75% of acute intestinal ischemia result from an arterial thrombus **(one-third of arterial occlusions)** or **embolus (two-thirds of arterial** occlusions) of the celiac or superior mesenteric arteries

- ❒ **Arterial embolus** occurs most commonly in patients with **chronic or recurrent atrial fibrillation, artificial heart valves, or valvular heart disease;** ☛
- ❒ **Arterial thrombosis** is usually associated with **extensive atherosclerosis or low cardiac output.**
- ❒ **Venous occlusion is rare**; it is occasionally seen in women taking oral contraceptives.
- ✓ The major clinical feature of acute **mesenteric ischemia** is **severe abdominal pain, often colicky and periumbilical at the onset**, later becoming diffuse and constant.
- ✓ **Superior mesenteric arteries** are commonly involved ☛
- ✓ **Vomiting, anorexia, diarrhea, and constipation** are also frequent
- ✓ Examination of the abdomen may reveal **tenderness and distention.**
- ✓ Bowel sounds are often normal even in the face of severe infarction. Some patients have a surprisingly normal abdominal examination in spite of severe pain.
- ✓ Mild gastrointestinal bleeding is often detected by examination of stool for occult blood; gross hemorrhage is unusual except in ischemic colitis. Leukocytosis is often present.
- ✓ Late in the course of the disease (24 to 72 h), **gangrene of the bowel occurs with diffuse peritonitis, sepsis, and shock.**
- ✓ Abdominal plain films in patients with **mesenteric ischemia** may reveal air-fluid levels and distention.
- ✓ Barium study of the small intestine reveals nonspecific dilation, poor motility, and evidence of thick mucosal folds **(thumbprinting)** ☛☛
- ✓ Acute **mesenteric ischemia** is a grave condition with a high morbidity and mortality.
- ✓ **Arteriography** is diagnostic ☛
- ✓ **Embolectomy** is the treatment

⇨ Chronic Intestinal Ischemia

- ❒ Called **abdominal angina.**
- ❒ Occurs under conditions of **increased demand for splanchnic blood flow.**
- ❒ The patient complains of **intermittent dull or cramping midabdominal pain 15 to 30 min after a meal,** lasting for several hours postprandially. ☛
- ❒ Significant weight loss due to decreased food intake **(food fear)** may be present. ☛
- ❒ Arteriographic studies should be performed to confirm the diagnosis
- ❒ The only definitive treatment is **vascular surgery or balloon angioplasty** to remove the thrombus or the **construction of bypass arterial grafts to the ischemic bowel.** ☛

➲ Appendix

- ❒ MC position is **retrocecal** ☛☛
- ❒ Appendicular artery is an **end artery.**
- ❒ **Mc Burneys point is in relation to appendicitis** ☛☛

⇨ Acute Appendicitis

- The peak incidence of acute **appendicitis** is in the second and third decades of life;
- It is relatively rare at the extremes of age.
- Infection with **Yersinia** organisms cause the disease, ☛☛ (PSEUDOAPPENDICITIS)
- Left sided appendicitis is diverticulosis. **APPGE 2005**
- Most commonly caused by a **fecalith**, which results from accumulation and inspissation of fecal matter around vegetable fibers.
- **Enlarged lymphoid follicles** associated with viral infections (e.g., measles), inspissated barium, worms (e.g., Oxy uris) **AI 1996**
- (Pinworms, Ascaris, and Taenia), andtumors (e.g. carcinoid or carcinoma) may also obstruct the lumen.
- **Tenderness at Mc Burneys point**
- **Retrocecal appendicitis : rigidity absent**
- **Pelvic and post ileal appendicitis : diarrhea (MISSED FREQUENTLY)** **AIIMS 1997**
- Gangrene and perforation occur. If the process evolves slowly, adjacent organs such as the terminal ileum, cecum, and omentum may wall off the appendiceal area so that a localized abscess will develop, whereas rapid progression of vascular impairment may cause perforation with free access to the peritoneal cavity.

Signs:

- ✓ **Pointing sign**☛☛
- ✓ **Rovsings sign**☛
- ✓ **Psoas sign**☛
- ✓ **Obturator** test☛

- Acute **appendicitis** may be the first manifestation of Crohn's disease.
- Fever greater than 102°F and leucocyte count greater than 18,000/mm^3 suggests **ruptured appendix**☛☛
- The history and sequence of symptoms are important diagnostic features of **appendicitis.**
- The initial symptom is almost invariably abdominal pain usually poorly localized in the periumbilical or epigastric region with an accompanying urge to defecate or pass flatus, neither of which relieves the distress.
- **Appendicitis** is the most common extrauterine condition requiring abdominal operation.
- **USG is helpful in diagnosis.** **PGI 2003**
- **USG AND CT Scan are confirmatory.** **PGI 2002**
- The treatment is early operation and appendectomy as soon as the patient can be prepared.
- The only circumstance in which operation is not indicated is the presence of a palpable mass 3 to 5 days after the onset of symptoms.

1

SURGERY

⇨ Remember for Extra Edge:

- ❒ **Rovsing's Sign:** Continuous deep palpation starting from the left iliac fossa upwards (anti clockwise along the colon) may cause pain in the right iliac fossa, by pushing bowel contents towards the ileocaecal valve and thus increasing pressure around the appendix.
- ❒ **Psoas Sign:** Psoas sign is right lower-quadrant pain that is produced with either the passive extension of the patient's right hip (patient laying on left side, with knee in flexion) or by the patient's active flexion of the right hip while supine. The pain elicited is due to inflammation of the peritoneum overlying the iliopsoas muscles and inflammation of the psoas muscles themselves. Straightening out the leg causes pain because it stretches these muscles, while flexing the hip activates the iliopsoas and therefore also causes pain.
- ❒ **Obturator Sign:** If an inflamed appendix is in contact with the obturator internus, spasm of the muscle can be demonstrated by flexing and internal rotation of the hip. This maneuver will cause pain in the hypogastrium.
- ❒ **Dunphy's Sign:** Increased pain in the right lower quadrant with coughing.
- ❒ **Sitkovskiy (Rosenstein)'s sign:** Increased pain in the right iliac region as patient lies on his/her left side.
- ❒ **Bartomier-Michelson's Sign:** Increased pain on palpation at the right iliac region as patient lies on his/her left side compared to when patient was on supine position.
- ❒ **Aure-Rozanova's Sign:** Increase pain on palpation with finger in right Petit triangle (can be a positive Shchetkin-Bloomberg's sign) - typical in retroceacal position of the appendix.
- ❒ **Blumberg Sign:** Also referred as rebound tenderness. Deep palpation of the viscera over the suspected inflamed appendix followed by sudden release of the pressure causes the severe pain on the site.

A number of clinical and laboratory based scoring systems have been devised to assist diagnosis. The most widely used is Alvarado score.

Symptoms

Migratory right iliac fossa pain: 1 point

Anorexia: 1 point

Nausea and vomiting: 1 point

Signs

Right iliac fossa tenderness: 2 points

Rebound tenderness: 1 point

Fever: 1 point

Laboratory

Leucocytosis: 2 points

Shift to left (segmented neutrophils): 1 point

⇨ Mucocele of Appendix

Mucocele of Appendix:

- ► **Is a benign tumor/retention cyst** — **AI 1989**
- ► **Can progress to malignancy.**

Appendicular Carcinoid:

- **Mc malignant tumor of appendix.** PGI 2007
- **Adeno carcinoma of appendix is rare.**
- **Treated by right hemicolectomy.**

⇨ Peritoneal Cavity

- **Is the largest cavity in the body**
- Mc causative organism of **acute bacterial peritonitis** is E. coli followed by klibessela. **AI 2006**
- **Peritoneal mesotheliomas** are associated with asbestos exposure. **AI 1996**
- Lymphoma and **retroperitoneal sarcoma are the most common malignant lesions of retroperitoneum.** **AIIMS 1998**
- **"Ormonds disease" is idiopathic retroperitoneal fibrosis.** **KERALA 1998**
- **"Peritoneal mice" is Appendicis epiploicae.** **AP 1997**
- **Commonest site of intraperitoneal abscess is "pelvic."** **JIPMER 1987**

Pneumococcal Peritonitis

There are two forms of this disease: (1) primary, and (2) secondary to pneumonia.

- ✓ **Primary** pneumococcal peritonitis is more common.
- ✓ The patient is often an undernourished girl between 3 and 6 years of age, and it is probable that the infection sometimes occurs via the vagina and Fallopian tubes, for pneumococci have been cultured from patients' vaginas. ☛
- ✓ In males, the infection is blood-borne from the upper respiratory tract or the middle ear. After the age of 10 years pneumococcal peritonitis is most unusual.
- ✓ Associated with nephritic syndrome. **JIPMER 1989**
- ✓ Children with nephritis are more liable to this condition than others.

Familial Mediterranean fever (periodic peritonitis) ☛☛

- ❒ Characterized by **abdominal pain and tenderness, mild pyrexia, polymorphonuclear leukocytosis and occasionally pain in the thorax and joints.** ☛
- ❒ The duration of an attack is 24-72 hours, when it is followed by complete remission but exacerbations recur at regular intervals.
- ❒ Most of the patients have undergone appendicectomy in childhood.
- ❒ This disease, often **familial**, is limited principally to **Arabs, Armenians and Jews**; other races are occasionally affected. ☛
- ❒ The peritoneum – **particularly in the vicinity of the spleen and the gallbladder – is inflamed.**
- ❒ There is no evidence that the interior of these organs is abnormal. Colchicine may prevent recurrent attacks.

Peritoneal bands and adhesions

Congenital bands and membranes. Intestinal obstruction is rarely seen except by an obliterated vitellointestinal duct.

1

SURGERY

Peritoneal Adhesions DNB 2011

- Peritoneal adhesions are abnormal deposits of fibrous tissue that form after peritoneal injury.
- They follow operation or peritonitis
- Are the commonest cause of small bowel obstruction and secondary female infertility in developed countries.

Mechanical intestinal obstruction is most often caused by postoperative adhesions or an internal hernia. The majority of postoperative patients with mechanical obstruction experience a short period of apparently normal recovery of intestinal function before manifestations of obstruction supervene.

Adhesion formation after abdominal and pelvic operations remains extremely common and is a source of considerable morbidity. The incidence of intra-abdominal adhesions in clinical and autopsy studies of patients who had prior laparotomies is high.

Adhesions are the most common cause of small bowel obstruction in Western countries and account for approximately one third of all intestinal obstructions. Pelvic adhesions account for infertility. Adhesions may also cause chronic abdominal and pelvic pain that may severely impair a person's quality of life. Abdominal adhesions account for major dangers of reoperative abdominal operations, including visceral damage and intestinal perforation.

Talc Granuloma

Talc (silicate of magnesium) should never be used as a **lubricant for rubber gloves** for it is a cause of peritoneal adhesions and granulomas in the Fallopian tubes.

Starch peritonitis

- Like talc, starch powder has found disfavor as a surgical glove lubricant.
- In a few starch-sensitive patients it causes a painful ascites, fortunately of limited duration.

Peritonitis

Is inflammation of the peritoneum

Primary Peritonitis:

- Inflammation of the peritoneal cavity without a documented source of contamination.
- It occurs more commonly in children than in adults and in women more than in men.
- This latter distribution is thought to be explained by entry of organisms into the peritoneal cavity through the fallopian tubes.
- In children, incidence peaks in the neonatal period and again, at age 4 to 5 years.
- The patients present with an acutely tender abdomen, fever, and leukocytosis.
- There may be a history of antecedent ear or upper respiratory tract infection.

Tuberculous Peritonitis:

The tubercle bacillus presumably gains entry to the peritoneal cavity by one of three mechanisms:

- **Transmurally from diseased bowel,**
- **From tuberculous salpingitis, or**
- **From the bloodstream.**

- The majority of patients **do not have radiographic evidence** of pulmonary or gastrointestinal tuberculosis, but nearly all have such a focus identified at autopsy.

- All have **positive tuberculin skin tests** even if the tuberculosis is confined to the peritoneum.
- The symptoms consists of fever, ascites, abdominal pain, and weakness. The ascites is progressive and may become massive.
- **Extensive adhesions** within the peritoneal cavity result in a matted feeling on physical examination.
- The ascitic fluid in the moist form is an **exudate.**
- On smear examination, lymphocytes are mainly present and rarely acid-fast bacilli are seen. Cultures of the fluid are positive in fewer than half the cases.
- Treatment is **generally nonoperative** and includes appropriate antibiotics.
- Operation should be reserved for diagnosis if needle biopsy fails or for complications such as fecal fistula.

⇨ Aseptic Peritonitis

- ✓ Is generally due to **chemical or foreign body irritants.**
- ✓ It may be followed by **secondary bacterial peritonitis.**
- ✓ Most chemical peritonitis is due to **various irritative body fluids** (bile, meconium, gastric contents).
- ✓ Foreign bodies may result from external trauma or may be acquired at the time of operation in the form of sutures, sponges, or starch granules.

⇨ Abdominal Cocoon/Sclerosing Encapsulating Peritonitis

Is a rare condition of unknown cause in which intestinal obstructions results from the encasement of variable lengths of bowel by a <u>dense fibrocollagenous membrane that gives the appearance of a cocoon.</u> This condition is not often suspected preoperatively, and therefore the diagnosis is usually made at laparotomy. **PGI 2009**

Secondary cocoon is caused by:

- ✓ **Previous abdominal surgery of peritonitis,**
- ✓ **Chronic ambulatory peritoneal dialysis,**
- ✓ **Prolonged use of Practolol**
- ✓ **Use of Providone Iodine for abdominal washout**
- ✓ **Placement of Lee Veen shunt for refractory ascites**
- ✓ **SLE**

History of similar episodes that resolved spontaneously <u>Presentations can be:</u>

- **Presentation with abdominal pain and vomiting**
- **Presence of a non tender soft mass on abdominal palpation.**
- **Features of increasing abdominal distension jaundice & features suggestive of liver pathology.**

➲ Frequently Asked

Subphrenic abscess

Anatomy

The complicated arrangement of the peritoneum results in the formation of four peritoneal and three extraperitoneal spaces in which pus may collect. Three of these spaces are on either side of the body, and one is approximately in the midline.

Left superior (Anterior) Intraperitoneal (Left Subphrenic)
✓ Is bounded above by the diaphragm, and behind by the left triangular ligament and the left lobe of the liver, the gastrohepatic omentum and anterior surface of the stomach. To the right is the falciform ligament and to the left the spleen, gastrosplenic omentum and diaphragm.
✓ Patient is toxic. **PGI 1986**
✓ The common cause of an abscess here is an **operation on the stomach, the tail of the pancreas, the spleen or the splenic flexure of the colon.**
Left inferior (Posterior) intraperitoneal (Left Subhepatic)
✓ Is another name for the 'lesser' sac.
✓ The commonest cause of infection here is complicated **acute pancreatitis**. In practice a perforated gastric ulcer rarely causes a collection here because the potential space is obliterated by adhesions.
Right superior (Anterior) intraperitoneal (Right Subphrenic)
✓ Lies between the right lobe of the liver and the diaphragm. It is limited posteriorly by the anterior layer of the coronary and the right triangular ligaments, and to the left by the falciform ligament.
✓ Common causes here are perforating cholecystitis, a perforated duodenal ulcer, a duodenal cap 'blow out' following gastrectomy and appendicitis.
Right inferior (Posterior) intraperitoneal (Right Subhepatic)
✓ Lies transversely beneath the right lobe of the liver in Rutherford Morison's pouch.
✓ It is bounded on the right by the right lobe of the liver and the diaphragm. To the left is situated the foramen of Winslow and below this lies the duodenum. In front are the liver and the gallbladder, and behind, the upper part of the right kidney and diaphragm.
✓ The space is bounded above by the liver, and below by the transverse colon and hepatic flexure. It is the deepest space of the four and the commonest site of a subphrenic abscess which usually arises from appendicitis, cholecystitis, a perforated duodenal ulcer or following upper abdominal surgery.

⇨ Syndromes Associated with Small Intestinal Neoplasms ☛☛☛☛

✓ **Bessauds-Hillmand-Augier Syndrome.** Sexual infantilism associated with intestinal polyposis.
✓ **Carter-Horsley-Hughes Syndrome.** Diffuse polyposis of the small and large intestine. ☛
✓ **Cowden's Disease or Multiple Hamartoma Syndrome.** Hamartomatous, juvenile, lipomatous, or inflammatory polyps are present mainly in the stomach and colon but are also present in the small intestine. Benign and malignant breast and thyroid disease are also found in these patients, as well as mucocutaneous lesions, tricholemomas, acral keratoses, and oral papillomas. ☛
✓ **Cronkhite-Canada Syndrome.** This syndrome is characterized by generalized gastrointestinal polyposis and **"ectodermal defects," such as alopecia, excessive skin pigmentations, and nail atrophy.** In the intestinal polyps, dilated cystic glands are found in an edematous lamina propria. Loss of protein from the gut, along with calcium, magnesium, and potassium deficiencies, may occur. ☛☛☛
✓ **Familial Polyposis of the Colon.** This syndrome is customarily associated with polyps of the colon, but cases of generalized polyposis have been recorded, with associated malignancy. ☛☛

✓	**Gardner's Syndrome:** This syndrome is generally characterized by **rectal and colonic polyposis**, but generalized polyposis has been recorded. These polyps are involved in the development of adenocarcinoma. The syndrome also includes **cysts of the skin, osteomas, fibrous and fatty tumors of the skin and mesentery, follicular odontomas, and dentigerous cysts and changes in the bony structures of the jaws.** This syndrome is familial and is transmitted as an autosomal dominant trait. AIIMS 2001
✓	**Gordon's Disease:** This is a **protein-losing gastroenteropathy, usually manifested as Ménétrier's disease**, which involves mucosal hypertrophy, hyperplasia of the superficial epithelium, degeneration in the glandular layer, and hypoproteinemia due to leakage of proteins through the mucous membranes. A diffuse gastrointestinal polyposis associated with protein loss has also been reported.
✓	**Juvenile Polyposis:** Juvenile polyposis is most commonly found in the colon and rectum, but isolated examples of generalized gastrointestinal polyposis have been reported with and without family history or other congenital abnormalities.

✓	**Muir-Torre Syndrome:** This syndrome was described to include **sebaceous adenomas, epidermoid cysts, fibromas, desmoids, lipomas, fibrosarcomas, and leiomyomas with visceral cancers.** 2011
✓	**Peutz-Jeghers Syndrome:** This syndrome is characterized by **hamartomatous polyps** of the gastrointestinal tract (stomach, small bowel, colon) that are associated with mucocutaneous pigmentation (lips, oral mucosa, fingers, forearm, toes, umbilical area). The skin pigmentation may fade after puberty, but that of the mucous membrane is retained. AIIMS 2001
✓	**Pseudoxanthoma Elasticum:** Benign **vascular lesions of the intestinal tract** have been reported in association with this disease.
✓	**Rendu-Osler-Weber Disease:** This disease is described as **telangiectasia** of the nasopharynx or gastrointestinal tract.
✓	**Turcot's Syndrome: Malignant brain tumors** are associated with inherited intestinal adenomatous polyposis. PGI 2002
✓	**Von Recklinghausen's Disease: Generalized neurofibromatosis** with café au lait skin pigmentation may also include **neurofibromas of the gastrointestinal tract.**

⇨ Peutz-Jeghers Syndrome

Is an autosomal dominant syndrome characterized by the **combination of hamartomatours polyps of the intestinal tract + hyperpigmentation of the buccal mucosa, lips and digits.**

The syndrome is associated with an increased 2-10% risk for cancer of the intestinal tract, with cancers reported throughout the intestinal tract, from the stomach to the rectum. The malignant potential is not that high.

DNB 2011

There is also an increased risk for extraintestinal maliganancies including:

- Carcinoma breast
- Carcinoma ovary
- Carcinoma cervix
- Carcinoma fallopian tubes
- Carcinoma thyroid
- Carcinoma lung, gall bladder, bile ducts, pancreas and testicles.

1

SURGERY

Treatment: The polypys may cause bleeding or intestinal obstruction (from intussusceptions). If surgery is required for these symptoms, an attempt should be made to remove as many polyps as possible with the aid of intraoperative endoscopy and polypectomy. Any polyp larger than 6.5 cm should be removed if possible.

It is reasobable to survey the **colon endoscopically every 2 years** and patients should be screened periodically for malignancies of th breast, cervix, ovary, testicles, stomach & pancreas.

⇨ Differentiate

GARDNERS SYNDROME	TURCOTS SYNDROME
❒ Intestial polps	❒ Intestinal polyps
❒ multiple osteomas	❒ CNS tumors mostly gliomas
❒ epidermal cysts	
❒ Fibromatosis	
❒ Abnormalities of teeth	
❒ High frequency of duodenal	
❒ Thyroid carcinomas	

➲ HNPCC

- ❒ **The increased risk for these cancers is due to inherited mutations that impair DNA mismatch repair**
- ❒ **HNPCC defects in DNA mismatch repair lead to microsatellite instability, also known as MSI-H, which is a hallmark of HNPCC. HNPCC is known to be associated with mutations in genes involved in the DNA mismatch repair pathway**
- ❒ **Amsterdam criteria**
- ❒ **The following are the Amsterdam criteria in identifying high-risk candidates for molecular genetic testing:**

Amsterdam Criteria:

- ❒ Three or more family members with a confirmed diagnosis of colorectal cancer, one of whom is a first degree (parent, child, sibling) relative of the other two
- ❒ Two successive affected generations
- ❒ One or more colon cancers diagnosed under age 50 years
- ❒ Familial adenomatous polyposis (FAP) has been excluded

Amsterdam Criteria II:

- ➦ Three or more family members with HNPCC-related cancers, one of whom is a first degree relative of the other two
- ➦ Two successive affected generations
- ➦ One or more of the HNPCC-related cancers diagnosed under age 50 years
- ➦ Familial adenomatous polyposis (FAP) has been excluded
- ➦ HNPCC defects in DNA mismatch repair lead to microsatellite instability, also known as MSI-H, which is a hallmark of HNPCC. MSI is identifiable in cancer specimens in the pathology laboratory.
- ➦ HNPCC is known to be associated with mutations in genes involved in the DNA mismatch repair pathway

➲ Non Neoplastic Polyps

Genes implicated in HNPCC

HNPCC1 **MSH2**

HNPCC2 **MLH1**

HNPCC5 **MSH6**

HNPCC4 **PMS2**

HNPCC3 **PMS1**

HNPCC6 **TGFBR2**

HNPCC7 **MLH3**

▶ Hyperplastic polyps	AIIMS 2006
▶ Hamartomatous polyp	AIIMS 2007
▶ Inflammatory polyp	AI 2006
▶ Almost all other polyps are malignant.	
▶ Juvenile polyp is most common in children.	PGI 1998
▶ **Villous adenoma has highest malignant potential than other histological types.**	PGI 1999

⇨ Meckel's Diverticulum

❒ A **true congenital diverticulum.**	PGI 2005
❒ It is a **vestigial remnant of the omphalomesenteric duct** (also called the **vitelline duct**), and is the most frequent malformation of the gastrointestinal tract	AIIMS 2005
❒ Meckel's diverticulum is located in the **distal ileum**, usually within about 60-100 cm of the ileocecal valve.	
❒ It is typically **3-5 cm long**, runs **antimesenterically** and has its own blood supply.	
❒ It is a remnant of the connection from the umbilical cord to the small intestine present during embryonic development.	

A Memory Aid is the Rule of 2's:

❒ 2% (of the population)	
❒ 2 feet (from the ileocecal valve)	PGI 2006
❒ 2 inches (in length)	
❒ 2% are symptomatic	
❒ 2 types of common ectopic tissue (gastric and pancreatic)	PGI 2005
❒ Most common age at clinical presentation is 2,	
❒ Males are **2** times as likely to be affected.	

1

SURGERY

- It can also be present as an indirect hernia, where it is known as a "**Hernia of Littre.**"
- Furthermore, it can be attached to the umbilical region by the vitelline ligament, with the possibility of vitelline cysts, or even a patent vitelline canal forming a vitelline fistula when the umbilical cord is cut.
- Torsions of intestine around the intestinal stalk may also occur, leading to **obstruction, ischemia, and necrosis.** NIMHANS 1986
- Symptoms
- The majority of people afflicted with Meckel's diverticulum are **asymptomatic**. If symptoms do occur, they typically appear before the age of two.
- The most common presenting symptom is **painless rectal bleeding,** followed by intestinal obstruction, volvulus and intussusception. Occasionally, Meckel's diverticulitis may present with all the features of acute appendicitis.
- A **technetium-99m (99mTc) pertechnetate scan** is the investigation of choice to diagnose Meckel's diverticula. AIIMS 1999
- Other tests such as colonoscopy and screenings for bleeding disorders should be performed, and angiography can assist in determining the location and severity of bleeding. Meckel's occurs more often in males
- Can be a leading point of intussusception. PGI 2001

Omphalomesenteric Duct Remnants

- Remnants of the omphalomesenteric (vitelline) duct may present as abnormalities related to the abdominal wall.
- In the fetus, the omphalomesenteric duct connects the fetal midgut to the yolk sac. This normally obliterates and disappears completely. However, any or all of the fetal duct may persist.

- An **umbilical polyp** is a small excrescence of **omphalomesenteric duct mucosa** that is retained in the umbilicus. Such polyps resemble umbilical granulomas except that they do not disappear after silver nitrate cauterization.
- **Umbilical sinuses** result from the continued presence of the **umbilical end of the omphalomesenteric duct.** These resemble umbilical polyps, but close inspection reveals the presence of a sinus tract deep to the umbilicus.
- Persistence of the **entire omphalomesenteric duct** is heralded by the passage of enteric contents from the umbilicus.
- **Cystic remnants of the omphalomesenteric duct** may persist and be asymptomatic for long periods of time. The **cysts** may be connected to the ileum with a fibrous band that is a remnant of the obliterated omphalomesenteric duct. Patients may present with acute volvulus and intestinal obstruction or with acute abdomen because of cyst infection.
- **Meckel's diverticulum** results when **the intestinal end of the omphalomesenteric duct persists.** This is a true diverticulum of the intestine with all layers of the intestinal wall represented.

Omphalocele

May be seen in the neonate and represents a defect in the closure of the umbilical ring. The herniated viscera are usually covered with a sac composed of amnion. **DNB 2011**

Gastroschisis

Is a defect of the abdominal wall that is located lateral to the umbilicus. It is caused by a failureof closure of the body wall in which abdominal viscera protrude through the defect. No sac is present to cover the herniated intestine

Anomalies of the Midgut

- Congenital abnormalities of the intestine are common;
- Most of them are anomalies of gut rotation-**nonrotation or malrotation of the gut**-that result from incomplete rotation and/or fixation of the intestines.
- **Nonrotation** occurs when the intestine does not rotate as it reenters the abdomen. As a result, the caudal limb of the midgut loop returns to the abdomen first and the small intestines lie on the right side of the abdomen and the entire large intestine is on the left. The usual 270-degree counterclockwise rotation is not completed, and the cecum lies just inferior to the pylorus of the stomach.
- **The cecum is fixed to the posterolateral abdominal wall (In midline) by peritoneal bands that pass over the duodenum.** These bands and the volvulus (twisting) of the intestines cause **duodenal obstruction.** AIPGME 2012
- This type of malrotation results from failure of the midgut loop to complete the final 90 degrees of rotation only two parts of the intestine are attached to the posterior abdominal wall: the duodenum and proximal colon. This improperly positioned and incompletely fixed intestine may lead to a catastrophic twisting of the midgut-**midgut volvulus.** The small intestine hangs by a narrow stalk that contains the superior mesenteric artery and vein.
- When midgut volvulus occurs, the superior mesenteric artery may be obstructed, resulting in infarction and **gangrene of the intestine** supplied by it Infants with intestinal malrotation are prone to volvulus and present with **bilious emesis** (vomiting bile).

Reversed Rotation

- In very unusual cases, the midgut loop rotates in a clockwise rather than a counterclockwise direction.
- As a result, the duodenum lies anterior to the superior mesenteric artery rather than posterior to it, and the transverse colon lies posterior instead of anterior to it.
- In these infants, the transverse colon may be obstructed by pressure from the superior mesenteric artery.
- In more unusual cases, the small intestine lies on the left side of the abdomen and the large intestine lies on the right side, with the cecum in the center.
- This unusual situation results from malrotation of the midgut followed by failure of fixation of the intestines.

1

SURGERY

⇨ Blind Loop Syndrome

- Overgrowth of bacteria within the small intestine accompanied by nutrient malabsorption is called the **stasis, stagnant loop, or blind loop syndrome.**
- In the stasis syndrome, the proximal small intestinal flora resembles that of the colon and the overgrowth flora competes with the human host for ingested nutrients. The resultant malabsorption is due to a disturbed intraluminal environment (catabolism of carbohydrate by gram-negative aerobes, deconjugation of bile salts by anaerobes, binding of cobalamin by anaerobes) and patchy damage to the small intestinal enterocyte.
- **Hematologically, blind loop syndrome involves mainly vitamin B12 deficiency, although there may also be a deficiency in folic acid.** **MAH 2012**
- The diagnosis of blind loop syndrome can be confirmed by the **Schilling test**, demonstrating intrinsic factor-resistant vitamin B 12 malabsorption.
- There are two main hypotheses for the development of vitamin B12 deficiency: **bacteria in the stagnant area use vitamin B12, leaving an inadequate amount for absorption, or the bacteria produce a toxin that inhibits absorption of vitamin B12.**
- **Steatorrhea** most likely occurs when the bacteria present in the blind loop structurally alter bile salts, interfering with absorption of fat. **AIIMS 2010**

⇨ Meckel's Diverticulum: Asked Frequently: Provided in Detail. Kindly read fully

- Is an embryologic derivative of **the vitelline duct.**
- Developmental anomalies related to persistence of the vitelline duct are among the most common abnormalities of digestive tract development Persistence of the vitelline duct may lead to
  - **Fistula between the umbilicus and the ileum when the entire duct remains patent;**
  - **Meckel's diverticulum due to failure of closure of the intestinal end of the duct;**
  - **An umbilical sinus when the umbilical side of the duct is not obliterated;**
  - **Fibrous cord between the umbilicus and the ileum representing an obliterated duct and its vessels;**

Important points:

- As many as 25% of Meckel's diverticula are connected to the umbilicus by a fibrous strand.
- Meckel's diverticulum is a **true diverticulum** containing all layers of the intestinal wall, usually arising from the **antimesenteric border of the ileum 45 to 90 cm. proximal to the ileocecal valve**
- It varies in length and diameter, ranging from **1 to 12 cm.**
- As the cells lining the vitelline duct are **pluripotent**, it is not uncommon to find heterotopic tissue within a Meckel's diverticulum.
- **Gastric mucosa** is present in 50% of all Meckel's diverticula, but in more than 75% of symptomatic patients.
- **Pancreatic mucosa** is encountered in approximately 5% of diverticula.
- Less commonly, these diverticula may harbor **colonic mucosa.**
- Tumors are an uncommon finding in a Meckel's diverticulum and include the benign entities **lipoma, leiomyoma, neurofibroma, and angioma.**

- **Malignant lesions**, including **leiomyosarcoma, carcinoid, and, less commonly, adenocarcinoma** can occur
- **Hemorrhage** is the **most common clinical problems** associated with Meckel's diverticulum is gastrointestinal bleeding presenting as bright red blood per rectum. Diagnosis of a Meckel's diverticulum possessing gastric mucosa can be made using **99mTc-pertechnetate** radioisotope scanning.
- **Intestinal Obstruction**. The cause of this obstruction may be volvulus of the small bowel around a diverticulum associated with a fibrotic band attached to the abdominal wall, intussusception, or, rarely, incarceration of the diverticulum in an inguinal hernia **(Littre's hernia).**
- **Diverticulitis.**

Umbilical Anomalies: These include fistulas, cysts, sinuses, and fibrous bands between the diverticulum and the umbilicus (filum enterale).

Colonic Polyposis Syndromes

Gardeners Syndrome	✓ Colonic cancer associated with soft tissue tumors (osteomas, lipomas, cysts, fibrosarcomas)
Turcots Syndrome	✓ Colonic cancer associated with central nervous system malignancies
Cronkhite Canada Syndrome	✓ Intestinal polyps, hyperpigmentation with alopecia and absence of finger nails.
Hereditary Polyposis Coli Syndrome or APC (Adenomatous Polyposis Coli)	✓ Most important presenting with hundreds of polyps. ✓ 100 % chances of malignant transformation. ✓ **autosomal dominant with involvement of chromosome 5** **KCET 2012**
Hereditary <u>Non</u> Polyposis Coli Syndrome (Lynch Syndrome)	✓ This consists of three family members having at leat two generations with colonic cancer. ✓ There is a high-risk of associated ovarian and endometrial cancer in this syndrome.
Cowdens Syndrome	✓ Hamartomas with increased risk of bleeding especially in a child presenting with rectal bleeding.

Remember: **DNB 2011**

- **In Lynch syndrome I (site-specific colon cancer) only inherited colonic neoplasms occur, whereas Lynch syndrome II (cancer family syndrome) includes female genital (uterine, ovarian) and breast cancer.**
- **Individuals in families with hereditary nonpolyposis colorectal cancer should have colonoscopy every 2 years beginning at an age 5 years younger than the age of the earliest colon cancer diagnosed in the family.**

1

SURGERY

Colonic Diverticula

- Herniations or sac like **protrusions of the mucosa** through the muscularis, at the point where a nutrient artery penetrates the muscularis.
- Most commonly in the **sigmoid colon** and decrease in frequency in the proximal colon.
- They **increase with age**
- Related to an **increase in intraluminal pressure.**
- Diet, deficient in dietary fiber or roughage. Result in decreased fecal bulk, narrowing of the colon, and an increase in intraluminal pressure in order to move the smaller fecal mass.
- Colonic diverticula are usually asymptomatic and are an incidental finding on barium enema or colonoscopy.

Diverticulitis

- Inflammation can occur in diverticular sac.
- The cause is mechanical, related to retention in the diverticula of undigested food residue and bacteria, which may form a hard mass called a fecalith. ☚
- More often in the left as in the right colon. ☚
- Acute colonic diverticulitis is a disease of variable severity characterized by **fever, left lower quadrant abdominal pain, and signs of peritoneal irritation muscle spasm, guarding, rebound tenderness.**
- Rectal bleeding, usually microscopic, is noted in 25% of cases; it is rarely massive. Polymorphonuclear leukocytosis is common.
- Massive hemorrhage from colonic diverticula is one of the most common causes of hematochezia in patients over age 60. ☚
- Complications include free perforation, which results in acute peritonitis, sepsis, and shock, particularly in the elderly.
- Abscess formation or fistulas then occur as the inflammatory mass burrows into other organs. Severe pericolitis may cause a fibrous stricture around the bowel, which can be associated with colonic obstruction and may mimic a neoplasm.
- **Diagnosis** During the acute phase of diverticulitis, barium enema and sigmoidoscopy may be hazardous, since contrast material or air under pressure may lead to rupture of an inflamed diverticulum and convert a walled-off inflammatory lesion to a free perforation.
- Colonoscopy or surgical excision may be required for accurate diagnosis. Abdominal computed tomography scan may demonstrate the presence of a pericolic abscess.

Aganglionic Megacolon (Hirschsprung's Disease)

- Congenital disorder due to **absence of enteric neurons** (ganglions) in the distal colon and rectum.
- Some patients have an autosomal dominant form of the disease with mutations in the RET gene;
- The aganglionic and contracted segment of bowel is unable to relax to permit passage of stool, causing the **normal proximal colon to become greatly dilated**☚☚

- **(Hirschsprung's disease is the congenital absence of enteric neurons in the submucosal and myenteric Plexuses, due to an arrest of the embryonic caudad migration of the enteric neurons along the gut. The aganglionic segment remains contracted, dilating the proximal normal bowel. The severity of symptoms and the age at diagnosis are related to the length of the aganglionic segment. Involvement of the rectum or additional parts of the colon results in constipation or obstipation in infancy, requiring emergent resection of the aganglionic bowel and a pull-through anastomosis to the anus.)** **AIIMS 2011**

- Barium enema reveals a narrowed segment in the rectosigmoid, with **massive dilation above. (Never forget)**
- Diagnosis is made by **full-thickness surgical biopsy**
- The treatment of choice is a **pull-through procedure** in which normally innervated colon is anastomosed to the distal rectum just above the internal sphincter, thus bypassing the contracted aganglionic segment and restoring normal defecation.

Acquired Megacolon

- In **Central and South America,**
- Infection with **Trypanosoma cruzi (Chagas' disease)**
- Result in **destruction of the ganglion cells of the colon**

Onset is in adult life:

- ✓ Schizophrenia
- ✓ Depression,
- ✓ Cerebral atrophy,
- ✓ Spinal cord injury, and
- ✓ Parkinsonism also may cause megacolon.
- ✓ Myxedema, and primary systemic sclerosis also can reduce colonic motility and produce marked colonic distention.

Postoperative Ileus

- The term **"ileus"** is **"misleading"** because **small bowel motility rapidly returns**
- After laparotomy, the normal propulsive activity of the gastrointestinal tract is temporarily depressed, a condition termed postoperative ileus. **AIIMS 2011**
- It probably follows trauma to the intestine if a laparotomy was performed or, in other procedures, increased sympathetic discharge from splanchnic nerves. Postoperative ileus is a predictable consequence of both **abdominal and extra-abdominal procedures.** Ileus is often the major factor in prolonging the hospital stay. The cause of postoperative ileus is thought to be a **sympathetically mediated inhibition of motility** that most significantly affects the colon. Other proposed inhibitory mechanisms include **bowel manipulation, stress-related hormones other than catecholamines (e.g. vasopressin), and postoperative narcotic usage.**

1

SURGERY

- Gastric peristalsis returns 24 to 48 hours after operation, and colonic activity usually returns after 48 hours, beginning at the cecum and progressing caudally. This postoperative ileus leads to mild abdominal distention (primarily from a distended colon) and absent bowel sounds in the first 48 to 72 hours. Return of normal peristaltic activity is often noted by mild cramps, passage of flatus, and return of appetite. **AIIMS 2011**

Ileus may be prolonged in patients with:

- **Metabolic disturbances (hypokalemia, uremia, diabetes),** **PGI 2009**
- **Intraperitoneal or retroperitoneal inflammation or hematomas, and**
- **Mesenteric vascular insufficiency and in those taking tricyclic antidepressant drugs.**
- **Acute colonic pseudo-obstruction (Ogilvie's syndrome) is a localized form of paralytic ileus affecting the large bowel, most frequently the proximal colon.**

⇨ Acute Intestinal Pseudo Obstruction

- Referred to as **Ogilvie's syndrome** **AIIMS 2007**
- Involving primarily the **colon** but occasionally also the small intestine.

Examination reveals a

- ✓ **Distended, tympanitic abdomen**
- ✓ **Reduced or absent bowel sounds.**
- ✓ **Localized tenderness** over the distended colon is common
- ✓ Abdominal films reveal **massive dilation of the colon and small intestine, occasionally with the presence of air-fluid levels.**

- **The cecum**, being the most capacious part of the colon, is often massively dilated and tender.
- Management requires careful correction of fluid and electrolyte abnormalities, intubation of the stomach or small intestine for decompression, and avoidance of drugs that depress intestinal motility.
- **Barium enema may be hazardous** because of the risk of perforating the already dilated bowel.

➲ Intussusception

- **Outer** tube Intussucipiens☛☛☛ **PGI 1997**
- **Inner** Tube Intussuseptum☛☛
- Stool **Red currant jelly**☛
- Lump Sausage shaped☛
- Emptiness in Iliac Fossa **Sign de dance**☛ **PGI 2001**
- **Target sign**
- **Coiled spring sign** **PGI 2000**
- Barium enema **Claw sign**☛

- **Volvolus of gut is usually clockwise**☛
- **Volvolus of sigmoid colon** is usually **anticlockwise**☛
- Intussusception is usually of type **Ileo colic**☛ **AI 1999**

⇨ Intussusception:

DNB 2011

The invagination of one portion of the intestine into an adjacent segment, is uncommon but may be life threatening.

Types:

- **In children more than 80% are ileo-colic**
- **Colo-colic is most common in elderly patients**

Causes:

- ✓ **Change in diet during weaning**
- ✓ **Upper respiratory tract viral infection**
- ✓ **Intestinal polyps**
- ✓ **submucous lipoma**
- ✓ **Leiomyoma of intestine**
- ✓ **Meckel's diverticulum**
- ✓ **Carcinoma**
- ✓ **Purpuric submucosal hemorrhages**

Treatment:

(A) Non-Operative: **Reduction by hydrostatic pressure using either saline or microbarium sulphate solution or air.**

(B) Surgery Indications:

- More than 48 hrs duration
- Features of perforation, strangulation, peritonitis
- Recurrent intussusceptions
- In adults, commonly resection is required.

⊃ Ischemic Colitis

- ❒ Most often affects the **elderly**
- ❒ Ischemic colitis is almost always **nonocclusive.**
- ❒ **In acute fulminant ischemic colitis**, the major manifestations are **severe lower abdominal pain, rectal bleeding, and hypotension.**
- ❒ Dilation of the colon and physical signs of peritonitis are seen in severe cases.
- ❒ Abdominal films may reveal **thumbprinting from submucosal hemorrhage and edema.**
- ❒ **Barium enema is hazardous** in the acute situation because of the risk of perforation. Sigmoidoscopy or colonoscopy may detect ulcerations, friability, and bulging folds from submucosal hemorrhage.
- ❒ **Surgical resection may be required** in some patients with fulminant ischemic colitis to remove gangrenous bowel; others with lesser degrees of ischemia may respond to **conservative medical management.**
- ❒ **Subacute ischemic colitis** is the most common clinical variant of ischemic colonic disease. It produces lesser degrees of pain and bleeding, often occurring over several days or weeks.

⇨ Angiodysplasia of the Colon

- ❒ **Vascular ectasias or arteriovenous malformations (AVMs)** that occur in the right colon of many older individuals and may cause bleeding.
- ❒ Angiodysplasia is a degenerative lesion consisting of **dilated, distorted, thin-walled vessels lined by vascular endothelium.**

1

SURGERY

- Lesions are **usually multiple and are found primarily in the cecum** and ascending colon, but in some patients they may be distributed from the stomach to rectum.
- **Colonoscopy** is diagnostic which allows treatment by laser photocoagulation, electrocautery, or injection with sclerosant.
- Some patients with massive uncontrolled bleeding or multiple sites of angiodysplasia may require **right hemicolectomy.**
- Angiodysplasias may also respond to **chronic estrogen-progesterone therapy.**

⇨ Colonoscopy

- A lighted probe called a colonoscope is inserted into the rectum and the entire colon to look for polyps and other abnormalities that may be caused by cancer.
- A colonoscopy has the advantage that if polyps are found during the procedure they can be immediately removed.
- Tissue can also be taken for biopsy, colonoscopy or FOBT plus sigmoidoscopy are the preferred screening options.
- **In a patient 50 years age comes with weakness for 5-6 months, with anemia, occult blood in stool present. the best initial investigation for him is:** Colonoscopy. **AIPGME 2010**

Is the most accurate method of assessing colonic disease.

General indications for flexible sigmoidoscopy or for colonoscopy include

- **Diagnosis,**
- **Biopsy to confirm or establish the nature of a disease process or malignant lesion,**
- **Therapeutic removal of polyps,**
- **Management of bleeding lesions,**
- **Surveillance and follow-up of lesions previously removed endoscopically or surgically,**
- **Detection and removal of foreign bodies, and**
- **Early cancer detection or another screening process.**

In addition, colonoscopy has also been used to facilitate endoscopic dilatation of anastomotic strictures. **Contraindications** should be considered. These include

- Suspected colonic perforation,
- Acute fulminating inflammatory bowel disease,
- Peritonitis with secondary paralytic ileus, and
- Acute inflammatory disease of the anus.

The efficacy and safety of diagnostic and/or therapeutic colonoscopy depend on the presence of a well-cleansed bowel. **A satisfactory bowel preparation** can be achieved by means of

- **Enemas and simple irrigation of the gastrointestinal tract with saline, mannitol preparation, solutions containing polyethylene glycol**
- **Citrate of magnesia,**
- **Castor oil, and**
- **Tap water enemas.**

➲ Virtual Colonoscopy: High Yield for 2011-2012 AIPGME

- ▶ Is an imaging procedure which uses **x-rays and computers** to produce two- and three-dimensional images of the colon (large intestine) from the lowest part, the rectum, all the way to the lower end of the small intestine and display them on a screen.
- ▶ Is used to diagnose colon and bowel disease, including polyps, diverticulosis and cancer.
- ▶ VC is **performed via computed tomography (CT), sometimes called a CAT scan, or with magnetic resonance imaging**
- ▶ VC is **more comfortable** than conventional colonoscopy for some people because it does not use a colonoscope.
- ▶ **No sedation** is needed
- ▶ VC provides **clearer, more detailed images** than a conventional x-ray using a barium enema.
- ▶ It **takes less time** than either a conventional colonoscopy or a lower GI series.
- ▶ VC provides a **secondary benefit of revealing diseases or abnormalities outside the colon**

⇨ Virtual Colonoscopy: PGI 2009

- **Better image than conventional colonoscopy**
- **Performed by CT/MRI**
- **Helpful for pathology outside colon**

➲ Colorectal Cancer

- ❒ Most colorectal cancers, regardless of etiology, arise from **adenomatous polyps**
- ❒ Probability of an adenomatous polyp becoming a cancer depends on the gross appearance of the lesion, its histologic features, and its size.
- ❒ Adenomatous polyps may be **pedunculated (stalked) or sessile (flat-based).** Cancers develop more frequently in sessile polyps.
- ❒ Villous adenomas, most of which are sessile, become malignant more than three times as often as tubular adenomas.
- ❒ The likelihood that any polypoid lesion in the large bowel contains invasive cancer is related to the size of the polyp, being negligible (<2%) in lesions <1.5 cm, intermediate (2 to 10%) in lesions 1.5 to 2.5 cm in size, and substantial (10%) in lesions >2.5 cm
- ❒ MC site: **Rectum**☛☛
- ❒ MC site in colon: **Sigmoid colon**☛ PGI 2006
- ❒ Mc type: **Adeno carcinoma**☛ PGI 2007
- ❒ Rght sided common in females.
- ❒ Right sided presents as anemia. PGI 2006
- ❒ Left sided presents as obstruction/pain. PGI 2001

⇨ Etiology and Risk Factors

Risk factors for the development of **colorectal cancer**

- ❐ upper socioeconomic populations
- ❐ ↑meat protein ☛
- ❐ ↑dietary fat and oil as well as elevations in the serum cholesterol ☛ **PGI 2003**
- ❐ ↑alcohol
- ❐ Smoking
- ❐ Sedentary habbits
- ❐ Obesity
- ❐ Deficiency of antioxidants
- ❐ Family history of the disease
- ❐ Streptococcus bovis Bacteremia ☛☛☛
- ❐ Ureterosigmoidostomy
- ❐ UC **PGI 2006**
- ❐ Crohns disease. **PGI 2002**
- ❐ FAP **PGI 2006**

⇨ Protective Factors

- ✓ **Aspirin and other nonsteroidal anti-inflammatory drugs**, which are thought to suppress cell proliferation by inhibiting prostaglandin synthesis. ☛☛☛ **PGI 2002**
- ✓ **Oral folic acid supplements and oral calcium supplements** have been found to reduce the risk of adenomatous polyps and colorectal cancers in case-control studies.
- ✓ **Ascorbic acid, tocopherols, and b-carotene**
- ✓ **Estrogen replacement therapy**

⇨ Clinical Features

- ► **Lesions of the right colon** commonly ulcerate, leading to chronic, insidious blood loss without a change in the appearance of the stool. Patients with tumors of the ascending colon often present with symptoms such as **fatigue, palpitations, and even angina pectoris and are found to have a hypochromic, microcytic anemia indicative of iron deficiency.**
- ► Radiographs of the abdomen often reveal characteristic annular, constricting lesions (**"apple-core" or "napkin-ring")** ☛☛
- ► **Cancers arising in the recto sigmoid** are often associated with **hematochezia, tenesmus, and narrowing of the caliber of stool;** anemia is an infrequent finding.
- ► **Liver is the most common site of metastasis. (1/3) patients show hepatic metastasis.** **PGI 2002**
- ► **Surgery is treatment of choice.** **PGI 2005**
- ► **Anterior resection:** ☛ for tumors of upper 2/3 of rectum.
- ► **Combined abdomino perineal resection:** for extensive tumors of lower 1/3 of rectum.
- ► **Immunotherapy:** ☛☛ for disseminated carcinoma colon.

Treatment of carcinoma left colon with acute obstruction: PGI 2008

- Hartman's procedure
- Left colectomy with anastomosis
- Proximal colostomy
- Extended Right colectomy with ileoanal anastomosis

⇨ Anal Canal

Anal canal above Dentate Line	Anal Canal Below Dentate Line
❒ Endodermal☛☛	❒ Ectodermal
❒ Cuboidal epithelium	❒ Stratified squamous
❒ Superior Rectal artery☛☛	❒ Inferior Rectal artery
❒ Superior Rectal Vein	❒ Inferior Rectal Vein
❒ Internal Iliac group of Lymph Nodes ☛☛	❒ Superficial inguinal group of lymph nodes☛
❒ Pain insensitive☛☛	❒ Pain sensitive

The Anal Valves of Ball

✓ Are a series of transversely placed semilunar folds linking the columns of Morgagni. They lie along and actually constitute the waviness of the dentate line.

The Crypts of Morgagni (syn. anal crypts) ☛

✓ Are small pockets between the inferior extremities of the columns of Morgagni. Into several of these crypts, mostly those situated posteriorly, opens one anal gland by a narrow duct.

✓ Infection of an anal gland can give rise to an abscess, and infection of an anal gland is the most common cause of anorectal abscesses and fistulae.

The Anorectal Ring

✓ Marks the **junction between the rectum and the anal canal.**

✓ It is formed by the joining of the **puborectalis muscle, the deep external sphincter, conjoined longitudinal muscle and the highest part of the internal sphincter.**

✓ The anorectal ring can be **clearly felt digitally**, especially on its posterior and lateral aspects. ☛☛

✓ Division of the anorectal ring results in **permanent incontinence of feces.**

✓ The position and length of the anal canal, as well as the angle of the anorectal junction, depend to a major extent on the **integrity and strength of the puborectalis muscle sling.** ☛☛

Fistula in ano

✓ **A fistula in ano is a track, lined by granulation tissue, which connects deeply in the anal canal or rectum and superficially on the skin around the anus.**

✓ It usually results from an anorectal abscess which burst spontaneously or was opened inadequately

✓ The fistula continues to discharge and, because of constant reinfection from the anal canal or rectum, seldom, if ever, closes permanently without surgical aid.

✓ An anorectal abscess may produce a track, the orifice of which has the appearance of a fistula, but it does not communicate with the anal canal or the rectum. By definition this is not a fistula, but a sinus.
✓ **Most fistulas derive from sepsis originating in the glands of the anal canal at the dentate line, and the path of the fistula is determined by the local anatomy.** Most commonly, they track in the fascial or fatty planes, especially the intersphincteric space between the internal and external sphincters into the ischiorectal fascia. In such instances, the track passes directly to the perineal skin. **In some instances, circumferential spread may occur in the ischiorectal fossa, with the track passing from one fossa to the contralateral one via the posterior rectum (a horseshoe fistula).**
✓ **Goodsall's rule** is often helpful. **MAH 2012**
Types of anal fistulae
Low-level fistulae open into the anal canal below the anorectal ring. ☛
High-level fistulae open into the anal canal at or above the anorectal ring. ☛

⇨ Fistula in Ano

Signs and symptoms (In Order of Prevalence)
➨ Perianal discharge ➨ Pain ➨ Swelling ➨ Bleeding ➨ Diarrhea
Skin excoriation
External opening
Important points in the history that may suggest a complex fistula include the following:
➨ Inflammatory bowel disease ➨ Diverticulitis ➨ Previous radiation therapy for prostate or rectal cancer ➨ Tuberculosis ➨ Steroid therapy ➨ HIV infection

➲ Types:

Intersphincteric
❒ Common course - Via internal sphincter to the intersphincteric space and then to the perineum
❒ Seventy percent of all anal fistulae
❒ Other possible tracts - No perineal opening; high blind tract; high tract to lower rectum or pelvis
Transsphincteric
❒ Common course Low via internal and external sphincters into the ischiorectal fossa and then to the perineum
❒ Twenty-five percent of all anal fistulae
❒ Other possible tracts High tract with perineal opening; high blind tract

Suprasphincteric
❐ Common course Via intersphincteric space superiorly to above puborectalis muscle into ischiorectal fossa and then to perineum
❐ Five percent of all anal fistulae
❐ Other possible tracts High blind tract (i.e., palpable through rectal wall above dentate line)
Extrasphincteric
❐ Common course From perianal skin through levator ani muscles to the rectal wall completely outside sphincter mechanism
❐ One percent of all anal fistulae **(Rare)**

Malignant lesions of the anus and anal canal
❐ Squamous cell carcinoma (most common) **JKBOPEE 2012**
❐ Basaloid carcinoma
❐ Mucoepidermal carcinoma
❐ Basal cell carcinoma
❐ Malignant melanoma
❐ Anal intraepithelial neoplasia (AIN)

⇨ Treatment of Anal Cancer

- ► Tumor of carcinoma rectum **lesss than 3 cm** from the dentate line but not invading the sphincter usually can be resected via a trans-anal procedure.
- ► Tumors **5 cm from the dentate line** may need a transcoccygeal approach or trans-anal endoscopic microsurgery **(TEM).**
- ► Tumors **7-10 cm** from the denate line require TEM or should be considered for **Low anterior resection (LAR).**
- ► **Abdomino-perineal operation (APR)** is indicated when
  - Tumor involves the anal sphincters,
  - When the tumor is too close to the sphincters to obtain adequate margins
  - Or in patients in whom sphincter preserving surgery is not possible because of unfavourable body habitus or poor Sphincter control.
- ► Hartmann's operation is an excellent palliative procedure done in elderly people who are not fit for major surgery like APR and also in locally advanced tumors.
- ► Here rectal growth is resected and upper end of the rectum is closed completely.
- ► Proximal colon is brought out as an end colostomy.

1

SURGERY

⇨ Ogilvie Syndrome (Details)

- Is acute pseudo obstruction. UP 2007
- Massive colonic distention in the absence of mechanical obstruction
- Severe form of ileus
- May result from autonomic imbalance
- Aerophagia and impairment of colonic motility by drugs are contributing factors

- Most common in bedridden, elderly patients; following orthopedic injuries; in patients taking psychotropic medications or narcotics
- Associated with metabolic disorders:

✓ **Hypothyroidism**

✓ **Diabetes**

✓ **Renal failure**

- Associated with collagen vascular diseases:

✓ **Lupus**

✓ **Amyloidosis**

✓ **Scleroderma**

LABORATORY FINDINGS

- May reveal electrolyte abnormalities (especially magnesium and potassium)
- WBC count usually normal, but an elevation may indicate bowel compromise

IMAGING FINDINGS

- **Abdominal X-ray:** Marked gaseous distention of colon, especially right colon. **Contrast enema:** Absence of mechanical obstruction.

⇨ Most Common Sites

- Typhoid ulcer: Terminal ileum
- Tuberculous ulcer: Terminal ileum
- Crohns disease: Terminal Ileum
- Gallstone Ileus: Terminal Ileum
- Post operative ileus: Colon AIIMS 2011
- Ulcerative colitis: Rectum
- Ameobic colitis: Sigmoid colon
- Volvolus: Sigmoid colon
- Diverticulae Sigmoid colon

⇨ Referred Abdominal Pains

- Biliary colic to: Right shoulder
- Renal colic to: Groin
- Appendicitis to: Periumbilical to Right iliac fossa
- Pancreatitis to: Back
- Ruptured Aortic Aneurysm to: Back
- Hip pain to: Knee

Important Signs in Patients with Abdominal Pain

Sign	Finding	Association
Cullen's sign	Bluish periumbilical discoloration	Retroperitoneal hemorrhage (hemorrhagic pancreatitis, abdominal aortic aneurysm rupture)
Kehr's sign	Severe left shoulder pain	Splenic rupture Ectopic pregnancy rupture KCET 2012
McBurney's sign	Tenderness located 2/3 distance from anterior iliac spine to umbilicus on right side	Appendicitis
Murphy's sign	Abrupt interruption of inspiration on palpation of right upper quadrant	Acute cholecystitis
Iliopsoas sign	Hyperextension of right hip causing abdominal pain	Appendicitis
Obturator's sign	Internal rotation of flexed right hip causing abdominal pain	Appendicitis
Grey-Turner's sign	Discoloration of the flank	Retroperitoneal hemorrhage (hemorrhagic pancreatitis, abdominal aortic aneurysm rupture)
Chandelier sign	Manipulation of cervix causes patient to lift buttocks off table	Pelvic inflammatory disease
Rovsing's sign	Right lower quadrant pain with palpation of the left lower quadrant	Appendicitis

- Cork screw esophagus Diffuse Esophagal spasm☛☛
- Rosary esophagus Diffuse Esophagal spasm☛
- **"Double Bubble sign in X ray abdomen" Annular Pancreas, ☛Duodenal atresia☛** KCET 2012
- "Scalloping of sigmoid colon". Ulcerative colitis
- "Microcolon on barium enema." Ileal Atresia
- "Bird of prey sign". Sigmoid volvolus☛☛
- **"String sign." Crohns disease** KCET 2012
- "Pipe stem colon" Ulcerative colitis☛
- Saw tooth appearance of colon Diverticular disease☛
- Apple Core Lesion/Napkin Ring appearance Lt Colonic Ca.☛
- Coffee bean sign Volvolus☛
- Claw Sign/Signe de dance Intussception☛
- Thumb printing sign Ischemic colitis☛

⇨ Burst Abdomen

Burst Abdomen (Syn. Abdominal Dehiscence)

- A **serosanguinous (pink) discharge** from the wound is a forerunner of disruption ☛☛
- Most pathognomonic sign of impending wound disruption
- Signifies that intraperitoneal contents are lying extraperitoneally.
- Patients often volunteer the information that they **'felt something give way'.**
- If skin sutures have been removed, omentum or coils of intestine may be forced through the wound and will be found lying on the skin. Pain and shock are often absent.
- There may be symptoms and signs of intestinal obstruction.

⇨ Hernia

Composition of a hernia

As a rule, a hernia consists of three parts – the sac, the coverings of the sac and the contents of the sac.

The sac

The sac is a diverticulum of peritoneum consisting of mouth, neck, body and fundus. The neck is usually well defined, but in some direct inguinal hernias and in many incisional hernias there is no actual neck. The diameter of the neck is important because strangulation of bowel is a likely complication where the neck is narrow, as in femoral and paraumbilical hernias.

The body of the sac

The body of the sac varies greatly in size and is not necessarily occupied. In cases occurring in infancy and childhood the sac is gossamer thin. In long-standing cases the wall of the sac may be comparatively thick.

▶ The covering
Coverings are derived from the layers of the abdominal wall through which the sac passes. In long-standing cases they become atrophied from stretching and so amalgamated that they are indistinguishable from each other.
▶ Contents
These can be:
▶ **Omentum = omentocele (syn. epiplocele);**
▶ **Intestine = enterocele. More commonly small bowel, but may be large intestine or appendix;**
▶ **A portion of the circumference of the intestine Richter's hernia;**
▶ **A portion of the bladder (or a diverticulum);**
▶ **Ovary with or without the corresponding fallopian tube;**
▶ **A Meckel's diverticulum = a Littre's hernia;**
▶ **Fluid — as part of ascites or as a residuum thereof.**

⇨ Important Hernia to be Remembered

Maydls hernia☛☛	Strangulated loops of bowel like W in abdomen
Pantaloon/Saddle bag Hernia☛	Occurrence of both direct and indirect inguinal hernia in same patient
Sliding Hernia	Hernia with sigmoid colon on left and cecum on right side
Laugiers hernia KCET 2012	**Femoral hernia** through Lacunar ligament of Gimbernat
Naraths Hernia☛	Hernia with congenital dislocation of hip
Spigelian Hernia☛☛ JK BOPEE 2009	An interparietal usually subumblical hernia
Obturator hernia☛	Hernia through obturator canal
Epigastic hernia☛☛	Hernia through linea alba
Littres hernia	Hernia of meckels diverticulum **MAHE 2002**
Ritchers Hernia☛☛	Hernia of a portion of circumference of bowel.
Morgagnis hernia	Hernia between costal and sternal parts of diaphragm **AP 1998**

⇨ Obturator Hernia

Is a relaltively rare pelvic hernia and usully occurs in elderly, thin, multiparous women affected more often than man because of their broader pelvis, larger obturator canal and multiple pregnancies.

Predisposing factors:

- **Women with a wider pelvis and more triangular obturator canal**
- **Malnutrition**
- **Age 70-90 years**
- **Concomitant conditions like chronic constipation, COPD, ascites, kyphoscoliosis**
- **Multiparity**

Clinical Features:

- ✓ Features of intestinal obstruction
- ✓ Swelling in scarpa' triangle & movement of limb is painful
- ✓ Referred pain of knee joint; through the geniculate branch of obturator nerve which signifies not only obturator hernia but also strangulation- **"Howship-Romberg sign"**
- ✓ On vaginal and rectal examination, the hernia can sometimes present as a tender swelling in the region of the obturator foramen.

Treatment: Surgery is indicated PGI 2009

⇨ Hernia En Glissade

- Hernia en glissade is also called as **sliding hernia.**
- The contents of hernia on **left side** are sigmoid colon and mesentry. PGI 1995
- Most common content **is Sigmoid Colon.**
- The contents of hernia on **right side** are the cecum.
- Sliding hernia occurs mostly in **males.**
- Five out of every six cases occur on **left side.**
- The incidence of hernia increases with **increasing age.**

⇨ Spigelian Hernia

- Spigelian hernia is an **interparietal** hernia.
- It lies at the level of **arcuate line** mostly.
- The arcuate line lies below umbilicus, hence it is a **subumblical** hernia. PGI 2000
- **Lies lateral to rectus abdominis.** PGI 2000
- The **Spigelian Fascia** is present only below the umbilicus and most of the Spigelian hernias are present sub umblically.
- In addition to this the fibrous bands of spigelian fascia **run transversely with small defects** in between which are the sites of spigelian Hernia.
- The Spigelian hernia may **contain loops of bowel,** colon, omentum or a part of **circumference of bowel only.**

⇨ Other Hernias

- Beclards Hernia: Hernia through opening for saphenous vein
- Treitz Hernia: Duodenojujenal hernia
- Rokintaskis Hernia: Mucus membrane Herniation through muscular layer of bowel

⇨ Common in Hernias

- MC type of hernia in men: Indirect inguinal
- MC type of hernia in women: Indirect inguinal

▶ Femoral hernia is more common in: Women	AIIMS 1997
▶ Femoral hernia is common on: Right side	
▶ Inguinal hernia is common on: Right side	PGI 2003
▶ **Femoral hernia strangulates: Commonly.**	PGI 2000

- ▶ **Reducible hernia: contents can be replaced back**
- ▶ **Irreducible hernia: contents cannot be replaced back.**
- ▶ **Strangulated hernia: compromised blood supply.**
- ▶ **External hernia: protrudes through all layers of abdominsl wall**
- ▶ **Interparietal hernia: hernia sac contained within musculoaponeurotic layer of abdominal wall**

⇨ Saphena Varix

Saphena Varix.

- ❒ A saccular **enlargement of the termination of the long saphenous vein**, usually accompanied by other signs of varicose veins.
- ❒ The swelling **disappears completely when the patient lies flat,** while a femoral hernia sac is usually still palpable.
- ❒ In both, there is an **impulse on coughing.**
- ❒ A saphena varix will, however, **impart a fluid thrill to the examining fingers** when the patient coughs or when the saphenous vein below the varix is tapped with the fingers of the other hand. Sometimes a **venous hum** can be heard when a stethoscope is applied over a saphena varix.

⇨ Pancreas

- ❒ The pancreas occupies a **retroperitoneal position** in the abdomen, lying posterior to the stomach and lesser omentum.
- ❒ It extends obliquely from the **duodenal C loop** to a more cephalad position in the **hilum of the spleen**
- ❒ The gland is divided into four portions: **the head (which includes the uncinate process), the neck, the body, and the tail.**
- ❒ It includes the posteroinferior extension arising from the ventral primordium, designated the **uncinate process.**

⇨ Causes of Pancreatic Injury

- ▶ **During Spleenectomy**
- ▶ **During Billiroth II Gastrectomy**
- ▶ **During islet cell tumor surgeries**
- ▶ **During sphincterotomy**

1

SURGERY

⇨ Heterotopic Pancreas

- ✓ The **development of pancreatic tissue outside the confines of the main gland** is a congenital abnormality referred to as heterotopic pancreas.
- ✓ Most commonly, **heterotopic pancreatic tissue is found in the stomach, (MC)** **AIIMS 2007**
- ✓ **Duodenum, small bowel, or Meckel's diverticulum.**
- ✓ In most locations, heterotopic pancreatic tissue **resides in a submucosal location**, presenting as firm, yellow, irregular nodules that vary in size from millimeters to several centimeters.
- ✓ The clinical significance of heterotopic pancreas is dependent on resultant complications. **Intestinal obstruction** may ensue, rarely as a result of the size of the mass, and more commonly following **intussusception**, with the ectopic pancreatic tissue serving as the intussusceptum. Other complications of heterotopic pancreas include **ulceration and hemorrhage.**

⇨ Pancreas Divisum

- Follows **failure of fusion of the two primordial ductal systems.**
- The **major portion of the pancreas is drained via the duct of Santorini via the minor duodenal papilla.** ☛☛
- The **major duodenal papilla usually communicates with a small duct of Wirsung, which drains the ventral pancreas, consisting of the inferior head and uncinate process.**☛
- The significance of pancreas divisum remains **controversial.** It is unknown whether the ductal anomaly has any causal relationship to the pancreatitis. **Annular pancreas.**
- Normal pancreatic tissue completely or partially encircles the **second portion of the duodenum.** ☛

⇨ Annular Pancreas

- ❒ Annular pancreas is a rare condition in which the **second part of the duodenum** is surrounded by a ring of pancreatic tissue continuous with the head of the pancreas **KCET 2012**
- ❒ It is typically associated with abnormal embryological development, however adult cases can develop.
- ❒ Postnatal diagnostic procedures include abdominal X-ray and ultrasound, CT scan, and upper GI and small bowel series.
- ❒ Treatment usually is bypassing the obstructed segment of duodenum by **Duodenostomy** **AIPGME 2010**

- ► Annular pancreas is thought to arise from failure of normal clockwise rotation of the **ventral pancreatic bud**
- ► Varying degrees of **duodenal obstructive symptoms** may be observed in this condition.
- ► There is a common association with other serious congenital anomalies such as **intracardiac defects, Down's syndrome, and intestinal malrotation.**
- ► In adults, symptoms may appear to be those of **upper gastrointestinal obstruction, chronic pancreatitis, or peptic ulcer.**
- ► **Obstructive symptoms** are an indication for operation.
- ► Retrocolic **duodenojejunostomy** is treatment of choice.☛☛

⇨ Acute Pancreatitis

Acute pancreatitis: Causes PGI 85, 87, TN 87, PGI 88

The vast majority of cases in the UK are caused by gallstones and alcohol Popular mnemonic is **GET SMASHED**

- Gallstones (MC cause) PGI 2000
- Ethanol
- Trauma
- Steroids
- Mumps (other viruses include Coxsackie B)
- Autoimmune (e.g. polyarteritis nodosa), Ascaris infection
- Scorpion venom
- Hypertriglyceridaemia, Hyperchylomicronaemia, **Hypercalcaemia**, Hypothermia
- ERCP
- Drugs (azathioprine, sulfasalazine, didanosine, bendroflume**thiazide**, frusemide, pentamidine, steroids, sodium valproate) PGP

Pain in a band form radiating to back with relief on sitting is a feature.

Hypercalcemia causes pancreatitis but Pancreatitis causes hypocalcemia. MAH 2012

A pancreatic pseudocyst may be palpable in the upper abdomen.

- **Grey turners sign (flanks)** PGI 2004
- **Cullens sign (umbilicus)**

A faint blue discoloration around the umbilicus (Cullen's sign) may occur as the result of hemoperitoneum, and a blue-red-purple or green-brown discoloration of the flanks (Turner's sign) reflects tissue catabolism of hemoglobin.

The diagnosis of acute pancreatitis

- ↑**level of serum amylase.** Values threefold or more above normal virtually clinch the diagnosis if overt salivary gland disease and gut perforation or infarctions are excluded.
- There is no definite correlation between the severity of pancreatitis and the degree of serum amylase elevation. After 48 to 72 h, even with continuing evidence of pancreatitis, total serum amylase values tend to return to normal.
- However, **pancreatic isoamylase and lipase levels** may remain elevated for 7 to 14 days.
- **Fetal fat estimation** diagnoses **insufficency** AIIMS 91
- **Gall stone pancreatitis has best prognosis.** AI 2004

Plain Abdominal X-ray shows:

- **Sentinel loop,**
- **Colon cut off sign,**
- **Renal halo sign**
- **CT Scan is the diagnostic modality of choice.** JK BOPEE 2011

Purtscher's Retinopathy, a relatively unusual complication, is manifested by a sudden and severe loss of vision in a patient with **acute pancreatitis**. It is characterized by a peculiar funduscopic appearance with cotton-wool spots and hemorrhages confined to an area limited by the optic disk and macula; it is believed to be due to occlusion of the posterior retinal artery with aggregated granulocytes.

Pancreatitis in Patients with AIDS The incidence of **acute** pancreatitis is increased in patients with AIDS for two reasons: (1) the high incidence of infections involving the pancreas, such as infections with **cytomegalovirus, Cryptosporidium, and the Mycobacterium avium complex**; and (2) the frequent use by patients with AIDS of medications such as **didanosine, pentamidine, and trimethoprim-sulfamethoxazole.**

⇨ Chronic Pancreatitis

- The **classic triad of "Pancreatic calcification, Steatorrhea, and Diabetes mellitus"** usually establishes the diagnosis of chronic pancreatitis and exocrine pancreatic insufficiency but is found in less than one-third of chronic pancreatitis patients.
- The **secretin stimulation test**, which usually gives abnormal results when 60% or more of pancreatic exocrine function has been lost. The radiographic hallmark of chronic pancreatitis is the presence of scattered calcification throughout the pancreas.

⇨ Hereditary Pancreatitis

Hereditary pancreatitis is a rare disease that is **similar to chronic pancreatitis** except for an early age of onset and **evidence of hereditary factors** (involving an autosomal dominant gene with incomplete penetrance). Genetic linkage analysis identified the hereditary pancreatitis gene on **chromosome.**

➲ Ranson's Criteria in Acute Pancreatitis

⇨ Prognostic Implications

Ranson's Criteria on Admission: MAH 2012

- Age > 55 years
- WBC > 16,000/uL
- Glucose >200 mg/dL (>11 mmol/L)
- LDH > 350 IU/L AIIMS 2010
- SGOT (AST) > 250 IU/L

Ranson's Criteria after 48 hr of Admission: AIPGME 2011

- Fall in hematocrit >10%
- Increase in BUN to > 5 mg/dL (>1.98 mmol/L)
- Calcium < 8 mg/dL (<2 mmol/L) AIIMS 2011
- PO2 < 60 mm Hg
- Base deficit > 4 meq/L (>4 mmol/L)
- Fluid sequestration > 6 Liters

⇨ Macroamylasemia

- In macroamylasemia, amylase circulates in the blood in a polymer form too large to be easily excreted by the kidney.
- Patients with this condition demonstrate an elevated serum amylase value, a low urinary amylase value, and a C_{am}/C_{cr} ratio of less than 1%.
- Usually macroamylasemia is an incidental finding and is not related to disease of the pancreas or other organs.
- Macrolipasemia has been documented in a few patients with cirrhosis or non-Hodgkin's lymphoma

Reurrent Pancreatitis Cccurs in Methyl Malonic Academia COMED 2008

Causes of Hyperamylasia:

- **Pancreas:**
- **Pancreatitis**
- **Complications of pancreatitis: pseudocyst, ascites, abscess, necrosis.**
- **Pancreatic trauma**
- **Ca pancreas**
- **Carcinoma lung, ovary, breast, esophagus** PGI 2011
- **Mumps, sialolithiasis, siadenitis**
- **Burns**
- **Pregnancy**
- **Cholelithiasis**
- **Choledocholithiasis**
- **Perforated peptic ulcer** PGI 2011
- **Ruptured ectopic**
- **Peritonitis** PGI 2011

⇨ Pancreatic Pseudocyst

- Pancreatic pseudocysts are localized collections of pancreatic secretions in a cystic structure that **lack an epithelial lining.**
  - Mc site body or tail.
  - Mc cause: pancreatitis (adults) AI 94
  - **Mc cause: trauma (children)** AI 1991
- Pseudocysts contain high concentrations of pancreatic enzymes, including amylase, lipase, and trypsin.
- Pancreatic pseudocysts develop in up to patients after an attack of acute alcoholic pancreatitis.
- Pseudocysts are also associated with acute pancreatitis with other causes, as well as with **chronic pancreatitis, pancreatic trauma, and pancreatic neoplasm**
- Most often present with upper abdominal pain AI 98
- Physical examination reveals abdominal tenderness in the majority of patients
- A CT scan of the abdomen is the favored study in an initial assessment for determining the presence of a pancreatic pseudocyst

1

SURGERY

- Complications: Infection, **MC PGI 2000**
- Rupture, haemmorage,
- < 5 cm managed conservatively
- **> 5 cm, cyst > 6 weeks, infection, complication:** Surgery
- Treatment of choice is **internal drainage (Cysteoduodenostomy).**

⇨ Pancreatic Carcinoma

- **More common in males than in females and in blacks than in whites.**
- **Cigarette smoking is the most consistent risk factor** **PGI 2000**
- **Chronic pancreatitis**
- **Diabetes mellitus.**
- **Alcohol abuse or cholelithiasis are not risk factors for pancreatic cancer.**
- **Heridetray pancreatitis, peutz jeughers syndrome, VHL, Ataxia telengectasia, Gardeners syndrome and Lynch syndrome II**
- **Mutations in K-ras genes**

CLINICAL FEATURES

Most common is: Ductal adenocarcinomas,

Most common in : Pancreatic head (70% of cases) **PGI 2000**

Most common symptom is: Pain and weight loss. **PGI 2000**

Most common physical sign is: Jaundice.

- Although the gallbladder is usually enlarged in patients with carcinoma of the head of the pancreas, it is palpable in 50% **(Courvoisier's sign)**
- Other initial manifestations include **venous thrombosis and migratory thrombophlebitis (Trousseau's sign), gastrointestinal hemorrhage** from varices due to compression of the portal venous system by tumor, and **splenomegaly** caused by cancerous encasement of the splenic vein.
- **CECT** is the most effective tecnique for diagnosis.
- **Whipples operation** is indicated for periampullary cancer or cancer head of pancreas.
- **"Gemcitabine"**, a **deoxycytidine analogue**, produces improvement in the quality of life for patients with advanced **pancreatic cancer.**

<u>The coexistence of peripheral venous thrombosis with visceral carcinoma, particularly pancreatic cancer, is called Trousseau's syndrome</u>. **DNB 2011**

Glucose intolerance, presumably a direct consequence of the tumor, often develops within 2 years of the clinical diagnosis. Other initial manifestations include

- **Venous thrombosis and Migratory Thrombophlebitis (Trousseau's Syndrome),**
- **Gastrointestinal hemorrhage** from varices due to compression of the portal venous system by tumor, and
- **Splenomegaly** caused by cancerous encasement of the splenic vein.

Zollinger-Ellison Syndrome/Gastrinoma

- ❐ **Mc site is duodenum followed by pancreas**
- ❐ **Mc malignant pancreatic endocrine tumor**
- ❐ **More common in males**
- ❐ **Non beta cell tumor** — AI 2002
- ❐ **Tumor of delta cells**

Zollinger Ellison syndrome is a **NET (Neuro endocrine tumor) secreting gastrin** — **PGI 2008**

- ❐ In ZES, CHARACTERISTICALLY **GASTRIC ACID HYPERSECRETION** IS PRESENT.
- ❐ This gastric acid hypersecretion causes **peptic ulcer** disease often **refractory and severe**, associated with diarrhea.
- ❐ The most common presenting symptom is **abdominal pain** (70-100%) Peptic ulcer can occur anywhere but the commonest location is the **duodenum** (50-70%) followed by pancreas. (20-40%)
- ❐ ZES occurs in association with **MEN 1**(Hyperparathyroidism, Peptic ulcer disease and Pituitary tumors). About 20-25% patients have associated MEN1 and in most cases Hyperparathyroidism is present before Hypergastrenemia.
- ❐ Diagnosis is based on **fasting hypergastrenemia and increased Basal acid output (BAO)**
- ❐ **Secretin injection test is used most important investigation.** — **AI 99**
- ❐ **Proton pump inhibitors** are the **drugs of choice.** — **AIIMS 95, AI 2007**
- ❐ Surgical cure is possible in only **30%** of patients.
- ❐ SOMATOSTATIN and Omperazole used. — **PGI 2001**
- ❐ Hepatic metastasis occurs in **one third** of patients. — **PGI 2008**

Gastrinoma Triangle:

90% of extrapancreatic gastrinomas lie here. — **AIIMS 2011**

Formed by:

- ❐ **3rd part of duodenum**
- ❐ **Cystic duct**
- ❐ **Pancreatic neck**

Ulcers in ZES

- ► Unusual location
- ► Ulcers in absence of predisposing factors.
- ► Ulcers in presence of hypercalcemia or family history of MEN 1
- ► Multiple ulcers
- ► Ulcers refractory to treatment
- ► Recurrence of ulcers
- ► Giant ulcers
- ► Ulcers with complications

1

SURGERY

➲ Insulinomas

- Insulinomas are MC **endocrine tumors** of the pancreas thought to be derived **from beta cells** that autonomously secrete insulin, which results in hypoglycemia **AIIMS 2004**
- The most common clinical symptoms are due to the effect of the hypoglycemia on the central nervous system (neuroglycemic symptoms) and include confusion, headache, disorientation, visual difficulties, irrational behavior, or even coma.
- Also, most patients have symptoms due to excess catecholamine release secondary to the hypoglycemia, including sweating, tremor, and palpitations. Characteristically these attacks are associated with fasting.
- Usually single. **AI, AIIMS**
- **Whipples triad is a feature.** **PGI 1997**
- **Weight gain occurs.**
- Insulinomas are **generally,** usually solitary (90%), and only 5 to 15% are malignant.
- They almost invariably occur only in the pancreas, **distributed equally in the pancreatic head, body and tail.** **AIIMS 2002**
- Insulinomas should be suspected in all patients with hypoglycemia, especially with a history suggesting attacks provoked by fasting or with a family history of MEN-1.
- In insulinomas, in addition to **elevated plasma insulin levels, elevated plasma proinsulin levels are found and C-peptide levels can be elevated.**
- Care should be taken to achieve total tumor capsule removal to prevent tumor recurrence. If enucleation is not possible, a larger pancreatic resection including pancreaticoduodenectomy may be necessary. **AIPGME 2010**

The biochemical diagnosis is established in 95% of patients during prolonged fasting (up to 72 h) when the following parameters are found:

- **Serum insulin levels of 10 μU/mL or more (normal <6 μU/mL)**
- **Glucose levels of less than 40 mg/dL**
- **C-peptide levels exceeding 2.5 ng/mL (normal <2 ng/mL)**
- **Proinsulin levels greater than 25% (or up to 90%) that of immunoreactive insulin**
- **Screening for sulfonylurea negative** **AIPGME 2010**

➲ Glucagonomas

- Glucagonomas are **endocrine tumors of the pancreas** that secrete **excessive amounts of glucagon that causes a distinct syndrome characterized by dermatitis, glucose intolerance or diabetes, and weight loss.**
- Glucagonomas mainly occur in persons between 45 and 70 years old. They are heralded clinically by a characteristic dermatitis (**migratory necrolytic erythema**; accompanied by glucose intolerance weight loss, anemia, diarrhea and thromboembolism
- The characteristic rash usually starts as an **annular erythema at intertriginous and periorificial sites,** especially in the groin or buttock. It subsequently becomes raised and bullae form; when the bullae rupture, eroded areas form. The lesions can wax and wane.

- A characteristic laboratory finding is **hypoaminoacidemia**
- Glucagonomas are generally large tumors at diagnosis, with an average size of 5 to 10 cm. Between 50 and 80% occur in the pancreatic tail and 50 to 82% have evidence of metastatic spread at presentation, usually to the liver. Glucagonomas are rarely extrapancreatic and usually occur singly.

⇨ Somatostatinoma Syndrome

- Somatostatinomas are **endocrine tumors that secrete excessive amounts of somatostatin**, which causes a syndrome characterized by **diabetes melitus, gallbladder disease, diarrhea, and steatorrhea.**
  COMED 2007
- Somatostatinomas occur primarily in the pancreas and small intestine, and the frequency of the symptoms differs in each.
- Somatostatinomas occur in the pancreas in 56 to 74% of cases, with the primary location being in the pancreatic head.

⇨ VIPomas AIIMS 1996

Are endocrine tumors that secrete excessive amounts of **VIP**, which causes a distinct syndrome characterized by **large-volume diarrhea, hypokalemia, and dehydration**. This syndrome is also called **Verner-Morrison syndrome, pancreatic cholera, or WDHA syndrome.**

- ✓ **Watery diarrhea,**
- ✓ **Hypokalemia, and**
- ✓ **Achlorhydria/hypochlorrydia**
- ✓ **Hypercalcemia**

⇨ Spleen

- **The gastrosplenic ligament**, contains the short gastric arteries and veins.
- **The splenorenal ligament** contains the splenic artery and vein, lymphatic structures, and often the tail of the pancreas.
- **The arterial supply to the spleen** is derived from the celiac artery from both the splenic artery and the short gastric arteries, which usually arise as branches of the gastroepiploic or the splenic arteries
- **The splenic vein** is formed by a coalescence of polar veins in the splenic hilum and courses with the splenic artery along the dorsal surface of the pancreas to enter the portal system.
- **The normal adult spleen** is a slightly concave, solid, dark red organ that measures approximately 3 × 8 × 14 cm.
- **MC cyst of spleen is pseudocyst.** AI 2010

⇨ Wandering (Ectopic) Spleen/Spleenosis

- Congenital deficiency or acquired laxity of the suspensory ligaments of the spleen may cause **extreme splenic mobility.**
- Palpable in the **lower abdomen or in the pelvis.**
- The majority of cases occur in **young and middle-aged women** in whom multiparity and laxity of the abdominal wall and splenic ligaments due to the hormonal effects.

- **An elongated splenic pedicle** predisposes a wandering spleen to torsion, leading either to development of acute symptoms due to splenic volvulus and infarction or to chronic and intermittent abdominal discomfort due to spontaneous torsion and detorsion.
- Splenic volvulus with infarction requires **emergency splenectomy.**

⇨ Pseudocyst of Spleen

- **Mc type** of cyst of spleen.
- Pseudocyst do not have epithelial lining and comprises of **70-80% of splenic cyst**.
- The are usually a **result of trauma** and represent resolution of a subscapular or intraparenchymal hematoma.
- Malaria, infectious mononucleosis, TB, and syphilis are all predisposing factors.
- Are **usually unilocular.**
- Occur commonly in women, children and young adult.
- The most frequent symptom is **left upper quadrant pain** radiating to left shoulder. AIPGME 2010

⇨ Splenic Artery Aneurysm

- Occur more frequently in **females,** ☛
- Medial dysplasia of the arterial wall. Atherosclerosis, pancreatitis, trauma or arteritis due to septic emboli, portal hypertension with splenomegaly.
- Most splenic artery aneurysms are asymptomatic, and characteristic **eggshell calcification** of an arteriosclerotic aneurysm may be an incidental finding on an abdominal radiograph.
- **Aneurysmal rupture** may occur, and the rupture initially may be contained within the lesser sac.
- Initial aneurysmal rupture into the **peritoneal cavity** or delayed rupture from the lesser sac are associated with findings of hemoperitoneum and exsanguinating hemorrhage. Rarely, a splenic artery aneurysm ruptures into the gastrointestinal tract, pancreatic duct, or splenic vein.

⇨ Splenic Abscess

Usually Results From

- ❒ Bacteremia associated with a primary septic focus such as bacterial endocarditis or lung abscess.
- ❒ Secondary infection in an area of the spleen damaged by infarction (sickle cell anemia or leukemia), trauma, or parasitic infestation.
- ❒ Clinical features of splenic abscess are those of **left subphrenic suppuration** and include fever, chills, left upper quadrant tenderness, and often splenomegaly.
- ❒ Ultrasonography and radionuclide and CT scans are useful.
- ❒ CT is the most direct way of evaluating the spleen.

⇨ Littoral Cell Angioma

- Littoral cell angioma is **a benign, vascular tumor** of spleen presenting as spleenomegaly.☛☛
- It may be associated with other malignancies and has malignant potential itself.
- The tumor arises from the **littoral cells in the splenic red pulp sinuses.** Littoral cell angioma affects both men and women equally with no specific age predilection. ☛

- It is **usually asymptomatic** and is discovered incidentally.
- Some of the patients with this entity may present with symptoms of **hypersplenism** such as anemia, thrombocytopenia, and splenomegaly, the latter seen in almost all patients with littoral cell angioma.

⇨ Splenunculi

These are single or multiple accessory spleens which are found

- **Near the hilum of the spleen** ☛☛ PGI 1995
- Splenic vessels and
- Behind the tail of the pancreas in 30 percent,
- In the splenic ligaments (Gastrocolic, greater omentum, spleenocolic)
- Mesocolon in the remainder.
- Up to 20 percent of people have such splenunculi and most are no larger than 2 cm in diameter.

Their importance lies in the fact that if not removed at the time of splenectomy they will undergo hyperplasia and may well be the site of persistent disease.

⇨ Situs Ambiguous

The 2 primary subtypes of **situs ambiguous include**

(1) **Right isomerism**, or asplenia syndrome, and AIPGEE 2011

(2) **Left isomerism**, or polysplenia syndrome.

In classic right isomerism, or asplenia,

- ✓ Bilateral right-sidedness occurs.
- ✓ These patients have bilateral right atria, a centrally located liver, and an absent spleen, and both lungs have 3 lobes.
- ✓ The descending aorta and inferior vena cava are on the same side of the spine.

In left isomerism, or polysplenia

- ✓ Bilateral left-sidedness occurs.
- ✓ These patients have bilateral left atria and multiple spleens, and both lungs have 2 lobes.

Interruption of the inferior vena cava with azygous or hemiazygous continuation is often present.

⇨ Spleenic Trauma

- **Kehrs sign is occurrence of pain in the tip of shoulder due to presence of blood/irritant in peritoneal cavity.** KCET 2012
- Kehrs sign in left shoulder is considered a **characteristic sign of splenic rupture.** ☛☛ AI 1995
- Kehrs sign is a **classic example** of referred pain (phrenic nerve)

Other important conditions causing Kehr's sign are:

- ✓ **Diaphragmatic lesions**
- ✓ **Ectopic pregnancy**
- ✓ **Renal calculi**
- ✓ **Hemoperitonium** MANIPAL

1

SURGERY

The signs and symptoms of splenic trauma are those of hemoperitoneum. Generalized and nonspecific abdominal pain in the left upper quadrant occurs in approximately one third of patients with splenic injury. Pain referred to the tip of the left shoulder (Kehr's sign) is inconstant, varying in incidence from 15% to 75%, and is unreliable for excluding splenic injury but is useful for enhancing the diagnostic probability if present. Kehr's sign is elicited by bimanual compression of the left upper quadrant after the patient has been in Trendelenburg's position for several minutes preceding the maneuver. On rare occasions, patients with splenic injury have a palpable tender mass in the left upper quadrant (Ballance's sign), caused by an extracapsular or subcapsular hematoma with omentum adherent to the injured spleen.

- Spleen is the most common organ injured in blunt abdominal injury.
- Contrast enhanced CT Scan is the investigation of choice for splenic injuries.

⇨ Features on X- ray Suggestive of Splenic Injury are

❐ **Obliteration of splenic shadow☛☛**	**JIPMER 1987**
❐ **Obliteration of psoas shadow**	**TN 1999**
❐ **Fracture of lower left ribs**	
❐ **Elevation of left diaphragm**	**TN 1999**
❐ **Indentation of stomach**	
❐ **Presence of fluid between coils of intestine.**	

⇨ Spleen

- **Felty's Syndrome: Rheumatoid arthritis with Hypersplenism**
- **Banti's Syndrome: Congestive spleenomegaly with Hypersplenism**
- **Egyptian Splenomegaly: Schistosomiasis**
- **Angiosarcoma: MC malignant Tumor of Spleen**
- **Splenosis: Rupture of spleen with dissemination into peritonium**
- **Spontaneous rupture is seen in Infectious mononucleosis typhoid, leukemia**

⇨ Splenic Artery Aneurysm: DNB 2011

- ❐ Aneurysms of the splenic artery are **rare** and occur more frequently in females.
- ❐ **Atherosclerosis** accounts for the majority of splenic artery aneurysms in males. Most splenic artery aneurysms are asymptomatic, and characteristic eggshellcalcification of an arteriosclerotic aneurysm may be an incidental finding on anabdominal radiograph.
- ❐ When symptoms are present, they are variable and consist primarily of vague **left hypochondriac discomfort.**
- ❐ Aneurysmal rupture may occur, and the rupture initially may be contained within the **lesser sac.** Initial aneurysmal rupture into the peritoneal cavity or delayed rupture from the lesser sac are associated with findings of **hemoperitoneum and exsanguinating hemorrhage**. Rarely, a splenic artery aneurysm ruptures into the **gastrointestinal tract, pancreatic duct, or splenic vein.**

⇨ **Splenectomy:**

➨ Mc indication for elective spleenectomy: ITP,	
➨ HS	AI 1999
➨ G6PD	
➨ Portal hypertension	PGI 2006
➨ Hyperspleenism	PGI 2006
➨ Autosplenectomy is seen in sickle cell anemia	
➨ Pneumococcal vaccine and N. meningitis vaccine given.	
➨ **Splenorraphy** is done in stable patient with lacerated spleen.	AI 2010

⇨ **Not Done for:**☛☛

➨ Asymptomatic	
➨ Splenomegaly with infection	
➨ Splenomegaly with ↑igm	
➨ Hereditary hemolytic anemia	AI 2000
➨ Acute leukemia	
➨ Agranulocytosis	
➨ Porphyria	AI 2005

⇨ **Complications:**

✓ Hemorrhage
✓ Hemetemesis
✓ Left basal atelectasis
✓ Pancreatitis, pancreatic abscess
✓ Risk of infections

⇨ **Spleenectomy Increases Risk for:**☛☛☛

❒ **Pneumococcal infections**	PGI 2005
❒ **H. influenza**	PGI 2005
❒ **Gram negative enteric organisms**	
❒ **Meningococcimeia**	
❒ **Babesia**	
❒ **Malaria**	

1

SURGERY

⇨ An Overwhelming Post-Splenectomy Infection (OPSI)

- ► An **overwhelming post-splenectomy infection** (OPSI) is a **rare but rapidly fatal infection** occurring in individuals following removal of the spleen. The infections are typically characterized by either meningitis or sepsis, and are caused by **Streptococcus pneumonia mostly.** **AIIMS 1999**
- ► The spleen contains many macrophages (part of the reticuloendothelial system), immune cells which phagocytose (eat) and destroy bacteria. In particular, these macrophages are activated when bacteria are bound by IgG antibodies (IgG1 or IgG3) or complement component C3b. These types of antibodies and complement are immune substances **called opsonizers,** molecules which bind to the surface of bacteria to make them easier for macrophages to phagocytose and destroy the bacteria.
- ► When the spleen is gone, IgG and complement component C3b are still bound to bacteria, but they cannot be removed from the blood circulation because the spleen, which contained the macrophages, is gone. The bacteria therefore are free to cause infection.
- ► Patients without spleens often need immunizations against pathogens that normally require opsonization and phagocytosis by macrophages in the spleen. These include common human pathogens with capsules
  - **Streptococcus pneumoniae** **PGI 2005**
  - **Salmonella typhi, Neisseria meningitidis, E. coli, Hemophilus influenzae, Streptococcus agalactiae, Klebsiella pneumonia** **AIIMS 1984**
  - **MC complication is left lower lobe atelectasis.** **JIPMER 1988**

⇨ Remember in Nutshell: About Overwhelming Post Splenectomy Infection

- ➢ Infection due to **encapsulated bacteria**
- ➢ Almost **50% due to strep. Pneumoniae**
- ➢ Other organisms include: Haemophilus influenzae, Neisseria meningitidis
- ➢ Occurs post splenectomy in **4% patients** without prophylaxis
- ➢ Mortality of OPSI is approximately **50%**
- ➢ Greatest risk in **first 2 years post op.**

► Acute hematological effects of splenectomy	► Chronic hematological effects of splenectomy
❒ **Leukocytosis**	➠ Anisocytosis
❒ Thrombocytosis	➠ Poikiolocytosis
❒ Heinz bodies	➠ Howell jolly bodies
❒ Basophilic stippling	➠ Nucleated erythrocytes

⇨ "<u>Massive</u>" Splenomegaly:

Causes are:	
✓ HAIRY CELL LEUKEMIA	PGI 2011
✓ CML	
✓ GAUCHERS DISEASE	PGI 2011

- ✓ MYELOFIBROSIS WITH MYELOID METAPLASIA
- ✓ CLL
- ✓ LYMPHOMAS
- ✓ POLYCYTHEMIA VERA
- ✓ DIFFUSE SPLEENIC HEMANGIOMATOSI

⇨ Liver

- 80% blood supply is from **portal vein.** 20% is from hepatic artery.
- Liver is divided into surgical right and left lobes by a line between gallbladder and middle hepatic vein. **Cantille line**
- Portal venous system lacks valves

⇨ "Caterpillar Turn" or "Moynihans Hump"

- Normally the arterial supply of gallbladder is from **cystic artery** which is a branch of **Right hepatic artery.**
- Sometimes an **accessory cystic artery** is also seen to arise from either **Gastroduodenal or right hepatic artery.** JK BOPEE 2009
- The Right hepatic artery takes a tortuous course called "**caterpillar turn**" or "**Moynihans hump.**" This can be a source of profuse bleeding.

- **Orthoptic liver transplant** is replacement of patient liver with donor liver.
- **Auxillary liver transplant** is transplanted along side of part of patients own liver.

⇨ Couinouds Segments of Liver: Nomenclature System for Hepatic Anatomy

- Was developed by **Soupault and Couinaud.**
- This system shows more consideration for the **hepatic venous drainage** and caudate lobe but also applies to the portal, biliary, and arterial anatomy.
- Instead of **four, there are eight segments:**
- **Four on the right, three on the left, and one corresponding to the topographic caudate lobe.**
- **Segment I** corresponds to the **caudate lobe;**
- **Segments II to IV** constitute the **left lobe;**
- **Segments V to VIII** the **right lobe.**
- The three main hepatic veins divide the liver into four sectors.
- The planes containing the right, middle, and left hepatic veins are called **portal scissurae,** while the planes containing portal pedicles are called **hepatic scissurae.**
- The caudate lobe is its own autonomous segment in the French system.

- Segment I: Caudate lobe. Rest of segments are clockwise: PGI 2007
- Segment II: Lateral segment left superior lobe.
- Segment III: Lateral segment left inferior lobe.

1

SURGERY

- Segment IV: Quadrate lobe — AIIMS 2007
- Segment V: Anterior segment right inferior lobe.
- Segment VI: Posterior segment right superior lobe.
- Segment VII: Posterior segment right superior lobe.
- Segment VIII: Anterior segment right superior lobe.
- Based on hepatic vein and portal vein division. — AI 2004
- **Segment I has independent vascular supply.** — UPSC 2002

Portal Vein

- Portal vein is an important vein formed behind the **neck of pancreas** by union of **Splenic vein and Superior Mesentric vein.** — JK BOPEE
- Drains blood from **GIT AND SPLEEN.**
- It is **8 cms in length.**
- It is the major source of **blood supply to liver.**
- It is **devoid of valves.**

Portal Hypertension

- **(>10 mm Hg)** most commonly results from increased resistance to portal blood flow. — COMED 2008
- Increased resistance can occur at three levels relative to the hepatic sinusoids:
  - **Presinusoidal,**
  - **Sinusoidal, and**
  - **Postsinudoidal.**
- **"Cirrhosis" is the most common cause of portal hypertension** in the United States
- Portal venous pressure may be measured directly by percutaneous transhepatic **"skinny needle"** catheterization or indirectly through transjugular cannulation of the hepatic veins

Sites of portosystemic anastomosis: involved in portal hypertension:

- **Umbilicus: caput medusa**
- **Lower end of esophagus: esophageal varices**
- **Rectum and anal canal: haemmoroids** — AI 2007
- **Bare area of liver** — AI 2007
- **Posterior abdominal wall.**

BLEEDING VARICES: Propranolol is the drug of choice for prophylaxis of bleeding.

Octerotide is the drug of choice for bleeding varices

Barium swallow shoes **string of beads** in esophagus.

TIPS is not an emergency procedure.

ESOPHAGEAL VARICES:

Varices in the distal esophagus and proximal stomach are a component of the collateral network that **diverts high pressure portal venous flow through the left and right gastric veins and the short gastric veins to the azygous system.** Variceal size, magnitude of portal pressure, and thickness of the epithelium overlying the varix are important factors. **LaPlace's law states that variceal wall tension is directly related to transmural pressure and varix radius and inversely related to variceal wall thickness, thus combining all three of these variables.** — DNB 2011

➲ Remember (Portal Vein): Frequently asked. High Yield Topic

- The portal venous system **carries all blood from the abdominal GI tract, spleen, pancreas, and gallbladder back to the heart through the liver.**
- The portal vein is **formed by the union of the superior mesenteric and splenic veins.**
- **At the porta hepatis it divides into the right and left branches,** which are segmentally distributed intrahepatically; the terminal portal venules drain into the sinusoids.
- In the resting state, the portal vein carries about 1 to 1.2 L/min of blood (about **75% of total hepatic blood flow**) and provides 2/3 of the liver's O2 supply.

The portal vein is valveless; thus, pressure in the portal system depends on the product of input from blood flow in the portal vein and total hepatic resistance to outflow.

Pathogenesis

Portal pressure can be defined by the equation P (portal pressure) = Q (blood flow in the portal venous system) X- R (hepatic resistance). Any condition causing increased portal venous flow, or increased hepatic resistance, can develop into portal hypertension.

Classification:

Portal hypertension has been subclassified traditionally according to the presumed site of resistance.

Presinusoidal hypertension can be either intra- or prehepatic:

Prehepatic (extrahepatic) causes include Portal veinThrombosis and splenic vein thromboses.

Intrahepatic presinusoidal hypertension occurs in

- **Schistosomiasis,**
- **Myelofibrosis and**
- **Leukemic liver infiltration,**
- **Idiopathic portal fibrosis,**
- **Nodular regenerative hyperplasia, and**
- **Granulomatous diseases (e.g., sarcoidosis and early stages of primary biliary cirrhosis).**

In all cases of presinusoidal hypertension, the directly measured portal venous pressure will greatly exceed the hepatic venous pressure gradient, which should be normal or near normal. The presinusoidal block prevents transmission of the elevated portal pressure to the wedged hepatic vein. **The overwhelming basis for sinusoidal and postsinusoidal portal hypertension is cirrhosis, particularly that due to alcohol.**

Postsinusoidal hypertension can again be divided into intrahepatic and posthepatic. Posthepatic causes include

- **Chronic heart failure,**
- **Constrictive pericarditis, and**
- **Obstruction of the hepatic venous outflow tract** by membranous webs in the inferior vena cava.

Intrahepatic postsinusoidal causes of portal hypertension include occlusive disease of the small veins and venules (veno-occlusive disease) and occlusions in large hepatic veins (Budd-Chiari syndrome). All cases of sinusoidal and postsinusoidal portal hypertension are associated with hepatic venous pressure gradients, which are about equal to the directly measured portal venous pressures. The resistance to flow extends from the hepatic venous system to the portal vein.

1

SURGERY

Splenomegaly may be the first evidence of portal hypertension of any cause or may reflect primary splenic pathology. AIPGME 2012

A portal pressure **above the normal level of 5 to 10 mm. Hg stimulates portosystemic collateralization.** Collateral vessels usually develop where the portal and systemic venous circulations are in close proximity Although the collateral network through the coronary and short gastric veins to the azygos vein is the most important one clinically, because it results in formation of

- ✓ **Esophagogastric varices**
- ✓ **Retroperitoneal collateral vessels,**
- ✓ **Hemorrhoidal venous plexus**
- ✓ **Bleeding from esophagogastric varices is the single most life-threatening complication of portal hypertension.**

⇨ The Child- Pugh Classification

- ❒ **MAH 2012,**
- ❒ **KCET 2012,**
- ❒ **AIIMS 2010,**
- ❒ **AIPGME 2010**

Is a means of assessing the severity of liver cirrhosis.Criterion are:

- ❒ **Bilirubin (Micromol/l)**
- ❒ **Albumin (g/l)**
- ❒ **PT (S prolonged)**
- ❒ **Encephalopathy**
- ❒ **Ascites**

⇨ The Individual Scores are Summed and then Grouped as:

- ➨ <7 = A
- ➨ 7-9 = B
- ➨ >9 = C

⇨ Amebic Liver Abscess

E. histolytica most often involves the **liver.**

- ➨ Mc in **right lobe. (postero superior surface)** PGI 2000
- ➨ Liquefaction necrosis is characteristic
- ➨ **Anchovy sauce pus: choclate colored pus due to RBC Lysis.** AI 1999
- ➨ Scant inflammatory response at margins.
- ➨ Some patients are febrile and have right-upper-quadrant pain, which may be dull or pleuritic in nature and radiate to the shoulder.

- Point tenderness over the liver and right-sided pleural effusion are common.
- Jaundice is rare.
- About one-third of patients with chronic presentations are febrile. Thus, the clinical diagnosis of an amebic **liver abscess** may be difficult to establish because the symptoms and signs are often nonspecific.
- **Complications of Amebic Liver Abscess**
  - ✓ Pleuropulmonary involvementManifestations include sterile effusions, contiguous spread from the liver, and rupture into the pleural space. **PGI 2000**
  - ✓ Rupture into the pleural space.
  - ✓ Rupture into the peritoneum.
  - ✓ Rupture into the pericardium, usually from abscesses of the left lobe of the liver.
- **DOC: Metronidazole**

⇨ Hydatid Disease

- **Echinococciosis** is also known as **hydatid disease.**☛
- Hydatid cyst is a **parasitic infection** of humans by the tapeworm of genus echinococcus.
- It is a **zoonosis.**
  - ✓ **Echinococcus granulosus** causes **Cystic Echinococcuosis**☛
  - ✓ **Echinococcus multilocularis** causing **Alveolar Echinococcuosis.**☛☛
  - ✓ **Echinococcus vogeli** causes **Polycystic disease**

Echinococcus Granulosus:

The **liver is the most common organ effected** followed by lungs, muscles, bones and kidneys.

Passage of hydatid membrane in emesis is called **hydatid emesia.**

Passage of hydatid membrane in stools is called **hydatid enterica.**

Flushing and urticaria occur in rupture of hydatid cyst.

1. **Abdominal tenderness** is the most common sign.
2. Tender hepatomegaly signifies secondary infection of the cyst.
3. Ascites is rare.
4. Spleenomegaly can be result of portal hypertension or splenic echinococciosis.

- **Brain involvement** depends on site of brain involved and may present as coma or herniation.
- **Bone and muscle** involvement presents as visible masses.
- Echinococciosis is caused by larval stages of parasite.
- Man is an **accidential intermediate host**. Other intermediate hosts are sheep and cattle.☛
- The **dog** is the **definitive host.**☛
- **Serological assay (Weinberg reaction)** is specific example of Complement fixation test used in detection
- ELISA is also sensitive, blood culture not useful. **PGI 2004**
- Eosinophilia is seen only in case of rupture of cysts.
- Detachment of cysts and their collapse leads to characteristic

1

SURGERY

- Water Lilly sign or floating membrane sign or camolottee sign. DNB 2011
- Other x ray signs of echinococcus are:
- Serpent sign/Rising sun sign
- Crumbled egg appearance. PGI 2007
- **Anaphylaxis, intrapleural rupture, intraperitoneal rupture** are secondary complications.
- **PAIR Technique** (Percutaneous Aspiration, injection of scolicidal agents and reaspiration of cyst contents) has also been used for treatment. PGI 2005
- **Albendazole** is the most effective drug most commonly used. PGI 2004

Hydatid Cyst of Lung AIIMS 2002

- ✓ Second most common site.
- ✓ Less often seen in association with liver cyst.
- ✓ Usually in lower lobes.
- ✓ Calcification uncommon.

Pyogenic Liver Abscess

- Has an increased incidence in **the elderly, diabetics and the immunosuppressed**, who usually present with anorexia, fevers and malaise accompanied by right upper quadrant discomfort.
- The diagnosis is suggested by the finding of a **multiloculated cystic mass** on ultrasound or CT scan) and is confirmed by aspiration for culture and sensitivity.
- Usually single and large. PGI 2001
- The most common organisms are **Escherichia coil and Streptococcus milleri** but other enteric organisms such as Streptococcus fecalis, Klebsiella and Proteus vulgaris also occur and mixed growths are common. Opportunistic pathogens include Staphylococci. Treatment is with antibiotics and ultrasound-guided aspiration. Percutaneous drainage without ultrasound guidance should be avoided as an empyema may follow drainage through the pleural space.
- Infection **through bile duct is the commonest route** followed by **hematogeneous route.** AIIMS 1998

Pyogenic Liver Abcess MC Cause is Billiary Tree Infections AIIMS 2011

The pathophysiology of liver abscess in general or pyogenic abscess in particular involves two basic elements: the presence of the organism and the vulnerability of the liver. The spread of bacterial or other organisms to the hepatic parenchyma may occur through

(1) The portal system;

(2) Ascension from the biliary tree;

(3) The hepatic artery during generalized septicemia;

(4) Direct extension from subhepatic or subdiaphragmatic infection; or

(5) A direct route following trauma.

The other most common sources are **cholecystitis, biliary or pancreatic cancer with obstruction, diverticulitis, regional enteritis, trauma, generalized sepsis, and pelvic inflammatory disease.** Patients receiving chemotherapy for hematologic or solid malignancies are at increased risk. Other important associations with hepatic abscess in adults include **colon cancer, diabetes, and cardiopulmonary disease. Bile ducts, biliary lymphatics, and periductal vascular channels** are the primary routes by which abscesses develop in association with biliary infection. Liver abscess occurs most commonly with **cholecystitis, choledocholithiasis, and malignant or benign biliary stricture.**

⇨ Bismuth-Strasberg Classification of Biliary Injury and Stricture

- Class A Injury to small ducts in continuity with the biliary system, cystic duct leak
- Class B Injury to sectoral ducts with consequent obstruction
- Class C Injury to sectoral duct with consequent bile leak
- Class D Lateral injury to extrahepatic ducts
- Class E1 Stricture > 2 cm distal to bifurcation
- Class E2 Stricture < 2 cm distal to bifurcation
- Class E3 Stricture at bifurcation
- Class E4 Stricture involving right and left ducts, ducts are not in continuity
- Class E5 Complete obstruction of bile buct

⇨ Hepatic Adenoma

- ✓ **Benign neoplasm.☛☛**
- ✓ **Derived from hepatocytes**
- ✓ **Seen in women taking OCPS☛**
- ✓ **Usually asymptomatic but may bleed intraabdominally.☛** **BHU 1988**
- ✓ **Seen as cold defects in hepatic syncitigraphy.☛**
- ✓ **Core biopsy contraindication.☛**
- ✓ **Aspiration biopsy can be done.**
- ✓ **>6 cm tumor should be excised.**

Focal nodular hyperplasia presents similarly but <u>without bleeding features</u>.☛☛☛

➲ Hepatocellular Carcinoma

⇨ Predisposing Factors

- Hepatitis B,☛ **JK BOPEE 2009**
- Hepatitis C,☛
- Alcoholic liver disease, **JK BOPEE**
- Alpha 1 antitrypsin deficiency,
- Hemachromatosis,
- Tyrosenemia,
- Aflatoxin B_1.☛
- Vinyl chloride, Thorium and Androgenic hormones are also implicated.☛

1

SURGERY

➠ AFP levels are raised. AFP is used as a **marker** for HCC.	**PGI 2000**
➠ Other markers are: Neurotensin, PIVKA 2	**AIIMS 2006**
➠ Early stage tumors are successfully treated. If untreated most patients die within 3-6 months of diagnosis.	
➠ Early resection helps in survival for 1-2 years and in selected cases may even prolong life.	
➠ Surgical resection offers the only chance for cure	

Ultrasound examination is **frequently used** to screen patients for HCC.	**PGI 2000**
Ultrasound examination should be the **first test** to be done.	
Ultrasound is less costly, sensitive and **can detect most tumors** greater than 3 cm.	

Remember:

- ❒ **Mc abdominal tumor. Mc solid tumor**☛
- ❒ **Mc in right lobe.**☛
- ❒ **Mc symptom is abdominal pain**

Hepatocellular carcinoma: The principal reason for the high incidence of hepatocellular carcinoma in parts of Asia and Africa is the frequency of chronic infection with **hepatitis B virus (HBV) and hepatitis C virus (HCV).**

"Chronic liver disease" of any type is a risk factor and predisposes to the development of liver cell carcinoma. These conditions include **alcoholic liver disease, a1-antitrypsin deficiency, hemochromatosis, and tyrosinemia.**

A small percentage of patients with hepatocellular carcinoma have a **paraneoplastic syndrome;**

Erythrocytosis may result from erythropoietin-like activity produced by the tumor;

Hypercalcemia may result from secretion of a parathyroid-like hormone. Other manifestations may include **hypercholesterolemia, hypoglycemia, acquired porphyria, dysfibrinogenemia, and cryofibrinogenemia.**☛

Imaging procedures to detect liver tumors **include ultrasound, CT, MRI, hepatic artery angiography, and technetium scans.**

Ultrasound is frequently used to screen high-risk populations and should be the first test if hepatocellular carcinoma is suspected; it is less costly than scans, is relatively sensitive, and can detect most tumors >3 cm.

Helical CT and MRI scans are being used with increasing frequency and have higher sensitivities.

AFP levels >500 ug/L are found in about 70 to 80% of patients with hepatocellular carcinoma. Lower levels may be found in patients with large metastases from gastric or colonic tumors and in some patients with acute or chronic hepatitis.

High levels of serum AFP (>500 to 1000 ug/L) in an adult with liver disease and without an obvious gastrointestinal tumor strongly suggest hepatocellular carcinoma.☛☛

Percutaneous liver biopsy can be diagnostic if the sample is taken from an area localized by ultrasound or CT. Because these tumors tend to be vascular, percutaneous biopsies should be done with caution. **PGI 2000**

Staging of hepatocellular carcinoma is based on **tumor size (< or > 50% of the liver), ascites (absent or present), bilirubin (< or > 3), and albumin (< or >3)** to establish **Okuda stages I, II, and III.** The natural history of each stage without treatment is: stage I, 8 months; stage II, 2 months; stage III, less than 1 month.

⇨ Fibrolamellar Carcinoma

Fibrolamellar carcinoma differs from the typical hepatocellular carcinoma in that it tends to occur in **young adults** without underlying cirrhosis.
NOT associated with cirrhosis — AIIMS 2001
This tumor **is nonencapsulated** but well circumscribed and contains fibrous lamellae;
It **grows slowly** and is associated with a longer survival if treated. — AIIMS 2001
Surgical resection has resulted in 5-year survivals >50%; if the lesion is nonresectable, liver transplantation is an option, and the outcome far exceeds that observed in the nonfibrolamellar variety of liver cancer.

Hepatoblastoma is a **tumor of infancy** that typically is associated with very high serum AFP levels.
The lesions are **usually solitary**, may be resectable, and have a better 5-year survival than that of hepatocellular carcinoma.

Angiosarcoma consists of vascular spaces lined by malignant endothelial cells. Etiologic factors include prior exposure to **thorium dioxide (Thorotrast), polyvinyl chloride, arsenic, and androgenic anabolic steroids.**

⇨ Epithelioid Hemangioendothelioma

Epithelioid hemangioendothelioma is of borderline malignancy;
Most cases are benign, but bone and lung metastases occur.
This tumor occurs in early adulthood, presents with right upper quadrant pain, is heterogeneous on sonography, hypodense on CT, and without neovascularity on angiography.
Immunohistochemical staining reveals expression of factor VIII antigen. In the absence of extrahepatic metastases, these lesions can be treated by surgical resection or liver transplantation.

⇨ Indications for Liver Transplantation

Children	Adults
❒ Biliary atresia — PGI 2005	❒ Primary biliary cirrhosis
❒ Neonatal hepatitis	❒ Secondary biliary cirrhosis
❒ Congenital hepatic fibrosis	❒ Primary sclerosing cholangitis — PGI 2004
❒ Alagille's disease	❒ Caroli's disease
❒ Byler's disease	❒ Cryptogenic cirrhosis
❒ α 1-Antitrypsin deficiency	❒ Chronic hepatitis with cirrhosis
❒ Inherited disorders of metabolism	❒ Hepatic vein thrombosis
❒ Wilson's disease	❒ Fulminant hepatitis — PGI 2005
❒ Tyrosinemia	❒ Alcoholic cirrhosis
❒ Glycogen storage diseases	❒ Chronic viral hepatitis
❒ Lysosomal storage diseases	❒ Primary hepatocellular malignancies
❒ Protoporphyria	❒ Hepatic adenomas
❒ Crigler-Najjar disease type I	
❒ Familial hypercholesterolemia	
❒ Hereditary oxalosis	
❒ Hemophilia	

1

SURGERY

⇨ Hepatic Dysfunction after Liver Transplantation

- Primary graft failure,
- Vascular compromise,
- Failure or obstruction of the biliary anastomoses, and
- Rejection.
- Postoperative jaundice may result from prehepatic, intrahepatic, and posthepatic sources. Prehepatic sources represent the massive hemoglobin pigment load from transfusions, hemolysis, hematomas, ecchymoses, and other collections of blood.
- Vascular compromise associated with thrombosis or stenosis of the portal vein or hepatic artery anastomoses; vascular anastomotic leak; stenosis, obstruction, or leakage of the anastomosed common bile duct;

➲ Meld

- The **"Model for End-Stage Liver Disease" (MELD) system** was implemented February 27, 2002 to **prioritize patients waiting for a liver transplant.** **JK BOPEE 2009**
- MELD is a numerical scale used for adult liver transplant candidates.
- The **range is from 6 (less ill) to 40 (gravely ill).** The individual score determines **how urgently a patient needs a liver transplant within the next three months.** The number is calculated using the most recent laboratory tests.
- Within the MELD continuous disease severity scale, there are four levels. As the MELD score increases, and the patient moves up to a new level, a new waiting time clock starts.
- Waiting time is carried backwards but not forward. If a patient moves to a lower MELD score, the waiting time accumulated at the higher score remains. When a patient moves to a higher MELD score, the waiting time at the lower level is not carried to the new level.

⇨ Primary Biliary Cirrhosis

- **Itch + Jaundice+ pruritus, and hepatomegaly** are common.
- Associated conditions include **thyroid dysfunction, Raynaud syndrome, and CREST syndrome.**
- **Hepatomegaly and, late in the disease, splenomegaly** are common findings.
- The liver function tests may show only a mild transaminitis or may display normal transaminase levels.
- The **alkaline phosphatase, however**, will be elevated strikingly,
- Whereas the **bilirubin** may be increased only slightly.
- The classic associated antibody is **anti-mitochondrial antibody.**

✓ **Try to remember like this. Along with examination prepration I would like you to develop concepts "simultaneously".**

➲ Carcinoid Syndrome

- ❐ Occurs in **less than 10% of patients with carcinoid tumors.**
- ❐ The carcinoid syndrome is encountered **when venous drainage from the tumor gains access to the systemic circulation so that vasoactive secretory substances escape hepatic degradation.**
- ❐ This situation obtains in three circumstances:
  - ► **When hepatic metastases are present,**
  - ► **When venous blood from extensive retroperitoneal metastases drains into paravertebral veins, and**
  - ► **When the primary carcinoid tumor is outside the gastrointestinal tract, e.g., a bronchial, ovarian, or testicular tumor.**

- ❐ The principal features of carcinoid syndrome include **flushing, sweating, wheezing, diarrhea, abdominal pain, cardiac valvular fibrosis, and pellagra dermatosis.**
- ❐ **Diarrhea is found in 83% of patients,** flushing in 49%, dyspnea in 20%, and bronchospasm in 6%.
- ❐ Many patients develop **right-sided cardiac valvular disease** with congestive heart failure. **Serotonin** and possibly other neurohumors produced by the tumor cause fibrosis, as well as eventual incompetence of the tricuspid and pulmonic valves.
- ❐ The lungs metabolize serotonin and the other mediators and protect the left heart from fibrosis. If one can establish that the tumor is slow growing, patients with carcinoid-induced cardiac lesions are candidates for valve replacement.
- ❐ Biochemical Mediators
- ❐ The specific etiologic agents for each of the protean manifestations of carcinoid tumors are not known. **Serotonin, prostaglandins, 5-hydroxytryptophan, substance P, kallikrein, histamine, dopamine, and neuropeptide K are thought to be involved in the clinical manifestations of carcinoid tumors**
- ❐ **Serotonin is thought to be largely responsible for both the diarrhea and the fibrosis.** The cardiac lesions and tricuspid and pulmonic insufficiency are components of this fibrosing phenomenon.
- ❐ Other substances, such as histamine, VIP, and prostaglandins, may also **contribute to the systemic manifestations in the carcinoid syndrome.**

Diagnosis

- ► **Urinary 5-HIAA or whole blood and platelet-poor plasma 5-HT is the most reliable test to confirm the diagnosis of carcinoid syndrome.**
- ► Occasionally, measurement of plasma levels of **substance P and neurotensin** by radioimmunoassay may also be helpful.
- ► Measurements of **neuron-specific enolase and chromogranins,** when available, provide nonspecific evidence of the presence of a neuroendocrine tumor.
- ► **A useful diagnostic aid is the pentagastrin provocative test,** which induces facial flushing, gastrointestinal symptoms, elevation in circulating 5-HT

1

SURGERY

Appendicular Carcinoids:

- ► Not the commonest site.
- ✓ Mc site: tip
- ✓ Presents as recurrent appendicitis
- ✓ Has good prognosis
- — Carcinoid tumors occur in ileum and appendix **AI 2010**
- — Rectum is rarely involved **AI 2010**
- — 5 year survival is more than 60%
- — Females are affected less

- ► The specific etiologic agents for manifestations of carcinoid tumors are: Serotonin, prostaglandins, 5-hydroxytryptophan, substance P, kallikrein, histamine, dopamine, and neuropeptide K are involved in the clinical manifestations of carcinoid tumors. Pancreatic polypeptide and motilin levels are often raised and may serve as markers of tumor activity and provide a means of monitoring tumor growth and response to therapy.
- ► Serotonin is thought to be largely responsible for both the diarrhea and the fibrosis. (Especially mid gut carcinoids) The cardiac lesions and tricuspid and pulmonic insufficiency are components of this fibrosing phenomenon. **PGI 2011**
- ► The vasomotor changes, however, are mediated by kinins and such vasoactive peptides as substance P, neuropeptide K, neurokinin A, and neurotensin.
- ► Other substances, such as histamine, VIP, and prostaglandins, may also contribute to the systemic manifestations in the carcinoid syndrome.

⇨ Congenital Abnormalities of the Gallbladder and Bile Ducts

Absence of the Gallbladder

Occasionally the gallbladder is absent. Failure to visualise the gallbladder is not necessarily a pathological problem.

The Phrygian Cap

The Phrygian cap is present in 2–6 percent of cholecystograms and may be mistaken for a pathological deformity of the organ. 'Phrygian cap' refers to hats worn by people of Phrygia, an ancient country of Asia Minor; it was rather like a liberte' cap of the French Revolution.

Floating Gallbladder

The organ may hang on a mesentery which makes it liable to undergo torsion.

Double Gallbladder

Rarely, the gallbladder is twinned. One of the twins may be intrahepatic.

Absence of the Cystic Duct

This is usually a pathological, as opposed to an anatomical anomaly and indicates the recent passage of a stone or the presence of a stone at the lower end of the cystic duct which is ulcerating into the common bile duct. The main danger at surgery is damage to the bile duct, and particular care to identify the correct anatomy is essential before division of any duct.

Low insertion of the Cystic Duct

The cystic duct opens into the common bile duct near the ampulla. All variations of this anomaly can occur. At operation they are not important. Dissection of a cystic duct which is inserted low in the bile duct should be avoided as removal will damage the blood supply to the common bile duct and can lead to stricture formation.

An accessory Cholecystohepatic Duct

Ducts passing directly into the gallbladder from the liver do occur and are probably not uncommon. Nevertheless, larger ducts should be closed but before doing so the precise anatomy should be carefully ascertained

Extrahepatic Biliary Atresia

Aetiology and Pathology

Atresia is present in one per 14, 000 live births, and affects male and females equally. The extrahepatic bile ducts are progressively destroyed by an inflammatory process which starts around the time of birth. Intrahepatic changes also occur and eventually result in biliary cirrhosis and portal hypertension. The untreated child dies before the age of 3 years of liver failure or Hemorrhage.

The inflammatory destruction of the bile ducts has been classified into three main types

- **Type I — Atresia restricted to the common bile duct;**
- **Type II — Atresia of the common hepatic duct;**
- **Ttype III — Atresia of the right and left hepatic ducts.**

Parasitic Infestation of the Biliary Tract

Biliary Ascariasis

- ✓ The round worm, **A. lumbnicoides**, commonly infests the intestine of inhabitants of Asia, Africa and Central America.
- ✓ It may enter the biliary tree through the ampulla of Vater and cause biliary pain.
- ✓ Complications include **strictures, suppurative cholangitis, liver abscesses and empyema of the gallbladder**. In the uncomplicated case, antispasmodics can be given to relax the sphincter of Oddi and the worm will return to the small intestine to be dealt with by antihelminthic drugs.
- ✓ Operation may be necessary to remove the worm or deal with complications. Worms can be extracted via the ampulla of Vater by ERCP.

Clonorchiasis (Asiatic Cholangiohepatis)

- ❒ The disease is **endemic in the Far East.**
- ❒ Fluke, up to 25 mm long and 5 mm wide, inhabits the bile ducts, including the intrahepatic ducts.
- ❒ **Fibrous thickening of the duct walls occur**. Many cases are asymptomatic. Complications include **biliary pain, stones, cholangitis, cirrhosis and bile-duct carcinoma.** **AI 2010**
- ❒ **Choledochotomy and T-tube drainage** and, in some cases, choledochoduodenostomy are required. Because a process of recurrent stone formation is set-up, a choledochojejunostomy with Roux loop affixed to the abdominal parietes is performed in some centres to allow easy subsequent access to the duct system.

Hydatid Disease

A large hydatid cyst may obstruct the hepatic ducts. Sometimes a cyst will rupture into the biliary tree and its contents cause obstructive jaundice or cholangitis, requiring appropriate surgery

1

SURGERY

➲ Cholelithiasis:

⇨ Predisposing Factors

Cholesterol and Mixed Stones

1. Familial disposition;
2. Hereditary aspects
3. Obesity
4. Weight loss
5. Female sex hormones
6. Ileal disease or resection **DNB 2011**
7. Increasing age
8. Gallbladder hypomotility leading to stasis and formation of sludge
   - Prolonged parenteral nutrition
   - Fasting
   - Pregnancy
   - Drugs such as octreotide
9. Clofibrate therapy
10. Decreased bile acid secretion
    - Primary biliary cirrhosis
    - Chronic intrahepatic cholestasis
    - Remember **fat, flatulent, female, fertile, forty/fifty**

Pigment Stones

1. Demographic/genetic factors: Asia, rural setting
2. Chronic hemolysis **PGI 1999**
3. Alcoholic cirrhosis **PGI 1999**
4. Chronic biliary tract infection, parasite infestation **PGI 1999**
5. Increasing age

⇨ Effects and Complications of Gallstones

- In the gallbladder:
  - Silent stones
  - Chronic cholecystitis
  - Acute cholecystitis **JKBOPEE 2012**
  - Gangrene
  - Perforation
  - Empyema
  - Mucocele
  - Carcinoma **JKBOPEE 2012**

- In the bile ducts:
  - Obstructive jaundice
  - Cholangitis
  - Acute pancreatitis JKBOPEE 2012
- In the intestine: Acute intestinal obstruction ('gallstone ileus) AI 1996

Remember:

- **Saint's Triad: Gall stones,Diverticulosis,Hiatus hernia** KCET 2012

Common Bile Duct (CBD) Stone

- **Seen in 15%patients with gallstones.**
- **Develop in gallbladder.**
- **Obstructive pattern seen.**
- **Mc cause of obstructive jaundice.** AI 2001
- **Can present with cholangitis.**
- **Bile duct diameter >6 mm on USG is suggestive.** AI 2006
- **ERCP, Sphincterotomy, with ballon clearance is standard treatment used.**
- **In cholangiography appears as meniscus sign.** AIIMS 1998

Gallstone Ileus: DNB 2011

- Gallstone Ileus refers to **Mechanical intestinal obstruction** resulting from passage of a large gall stone into bowel lumen.
- This particular complication follows internal fistulas in which a **gallstone or common duct stone gains entrance into the intestinal tract** through an internal biliary fistula.
- The usual potential complication is **ascending cholangitis.**
- A typical presentation of gallstone ileus is a **history of frequent previous episodes of partial bowel obstruction** that exacerbate and abate as the stone negotiates its way into a narrower region of the intestinal tract. This phenomenon is called a **tumbling obstruction.**
- Three fourths of the spontaneous fistulas underlying gallstone ileus occur between the gallbladder and the duodenum.
- Most gallstones that enter the gastrointestinal tract are either passed or vomited, but 10% to 15% may lead to gallstone ileus.
- The common site of obstruction, found in two thirds of patients, is the **ileum.** AI 1999
- The diagnosis is easily made if a **large mass lesion** is found at the site of bowel obstruction; this mass is readily identified if the gallstone is opaque. Sometimes, even if it is nonopaque, it can be observed because of surrounding intestinal air.
- In addition, the **finding of air in the biliary tree** makes the diagnosis almost certain.
- The proper treatment of gallstone ileus is relief of the intestinal obstruction, usually by the performance of an **enterotomy and removal of the stone.** PGI 2001
- Concomitant definitive correction of the internal fistula is advocated if the patient is in good condition and has sustained no prolonged.

1

SURGERY

⇨ **The Classical X-ray Description of Gallstone Ileus in "Riglers Triad":** **PGI 2011**

- Ectopic gallstone,
- Partial or complete bowel obstruction and
- Gas in the gallbladder or biliary tree.

➲ Acute and Chronic Cholecystitis

⇨ Acute Cholecystitis

- ❐ Usually follows obstruction of the cystic duct by a stone.
- ❐ **Mc agent: Escherichia coli, Klebsiella spp.**, group D Streptococcus, Staphylococcus spp., and Clostridium spp.
- ❐ Deep inspiration or cough during subcostal palpation of the RUQ usually produces increased pain and inspiratory arrest **(Murphy's Sign).**
- ❐ The **triad of sudden onset of RUQ tenderness, fever, and leukocytosis is highly suggestive.** Typically, leukocytosis in the range of 10,000 to 15,000 cells per microliter with a left shift on differential count is found.
- ❐ The radionuclide **(e.g., HIDA) biliary scan** is IOC **PGI 2005**
- ❐ **Ultrasound** will demonstrate calculi in 90 to 95% of cases.

⇨ Acalculous Cholecystitis

Especially Associated With

- ❐ **Serious Trauma or**
- ❐ **Burns,**
- ❐ **Diabetes** **PGI 2006**
- ❐ **TPN** **PGI 2006**
- ❐ With the **postpartum period** following prolonged labor, and
- ❐ **Orthopedic and other nonbiliary major surgical operations** in the postoperative period. Vasculitis, obstructing adenocarcinoma of the gallbladder, diabetes mellitus, torsion of the gallbladder, "unusual" bacterial infections of the gallbladder (e.g. Leptospira, Streptococcus, Salmonella, or Vibrio cholerae), and parasitic infestation of the gallbladder. **AIIMS 2005**
- ❐ Acalculous **cholecystitis** may also be seen with a variety of other systemic disease processes **(sarcoidosis, cardiovascular disease, tuberculosis, syphilis, actinomycosis, etc.)** and may possibly complicate periods of prolonged parenteral hyperalimentation.
- ❐ USG is IOC. **PGI 2006**

⇨ Emphysematous Cholecystitis

- ❐ Begin with acute **cholecystitis** (calculous or acalculous) followed by ischemia or gangrene of the gallbladder wall and infection by gas-producing organisms.
- ❐ Bacteria most frequently cultured in this setting include **anaerobes, such as C. welchii or C. perfringens, and aerobes, such as E.coli.**
- ❐ This condition occurs most frequently **in elderly men and in patients with diabetes mellitus.**

- ❒ The diagnosis is usually made on plain abdominal film by the finding of gas within the gallbladder lumen, dissecting within the gallbladder wall to form a gaseous ring, or in the pericholecystic tissues. The morbidity and mortality rates with emphysematous **cholecystitis** are considerable. Prompt surgical intervention coupled with appropriate antibiotics is mandatory.
- ❒ **The gas is produced by bacteria; Clostridium perfringens (MC), E. coli, Klebsiella, or a mixture of organisms is usually found. C. perfringens has been cultured in about half the reported cases. DNB 2011**

⇨ Choledochal Cysts

- ❒ The classic symptoms are **abdominal pain, jaundice, and an abdominal mass**, but not all children have a mass.
- ❒ In both children and adults, cholangitis is frequent, probably because of bile stasis and colonization with bacteria.
- ❒ Most cysts can be detected by ultrasonography or by radionuclide scanning, but the definitive diagnosis requires cholangiography.
- ❒ Choledochal cysts should be treated by **complete excision and Roux-en-Y hepaticojejunostomy** whenever possible.
- ❒ Recurrent pancreatitis , development of carcinoma in the cyst can occur,
- ❒ **Type 1 cyst is most common.** PGI 2011

⇨ Hemobilia

May Follow

- ✓ **Trauma**
- ✓ **Operative injury to the liver or bile ducts,**
- ✓ **Intraductal rupture of a hepatic abscess**
- ✓ **Aneurysm of the hepatic artery,**
- ✓ **Biliary or hepatic tumor hemorrhage, or**
- ✓ **Mechanical complications of choledocholithiasis or**
- ✓ **Hepatobiliary parasitism.**
- ✓ Diagnostic procedures such as **liver biopsy, percutaneous transhepatic cholangiography (PTHC),** and **transhepatic biliary drainage catheter placement** may also be complicated by hemobilia.

- **Patients often present with a classic triad of "biliary colic, obstructive jaundice, and melena or occult blood in the stools."** DNB 2011
- The diagnosis is sometimes made by cholangiographic evidence of blood clot in the biliary tree, but selective angiographic verification may be required. Although minor episodes of hemobilia may resolve without operative intervention, surgical ligation of the bleeding vessel is frequently required.

⇨ Acalculous Cholecystopathy

- Recurrent episodes of typical RUQ pain characteristic of biliary tract pain,
- Abnormal CCK cholescintigraphy demonstrating a gallbladder ejection fraction of less than 40%,
- Infusion of CCK reproduces the patient's pain. An additional clue would be the identification of a large gallbladder on ultrasound examination.

1

SURGERY

⇨ Chronic Cholecystitis

Chronic inflammation of the gallbladder wall is almost always associated with the presence of gallstones and is thought to result from repeated bouts of subacute or acute **cholecystitis** or from persistent mechanical irritation of the gallbladder wall. The presence of bacteria in the bile occurs in more than one-quarter of patients with chronic **cholecystitis.**

⇨ Empyema of the Gallbladder

- Usually results from progression of acute cholecystitis with persistent cystic duct obstruction to superinfection of the stagnant bile with a pus-forming bacterial organism.
- The clinical picture resembles that of cholangitis with high fever, severe RUQ pain, marked leukocytosis, and often, prostration.
- Empyema of the gallbladder carries a high-risk of gram-negative sepsis and/or perforation.
- Emergency surgical intervention with proper antibiotic coverage is required as soon as the diagnosis is suspected.

⇨ Hydrops or Mucocele of the Gallbladder

- May also result from prolonged obstruction of the cystic duct, usually by a large solitary calculus.
- In this instance, the obstructed gallbladder lumen is progressively distended, over a period of time, by mucus (mucocele) or by a clear transudate (hydrops) produced by mucosal epithelial cells. A visible, easily palpable, nontender mass sometimes extending from the RUQ into the right iliac fossa may be found on physical examination.
- The patient with hydrops of the gallbladder frequently remains asymptomatic, although chronic RUQ pain may also occur. Cholecystectomy is indicated, since empyema, perforation, or gangrene may complicate the condition.

⇨ Cholangitis

- ✓ The characteristic presentation of acute cholangitis involves **biliary colic+jaundice, + spiking fevers** with chills **AIPGMEE 2011**
- ✓ Blood cultures are frequently positive, and leukocytosis is typical.
- ✓ **Nonsuppurative acute cholangitis** is most common and may respond relatively rapidly to supportive measures and to treatment with antibiotics.
- ✓ **In suppurative acute cholangitis**, however, the presence of pus under pressure in a completely obstructed ductal system leads to symptoms of severe toxicity mental confusion, bacteremia, and septic shock.
- ✓ Response to antibiotics alone in this setting is relatively poor, multiple hepatic abscesses are often present, and the mortality rate approaches 100% unless prompt endoscopic or surgical relief of the obstruction and drainage of infected bile are carried out. Endoscopic management of bacterial cholangitis is as effective as surgical intervention.
- ✓ **ERCP with endoscopic sphincterotomy** is safe and the preferred initial procedure for both establishing a definitive diagnosis and providing effective therapy.

Remember:

Reynolds' Pentad: **Charcot's triad (fever, jaundice, and upper abdominal pain) plus hypotension and altered mental status changes (CNS depression).**

Charcot's Neurological triad is also seen in multiple sclerosis. Charcot's neurologic triad is the combination of nystagmus + intention tremor+ scanning or staccato speech. The triad is associated with Multiple Sclerosis where it was first described.

Cholangiocarcinoma

Adenocarcinoma of the extrahepatic ducts is more common. There is a slight male preponderance (60%), and the incidence peaks in the fifth to seventh decades.

Apparent predisposing factors include

- ✓ **Some chronic hepatobiliary parasitic infestations,**
- ✓ **Congenital anomalies with ectactic ducts,**
- ✓ **Sclerosing cholangitis, chronic ulcerative colitis,**
- ✓ **Occupational exposure to possible biliary tract carcinogens (employment in rubber or automotive plants).**
- ✓ **Perihilar mc location.** **AIIMS 2008**

Nodular lesions often arise at the bifurcation of the **common bile duct (Klatskin tumors)** and are usually associated with a collapsed gallbladder.

Patients with **cholangiocarcinoma** usually present with biliary obstruction, painless jaundice, pruritus, weight loss, and acholic stools.

The diagnosis is most frequently made by cholangiography following ultrasound demonstration of dilated intrahepatic bile ducts.

Klastkin Tumor

- Tumor of CBD between cystic duct and common hepatic duct.
- ↓metastasis
- Slow growth
- Shows sclerosing features

Carcinoma of the Papilla of Vater

- The ampulla of Vater may be involved by extension of tumor arising elsewhere in the duodenum or may itself be the site of origin of a sarcoma, carcinoid tumor, or adenocarcinoma.
- Papillary adenocarcinomas are associated with slow growth and a more favorable clinical prognosis than diffuse, infiltrative cancers of the ampulla, which are more frequently widely invasive.
- **The presenting clinical manifestation** is usually **obstructive jaundice.**
- **Endoscopic retrograde cannulation of the pancreatic duct is the preferred diagnostic technique** when ampullary carcinoma is suspected, because it allows for direct endoscopic inspection and biopsy of the ampulla and for pancreatography to exclude a pancreatic malignancy.
- **Cancer** of the papilla is usually treated by **wide surgical excision.**
- **Lymph node or other metastases are present** at the time of surgery in approximately 20% of cases

⇨ Cancer of the Gallbladder

- **Female/Male** ratio is 4:1,
- The clinical presentation is most often one of **unremitting right upper quadrant pain associated with weight loss, jaundice, and a palpable right upper quadrant mass.**
- Adenocarcinoma **most common type.**
- Fundus is the **most common site.**
- Biliary colic is the **most common presentation.**
- Gallstones are the **most common predisposition.** PGI 2002

➲ Risk Factors for GB CANCER

- The association between cancer of the **gallbladder and gallstones** is **well established.** AIIMS 1998
- A parallel exists between the epidemiology of cancer of the gallbladder and that of gallstones. There is no predilection for the development of carcinoma in a gallbladder containing single or multiple stones.
- It has been suggested that there may be some relationship between carcinoma and the **size of a stone.**
- A patient with a 3 cm gallstone is reportedly 10 times more likely to develop carcinoma than someone with a stone less than 1 cm.
- There are several other pathologic conditions of the gallbladder in addition to gallstones that are associated with the development of carcinoma.

There is believed to be a 15% incidence of carcinoma of the gallbladder in patients who have or have had a **cholecystoenteric fistula** and the tumor may develop as much as 16 years later.

The incidence of carcinoma in a **calcified or porcelain gallbladder** is reported to range from 12.5 to 61%.
PGI 2005

It is now generally accepted that **adenoma of the gallbladder** is a precancerous lesion. Adenomas present as polypoid lesions which are best detected by ultrasonography.

It has been suggested that **xanthogranulomatous cholecystitis** a rare form of chronic cholecystitis that may grossly mimic cancer of the gallbladder is also associated with a higher than expected incidence of carcinoma.

Cancer of the gallbladder is more frequent in the presence of **congenital biliary dilatation** in which case there appears to be a lower incidence of associated gallstones

- **Ulcerative colitis** has a well-known association with biliary tract malignancy.
- Although the majority of such malignancies involve the bile ducts as many as 13% originate in the gallbladder.

Rokintansky Aschoff sinuses Outpouching of Gallbladder Mucosa☛

- Mucosal Folds of Cystic Duct **Valves of Heister**☛
- Lymph node of GB **Cystic LN of Lund**☛
- **Monynihans Hump:** Tortuous course of Right Hepatic Artery in front of Cystic Duct. Also Called **Caterpillar Turn**☛
- **Callots Triangle Triangle Bounded above by Liver, Medially by Common Hepatic Duct, Below by cystic duct**☛
- **"Straw Berry" Gallbladder** Cholesterosis☛
- **Sea gull or Mercedes Benz Sign** Radiolucent Gall shadow in cholelithiasis **DNB 2011**
- **Murphys sign/Boas Sign:** Acute Cholecystitis☛☛

Ampulla of Vater Tumors

- **Adenoma and adenocarcinoma of the ampulla of Vater account for about 10% of neoplasms that obstruct the distal bile duct of primary tumors of the ampulla of Vater, 33% are adenomas and 67% are adenocarcinomas**
- **It is suspected that malignant change in an adenoma gives rise to most carcinomas, and adenomas may contain focus of adenocarcinoma**
- **Associated with familial adenomatous polyposis**
- **Partial or complete obstruction of the common bile duct and pancreatic duct at the ampulla of Vater**
- Exophytic mass at the ampulla visible on endoscopy
- Jaundice, abdominal pain, and weight loss may be presenting symptoms
- **Symptoms and signs**

✓ Jaundice

✓ GI bleeding from ampullary tumor

✓ Weight loss

✓ Abdominal pain

LABORATORY FINDINGS

✓ Elevated serum bilirubin

✓ Anemia

IMAGING FINDINGS

- **CT scan:** Dilation of the biliary tree and pancreatic duct; also for staging
- **Abdominal US:** Dilated biliary tree and pancreatic duct
- **ERCP:** Dilation of the biliary and pancreatic ducts
- In 75% of cases, the tumor is visible as an exophytic papillary lesion, an ulcerated tumor, or an infiltrating mass
- In 25% of cases, there is no intraduodenal growth, and endoscopic sphincterotomy is necessary to display the tumor
- An adequate biopsy specimen can usually be obtained from these lesions.

1

SURGERY

⇨ Acute Cholangitis (Nutshell Here)

- ❒ MC organisms: E. coli, Klibessela, Pseudomonas, Enterococcus — AI 2006
- ❒ **Obstruction of CBD** leading to bacterial stasis, bacterial overgrowth, suppuration, Biliary sepsis.
- ❒ **Charcots triad**: Fever+ RUQ pain+ Jaundice. — AIIMS 2007
- ❒ **Reynauds pentad**: Fever+ RUQ pain+ Jaundice.+ Shock+ Confusion
- ❒ **Suppurative cholangitis** has a high mortality rate

⇨ Sclerosing Cholangitis (Nutshell Here)

- ❒ **Progressive, inflammatory, sclerosing, and obliterative process affecting the "extrahepatic and/or the intrahepatic bile ducts".** ☛☛ — PGI 2005
- ❒ The disorder occurs in about 70% in association with **inflammatory bowel disease**, especially ulcerative colitis.
- ❒ Also associated (albeit rarely) with
- ❒ **Multifocal Fibrosclerosis Syndromes** such as
  - ▶ **Retroperitoneal, mediastinal, and/or periureteral fibrosis;**
  - ▶ **Riedel's struma; or**
  - ▶ **Pseudotumor of the orbit.**

Cholangiopancreatography may demonstrate a broad range of biliary tract changes as well as pancreatic duct obstruction and occasionally pancreatitis

- ❒ Often present with signs and symptoms of chronic or intermittent **biliary obstruction: jaundice, pruritus, RUQ abdominal pain, or acute cholangitis.**
- ❒ Late in the course, complete biliary obstruction, secondary biliary cirrhosis, hepatic failure, or portal hypertension with bleeding varices may occur.
- ❒ The diagnosis is established **beaded appearance on cholangiography** ☛

Complications

- ✓ Adenocarcinoma colon
- ✓ Adenocarcinoma bile ducts
- ✓ Cirrhosis

⇨ Hemobilia (Questions Asked)

Triad of

- ▶ Abdominal pain
- ▶ Obstructive jaundice — AI 1998
- ▶ Melana — AI 1998

Occurs as a result of bleeding into biliary tract.

Causes:

- ✓ Trauma — AIIMS 2000
- ✓ Gallstones — AIIMS 2000
- ✓ Cholangiohepatitis
- ✓ Neoplasms of hepatobiliary system
- ✓ Hepatic artery trauma

Kidney

UTI

- Patients with UTIs often present with **dysuria, frequency, and urgency.**
- Physical examination is often unremarkable, although there may be some suprapubic tenderness if a cystitis is the predominant infection rather than a urethritis.
- Urine "dip" will often be positive for **leukocyte esterase and nitrites.**
- Microscopic urinalysis will often show the **presence of white blood cells and red blood cells.**
- **Escherichia coli** is the offending organism in about 80% of cases.
- Treatment of an uncomplicated urinary tract infection is with a 3-day course of oral antibiotics.
- **Trimethoprim-sulfamethoxazole** has been shown to be safe, effective, and cost-effective in the treatment of uncomplicated UTIs.

Renal Tuberculosis **DNB 2011**

- Tuberculosis of the urinary tract arises from **haematogenous infection** from a distant focus which is often impossible to identify. The lesions are usually confined to one kidney.
- A group of tuberculous granulomas in a renal pyramid coalesces and forms an ulcer. Mycobacteria and pus cells are discharged into the urine.
- Sterile pyuria is a consistent feature. **PGI 1998**
- Untreated, the lesions enlarge and **a tuberculous abscess** may form in the parenchyma.
- The necks of the calyces and the renal pelvis stenosed by fibrosis confine the infection so that there is tuberculous pyonephrosis which is sometimes localised to one pole of the kidney.
- Extension of pyonephrosis or tuberculous renal abscess leads to perinephric abscess and the kidney is progressively replaced by caseous material **(putty kidney)** which may be calcified **(cement kidney).**
- At any stage the plain radiograph may show areas of calcification **(pseudocalculi).**
- Less commonly the kidneys may be bilaterally affected as part of the generalised process of miliary tuberculosis
- Renal tuberculosis is often associated with tuberculosis of the bladder and typical tuberculous granulomas may be visible in the bladder wall. In the male, tuberculous epididymo-orchitis may occur without apparent infection of the bladder.
- IVU is the most sensitive technique for detecting early renal TB. **AI 2006**

Renal Carbuncle

- An **abscess** in the **renal parenchyma** as the result of blood-borne spread of organisms, especially coliforms or Staphylococcus aureus, from a focus elsewhere in the body.
- Occasionally the condition results from infection of a haematoma following a blow to the kidney.
- Renal carbuncle is most commonly seen in **diabetic patients, intravenous drug abusers, those debilitated by chronic disease and patients with acquired immunodeficiency.**

1

SURGERY

Pathology. The renal parenchyma contains an encapsulated necrotic mass.
Clinical features. There is an ill-defined tender swelling in the loin, persistent pyrexia and leucocytosis, signs that closely simulate those of perinephric abscess. In early cases there is no pus or bacteria in the urine but they appear after a day or so. Urography shows a space occupying lesion in the kidney which may be confused with a renal adenocarcinoma on ultrasonography and CT.
Treatment. Resolution by antibiotic treatment alone is unusual. Formal open incision of the abscess may be necessary if the pus is too thick to be drained by percutaneous aspiration.
Idiopathic Retroperitoneal Fibrosis ☛

- Rare condition in which one or both ureters become bound up in a **progressive fibrosis of the retroperitoneal tissues.** ☛
- The cause is unknown although some cases may be drug related.
- The patient complains of backache which is unremitting for several months.
- The onset of anuria and renal failure prompts investigation of the renal tract which reveals hydronephrosis.
- The excretion urogram typically shows displacement of the obstructed ureters **towards the midline** and the appearances on CT are diagnostic. ☛
- The sedimentation rate is markedly raised.

Randall's Plaque and Microliths

- ❒ Initial lesion in some cases of kidney stone was an **erosion at the tip of a renal papilla.** ☛
- ❒ **Deposition of calcium** on this erosion produced a lesion which has been called **Randall's plaque.**
- ❒ Minute concretions **(microliths)** regularly occur in the renal parenchyma these particles are carried by lymphatics to the subendothelial region where they may accumulate.
- ❒ Ulceration of the epithelium exposes the potential calculus to the urine with the result that a stone forms. The importance of **Randall's plaques and Carr's microliths** is the pathogenesis for calculi.
- ❒ Renal calculi overlie spine on lateral view. AI 2001
- ❒ **Renal colic+swelling in lion+disappearance of swelling with micturation=Dielts crisis.** AI 1996
- ❒ **Pain in ureteric colic is due to ureteric peristalsis.** AI 2008
- ❒ **Noncontrast CT is the most sensitive diagnostic method for acute ureteric colic.** AI 2005

⇨ "Renal Calculi":

- ► **Calcium stones**: Calcium oxalate and calcium phosphate stones make up **75 to 85% of the total renal calculi** ☛
- ► **Most common.** AIIMS 2000
- ► Calcium stones are **more common in men**; the average age of onset is the third decade. Approximately 60% of people who form a single calcium stone eventually form another within the next 10 years.
- ► In the urine, calcium oxalate monohydrate crystals **(whewellite)** usually grow as biconcave ovals that resemble red blood cells in shape and size but may occur in a larger, "dumbbell" form.

- ► **Uric acid stones** are **radiolucent** and are also more common in men. AIIMS 2000
- ► Half of patients with uric acid stones have gout; **uric acid lithiasis** is usually familial whether or not gout is present. In urine, uric acid crystals are **red-orange in color** because they absorb the pigment uricine.
- ► Uric acid gravel appears like red dust, and the stones are also orange or red on some occasions.

- **Cystine stones** are uncommon , lemon yellow, and sparkle
- Radiopacity is due to the **sulfur content.**
- Cystine crystals appear in the urine as flat, **hexagonal plates.**

- **Struvite stones** are common and **potentially dangerous.**
- These stones occur mainly in **women** or patients who require chronic bladder catheterization and result from urinary tract infection with **urease-producing bacteria, usually Proteus species.** AI 1996
- Grow in **alkaline urine** AIIMS 2001
- **Grow in infected urine.** AI 1996
- The stones can grow to a large size and fill the renal pelvis and calyces to produce a **"staghorn" appearance.**
- They are **radiopaque** and have a variable internal density. In urine, struvite crystals are **rectangular prisms** said to resemble **coffin lids.**

Calcium Stones:

Calcium urate stones are associated with the following disorders:

- Hyperparathyroidism
- Increased gut absorbtion of calcium
- Renal calcium leak
- Renal phosphate leak
- Hyperuricosuria
- Hyperoxaluria
- Hypercitraturia
- Hypomagnesuria

Factors Influencing Stone Formation in Urine

Promoting Factors

- Hypercalciuria
- Hyperoxaluria
- Hyperuricemia
- Hypocitraturia
- Hypomagnesemia
- Low fluid intake

⇨ Inhibitors of Stone Formation

- Citrate
- Magnesium
- Tamm-horsfall protein
- High fluid intake

⇨ Important Points

- On X-ray lateral view renal stone is superimposed on shadow of vertebral column.
- CT scan is the invstigation of choice for emergency.
- Most of ureteric calculi originate in kidney.
- Sites of impaction of ureteric calculi:
  - ✓ **Pelvi uretreric junction**
  - ✓ **At crossing of iliac artery**
  - ✓ **Entering the bladder wall**
  - ✓ **Ureteric orifice.**
- Small (<2.5 cms) Stone in proximal ureter: **ESWL**
- (>2.5 cms) Stone in proximal ureter: **Nephrolithotomy**
- Small stone in distal ureter: **Ureteroscopic removal**
- Large/long standing stone in distal ureter: **Ureterolithotomy**
- **Stones hard to break in ESWL: Cysteine stones** **AI 2010**

⇨ Stones (Calculi)

- ❐ **Whewellite:** (Calcium oxalate Monohydrate crystals)☚
- ❐ **Weddilite:** (Calcium oxalate Dihydrate crystals)
- ❐ **Stag horn/coffin lid:** Struvite☚☚☚
- ❐ **Radiolucent:** Uric acid☚
- ❐ **Radiopaque:** Calcium, Struvite, Cysteine☚

⇨ Perinephric and Renal Abscesses

- The presentation of perinephric and renal abscesses is quite nonspecific.
- Flank pain and abdominal pain are common.
- At least 50% of patients are febrile.
- Pain may be referred to the groin or leg, particularly with extension of infection.
- **Perinephric or renal abscess should be most seriously considered when a patient presents with symptoms and signs of pyelonephritis and remains febrile after 4 or 5 days, by which time the fever should have resolved.**
- **Renal ultrasonography and abdominal CT are the most useful diagnostic modalities.**
- Treatment for perinephric or renal abscesses includes drainage of pus and antibiotic therapy directed at the organism(s) recovered.
- For perinephric abscesses, percutaneous drainage is usually successful.

⇨ Complication of PCNL

- Bleeding - Venous bleeding is most common, it can be managed by clamping the nephrostomy tube for 30 to 45 min. Arterial bleeding is more serious prolem, can occur either preoperative or in postoperative period.
- Extravasation - Normal saline should be used as the irrigation fluid to minimize adverse effect if extravasation occurs.
- Retained Fragments - on a post procedure film can be an unwanted finding. Reinsertion of the nephroscope will permit removal. Sometimes stones are extruded through the collecting system or noted in the perinephric tissues outside the kidney. It is not important to remove them.
- UPJ Obstruction
- Sepsis — AIPGME 2010

➲ Renal Cell Carcinoma — AIIMS 2001

SYNONYM: Hypernephroma, Adenocarcinoma, Grawitz tumor☛☛

✓ Accounts for 90 to 95% of malignant neoplasms arising from the kidney.

Unusual Features:

- ❒ Refractoriness to cytotoxic agents, ☛
- ❒ Propensity to invade renal vein JK BOPEE 2011
- ❒ Infrequent but reproducible responses to biologic response modifiers such as interferon and interleukin (IL) 2, ☛
- ❒ Spontaneous regression.☛

EPIDEMIOLOGY AND ETIOLOGY

- ✓ Cigarette smoking ☛
- ✓ Von Hippel-Lindau (VHL) syndrome. Tuberous sclerosis and polycystic kidney disease.☛ — COMED 2003
- ✓ Abnormalities on chromosome 3 are most frequent.
- ✓ Most of the cancers arise from the **epithelial cells of the proximal tubules.**
- ✓ Categories Include:

Clear cell carcinoma (60% of cases), ☛ — AIIMS 2005

HERE CLEAR CELLS ARE SEEN. — PGI 2011

Papillary (5 to 15%), chromophobic tumors (5 to 10%),

oncocytomas (5 to 10%), and

collecting or Bellini duct tumors (RARER)

➲ Clear Cells in Clear Cell Carcioima

Depending on the amounts of lipid and glycogen present, **the tumor cells of clear cell renal cell carcinoma may appear almost vacuolated or may be solid. The classic vacuolated (lipid-laden), or clear cells are demarcated only by their cell membranes. The nuclei are usually small and round.**

1

SURGERY

- ✓ The presenting signs and symptoms include **hematuria, abdominal pain, and a flank or abdominal mass.** This "**classic triad**" occurs in 10 to 20% of patients. Other symptoms are fever, weight loss, anemia, and a varicocele ☛
- ✓ Causes expansile osteolytic lesions. **AI 2006**
- ✓ A spectrum of paraneoplastic syndromes has been associated with these malignancies, including
  - **Erythrocytosis,** ☛
  - **Hypercalcemia,** **JIPMER 1995**
  - **Nonmetastatic hepatic dysfunction (Stauffers' syndrome)** ☛
  - **Accquired dysfibrinogenemia.**

Erythrocytosis is present at presentation in only about 3% of patients. ☛ **JIPMER 1995**

- **More frequently anemia, a sign of** advanced disease, ☛
- **Cushings syndrome** **JIPMER 1995**
- **Galactorrhea**
- **Amyloidosis**
- **Hypertension** ☛
- **PUO**

Staging by "Robson" staging ☛☛

- ✓ **Mc site of metastasis is lung,** soft tissue, bone, liver. **AIIMS 1997**
- ✓ **Secondaries are "expansile , osteolytic"**
- ➨ The standard management for stage I or II tumors and selected cases of stage III disease is **radical nephrectomy.** **JK BOPEE**
- ➨ There is no proven role for adjuvant chemotherapy, immunotherapy, or radiation therapy following successful surgical removal of the tumor, even in cases with a poor prognosis.
- ➨ **Surgery in the Setting of Metastases** Nephrectomy may be indicated in highly selected cases for the alleviation of symptoms, including pain or recurrent urinary hemorrhage, and particularly if the latter is severe or associated with obstruction.

⇨ Renal Cell Carcinoma: Important Points

- ❒ The **classic triad** of palpable **mass, hematuria, and flank pain** occurs in less than 15% of patients with renal cell carcinoma (RCC), but 10 to 40% of patients with this disease may develop a paraneoplastic syndrome.
- ❒ **Hypercalcemia** is the most common of the paraneoplastic syndromes in patients with RCC and of those with hypercalcemia and RCC, approximately 75% have high-stage lesions.
- ❒ Approximately 50% of all patients with hypercalcemia and RCC have bone metastases, hence this form of hypercalcemia is termed metastatic hypercalcemia.
- ❒ **Hypertension** is experienced by almost 40% of those with RCC and is typically associated with low-grade tumors of clear-cell histology.

- ❒ In up to one-third of cases, symptoms such as **fever, weight loss, and fatigue** are the first symptoms of RCC; fever is found in 20 to 30% of those with RCC and is the sole presenting complaint in approximately 2% of patients.
- ❒ Other conditions associated with RCC include
  - ✓ **Polycythemia,**
  - ✓ **Nonmetastatic hepatic dysfunction,**
  - ✓ **Galactorrhea,**
  - ✓ **Cushing's syndrome,**
  - ✓ **Hyper/hypoglycemia,**
  - ✓ **Amyloidosis**
  - ✓ **Neuromyopathies.**
  - ➢ Most paraneoplastic syndromes associated with localized RCC are definitively treated with nephrectomy only; the recurrence of a previous paraneoplastic syndrome should alert the physician to possible disease progression.

➲ Angiomyolipoma Kidney: High Yield for 2011-2012 AIPGME

- ❒ Is a **benign renal neoplasm composed of fat, vascular, and smooth muscle elements.**
- ❒ Two types are described: **isolated angiomyolipoma and angiomyolipoma that is associated with tuberous sclerosis.**
- ❒ Isolated angiomyolipoma occurs sporadically
- ❒ Angiomyolipoma that is associated with tuberous sclerosis accounts for 20% of angiomyolipomas. The lesions are typically larger than isolated angiomyolipomas, and they are often bilateral and multiple. Angiomyolipomas occur in 80% of patients with tuberous sclerosis. Angiomyolipomas occur in young women with **lymphangiomyomatosis**. Although angiomyolipomas are considered benign, rare cases that are possibly related to multicentric disease have been reported regarding extension into the **renal vein, the inferior vena cava (IVC), or both; deposits in the regional lymph nodes have also been reported.**
- ❒ Most small angiomyolipoma lesions are asymptomatic and are found incidentally on imaging studies.
- ❒ The **demonstration of fatty attenuation in renal tumor on computed tomography (CT) scanning studies is virtually diagnostic of angiomyolipomas.**
- ❒ The blood vessels in angiomyolipomas frequently have an angiomatous arrangement, wherein the vessels are tortuous and thick walled. The blood vessels do not have elastic tissue, but they do have a disorganized adventitial cuff of smooth muscle.
- ❒ The characteristic absence of elastic tissue in the tumor vessels **predisposes the patient to aneurysm formation and spontaneous hemorrhage.**

➲ Von Hippel-Lindau Disease High Yield for 2011-2012 AIPGME

Is an autosomal dominant syndrome that confers predisposition to a variety of neoplasms, including the following:

- **Renal cell carcinoma with clear cell histologic features**
- **Pheochromocytoma**
- **Pancreatic cysts and islet cell tumors**
- **Retinal angiomas**

- Central nervous system hemangioblastomas
- Endolymphatic sac tumors
- Epididymal cystadenomas

⇨ Birt-Hogg - Dube Syndrome

Is a hereditary cutaneous syndrome. Patients with Birt-Hogg-Dube syndrome have a dominantly inherited predisposition to develop benign tumors of the hair follicle (i.e., **fibrofolliculomas**), predominantly on the face, neck, and upper trunk, and are at risk of developing **renal tumors, colonic polyps or tumors, and pulmonary cysts.**

➲ Wilms Tumor

Associated With:

- ❒ Beckwith-Wiedemann syndrome (macroglossia, gigantism, visceromegaly, hypoglycemia, abdominal wall defects)
- ❒ WAGR Syndrome (Wilms, Aniridia, Ambiguous Genitalia, Mental Retardation)
- ❒ Neurofibromatosis
- ❒ Denys-Drash syndrome
- ❒ Perlman familial nephroblastomatosis
- ❒ Other genital abnormalities
  - 1-2% incidence of bilateral disease
  - As high as 7% multicentricity
  - Symptoms and signs

Abdominal Mass

- ✓ Pain
- ✓ Fever
- ✓ Hematuria

➲ Pheochromocytoma

- ❒ Tumor of chromaffin cells
- ❒ (Headache) Hypertension is a common symptom but not a reliable symptom of pheochromocytoma.
- ❒ Pheochromocytoma is a cause of "**Episodic/Paroxysmal "Hypertension** and not persistent Hypertension.☛
- ❒ Pheochromocytoma is also a cause of "**Orthostatic Hypotension.**"☛
- ❒ **Microscopically, pheochromocytomas are composed of polygonal to spindle-shaped chromaffin cells and their supporting cells, compartmentalized into small nests, or "Zellballen," by a rich vascular network.**

  KCET 2012
- ❒ The cytoplasm of the neoplastic cells often has a finely granular appearance, highlighted by a variety of silver stains, because of the presence of granules containing catecholamines. Electron microscopy reveals variable numbers of membra. Ne-bound, electron-dense granules, representing catecholamines and sometimes other peptides.

- ❒ NA production is ↑↑
  - ❒ **Bilateral in 10% cases**
  - ❒ **Extraadrenal in 10% cases**
  - ❒ **Familial in 10% cases**
  - ❒ **Malignant in 10% cases**
  - ❒ **Multiple in 10% cases**
- ❒ ↑Urinary VMA levels seen.
- ❒ ↑Urinary metanephrine
- ❒ MIBG Scan is **most specific and sensitive for diagnosis.**

Associated with

- ❒ **MEN 2 Syndromes**
- ❒ **Von-hippel Landau syndrome**
- ❒ **Neurofibromatosis**
- ❒ **Sturge-Weber syndrome**

⇨ Renal Artery Stenosis/Ischemic Renal Disease

- ❒ Accounts for 2 to 5% of hypertension.
- ❒ Commonest cause in the **middle-aged and elderly** is an atheromatous plaque at the origin of the **renal artery.**
- ❒ **In younger women**, fibromuscular dysplasia is the commonest cause.

Renal artery stenosis should be suspected when hypertension develops in a previously normotensive individual over 50 years of age or in the young (under 30 years) with suggestive features: symptoms of vascular insufficiency to other organs, high-pitched epigastric bruit on physical examination, symptoms of hypokalemia secondary to hyperaldosteronism (muscle weakness, tetany, polyuria), and metabolic alkalosis.

Understand the difference:

- ► The "**best initial screening test**" is a renal ultrasound
- ► A positive captopril test, which has a sensitivity and specificity of greater than 95%, constitutes an "**excellent follow-up procedure**" to assess the need for more invasive radiographic evaluation.
- ► Magnetic resonance angiography (MRA) is the "**most sensitive (100%) and specific**" **(95%)** test for the diagnosis of renal arterial stenosis.
- ► **The "most definitive diagnostic procedure" is bilateral arteriography with repeated bilateral renal vein and systemic renin determinations.**

TREATMENT

Interventional therapy (i.e., surgery or angioplasty) is superior to medical therapy, which, while controlling blood pressure, does little to salvage renal mass lost to ischemic injury.

1

SURGERY

⇨ Fibromuscular Dysplasia:

- Is characterized by **fibrous thickening** of the **intima**, **media**, **or adventitia** of the artery.
- Up to 75% of all patients with FMD will have disease in the **renal arteries**. The lesions cause narrowing of the artery lumen.
- The second most common artery affected is the **carotid artery**
- Less commonly, FMD affects the arteries in the abdomen (supplying the liver, spleen and intestines) and extremities (legs and arms).
- FMD is an angiopathy that affects **medium-sized arteries** predominantly in **young women of childbearing age.** FMD most commonly affects the renal arteries and can cause refractory renovascular hypertension.
- The **beadlike dilatations** observed within FMD lesions share gross and histologic characteristics of aneurysms. This wall weakness may allow for vessel dilation (**aneurysm formation and beading in FMD**) as well as injury, which then causes compensatory fibroplasias.

➲ Adult Polycystic Kidney Disease: High Yield for AIPGMEE, AIIMS, PGI 2012/2013

Is inherited as autosomal dominant in 90% cases. ADPKD commonly presents in 3rd - 4th decade of life. Clinical features:-

- ✓ Chronic flank pain,
- ✓ Gross and microscopic haematuria,
- ✓ Loss of Renal concentrating ability,
- ✓ Nephrolithiasis

⇨ Associations

- ❒ Hepatic cysts
- ❒ Cysts of spleen, pancreas, Ovaries
- ❒ Intracranial aneurysms
- ❒ Colonic diverticular disease (Most common)
- ❒ Mitral valve prolapse

⇨ Nut Crackers Phenomenon

- ❒ Is seen in varicocele.
- ❒ It refers to **nut inside a cracker** like image.
- ❒ The left renal vein is distended in varicocele on left side.
- ❒ As a result" **Left renal vein gets compressed"** in between superior mesenteric artery and the aorta leading to renal vein hypertension.
- ❒ The remedy is surgical transposition of left renal vein.

The two diseases most commonly leading to renal failure and treatable by kidney transplantation are **glomerulonephritis and insulin-dependent diabetes mellitus**
Other important causes include :
❒ **Polycystic kidney disease,**
❒ **Hypertensive nephrosclerosis,**
❒ **Alport's disease,**
❒ **IgA nephropathy,**
❒ **Systemic lupus erythematosus,**
❒ **Nephrosclerosis,**
❒ **Interstitial nephritis,**
❒ **Pyelonephritis,**
❒ **Obstructive uropathy, and**
❒ **Hypertensive nephrosclerosis.**

The left kidney is chosen, if possible, since its longer renal vein facilitates the recipient operation.
However, if the arteriogram shows multiple renal arteries on one side, the **kidney with a single artery** is usually selected to facilitate the anastomosis.
A flank incision is used. After Gerota's fascia is incised, the greater curvature of the kidney and the upper pole are mobilized, and the hilar structures are exposed.
On the left side, the adrenal and gonadal veins are ligated so that the full length of the renal vein can be utilized.
Traction on the renal artery should be avoided, since it causes spasm and decreased kidney perfusion, possibly compromising early function.
The ureter should be mobilized, along with its blood supply and a generous amount of periureteric tissue. It is divided close to the bladder after ligating the distal end.

⇨ Carcinoma of the Bladder (Urinary)

Carcinoma of the Bladder	
Carcinoma arising within the bladder may be of three cell types: **transitional, squamous and adenocarcinoma [or mixed owing to metaplasia in a transitional cell carcinoma (TCC)].**	
❒ Over 90 percent are **transitional cells in origin.**	PGI 1997
❒ Pure squamous carcinoma is uncommon **(Schistosomiasis, stones, irradiation, smoking)**	PGI 1997
❒ Primary adenocarcinoma, which arises either from the **urachal remnant** or from **areas of glandular metaplasia,** accounts for 1–2 percent of cases.	
❒ Mc site: **trigone and posterior wall.**	
❒ Mc symptom: **painless hematuria**	AIIMS 1996

1

SURGERY

Transitional Cell Carcinoma
Following compounds may be carcinogenic:
❒ 2-naphthylamine;
❒ 4-aminobiphenyl;
❒ Benzidine;
❒ Chlornaphazine;
❒ 4-chloro-o-toluidine;
❒ O-toluidine;
❒ 4,4'-methylene bis (2-choloraniline);
❒ Methylene dianiline;
❒ Benzidine-derived azo dyes.
Occupations: Significantly Excess Risk of Bladder Cancer
➨ Textile workers
➨ Dye workers
➨ Tyre rubber and cable workers
➨ Petrol workers
➨ Leather workers
➨ Shoe manufacturers and cleaners
➨ Painters
➨ Hairdressers
➨ Lorry drivers
➨ Drill press operators
➨ Chemical workers
➨ Rodent exterminators and sewage workers

❒ **Cystoscopy** is the main stay for evaluation.	
❒ Antigenic tests utilizing **NMP-22, MCM Proteins** are used.	
❒ **Filing defect on IVU** is the most common sign.	
❒ Much said about **intravesical BCG** is advised for initial stage (Ta).	**AIIMS 2005**
► Kiss cancer is benign tumor of bladder.	**AIIMS 1980**
► Tear drop bladder is pelvic haematoma.	**PGI 1999**
► Secondary vesical calculus is stone in bladder after infection.	**PGMEE 2006**

⇨ **Schistosomiasis**

- **Sch. Hematobonium** is causative agent.☛
- Resides in **vesical venous plexus.**☛
- Urticaria at site of penetration occurs **(swimmers itch)**☛
- **Calcifications with small contracted bladder** — AIIMS 2001

Intermittent	Painless	Terminal	Hematuria

- **Prizaqiental** is the DOC.

Surgery is done in case of:

- ✓ Secondary bacterial cystitis
- ✓ Urinary calculi
- ✓ Ureteric stricture
- ✓ Seminal vesiculitis
- ✓ Fibrosis of bladder and bladder neck
- ✓ Cancer

⇨ **Cystoscopic Features**

- **Pseudotubercles** on cystoscopy are the earliest specific features. The pseudo tubercles are larger, more prominent, more numerous, more yellow and more distinctly grouped.☛ — JK BOPEE 2009
- **"Nodules"** are due to fusion of Tubercles.
- **"Sandy patches"** are a result of calcified dead ova
- **"Ulceration"** is the result of sloughing of mucus membrane containing dead ova. Ulcers are shallow, Bleed readily.
- **"Carcinoma"** is the end result of neglected bilharziasis
- Carcinoma commences in ulcer and not papilloma.
- It is usually well-advanced and requires radical cystectomy.

➲ Red Urine:

⇨ **Can be caused by**

- Gross hematuria,
- Hemoglobinuria,
- Myoglobinuria,
- Certain foods/ medications (e.g., rifampin, nitrofurantoin, chloroquine, azo dyes, beets, blackberries), and
- Presence of urates.

- The strip-test for blood in a urinalysis does not test directly on red blood cells; rather it tests the **presence or absence of hemoglobin.**
- It is sensitive to **5-20 red blood** cells per high power field (hpf) in the urine, but it is even more sensitive to free hemoglobin. Because of the structural similarity of myoglobin and hemoglobin, the strip-test reagents also react to myoglobin.
- Therefore, a positive test for "blood" in a strip test of urinalysis can mean red blood cells, hemoglobin, or myoglobin.
- It is important to perform microscopic analysis of the urine to distinguish between these possibilities.
- In this case, the absence of a significant number of red blood cells (1 RBC/hpf) does not
- Qualify for hematuria, and the presence of 4 + blood on the strip test is consistent with myoglobinuria or hemoglobinuria.
- The fact that it happens abruptly after vigorous exercise further suggests that the red urine might be secondary to myoglobinuria, which happens not uncommonly after exercise.
- It is important to confirm with a quantitative test of urine myoglobin. The serum creatinine phosphokinase (CK) level should also be tested for possible rhabdomyolysis. If rhabdomyolysis is present with elevated creatinine phosphokinase, the patient should be admitted for aggressive IV hydration and treatment with sodium bicarbonate to alkalinize the urine to prevent precipitation of the myoglobin in the renal tubules.

⇨ Special Forms of Lower Urinary Tract Infection

Acute Abacterial Cystitis (Acute Hemorrhagic Cystitis)

- The patient presents with symptoms of severe UTI.
- Pus is present in the urine, but no organism can be cultured.
- It is sometimes associated with abacterial urethritis and is commonly sexually acquired. Tuberculous infection and carcinoma in situ must be ruled out.
- The underlying causative organism may be **mycoplasma or herpes.**

Frequency-Dysuria Syndrome (Urethral Syndrome)

- This is common in women.
- It consists of symptoms suggestive of urinary infection, but with negative urine cultures and absent pus cells.
- Carcinoma in situ, tuberculosis and interstitial cystitis should be excluded.
- Adopt general measures such as wearing cotton underwear, using simple soaps, general perineal hygiene and voiding after intercourse.
- Other treatments include cystoscopy and urethral dilatation, although the benefits remain doubtful.

Tuberculous Urinary Infection	
▶ Tuberculous urinary infection is **secondary to renal tuberculosis.**	
▶ Cystoscopy shows that early tuberculosis of the bladder **commences around the ureteric orifice or trigone**	
▶ The earliest evidence being **pallor of the mucosa** due to submucous edema.	
▶ Subsequently tubercles may be seen **cobble stone appearance**	**PGI 1997**
▶ Long-standing cases there is much fibrosis and the capacity of the bladder is greatly reduced sacrred, fibrosed, small capacity **(thimble bladder)**	**AI 1991**
▶ Rigid wide mouthed ureter(**golf hole ureter)**	**PGI 1997**

⇨ Other Conditions Affecting Urinary Bladder

Genuine stress incontinence is defined as urinary leakage occurring during increased bladder pressure when this is solely due to increased abdominal pressure and not due to increased true detrusor pressure It is caused by sphincter weakness. The commonest cause of leakage of urine in women is genuine stress incontinence (GSI), although in some parts of the world vesicourethral fistulae owing to neglected labour are very common. GSI occurs secondary to weakness of the distal sphincter mechanism associated with laxity of the pelvic floor. It is usually found in multiparous women with a history of difficult labour often accompanied by the use of forceps.

Chronic urinary retention with overflow incontinence. This is recognised by a large residual volume of urine and is usually associated with high pressures during bladder filling.

- **Neurogenic incontinence** The common causes include:
- **Myelodysplasia;**
- **Multiple sclerosis;**
- **Spinal cord injuries;**
- **Cerebral dysfunction [cerebrovascular accident (CVA), dementia);**
- **Parkinson's disease (paralysis agitans).**

These conditions lead to a combination of neurogenic vesical dysfunction often associated with loss of mobility. Careful investigation of the whole urinary tract is always required, and the treatment needs to strike a fine balance between preventing hydronephrosis from abnormally high bladder pressures yet at the same time maintaining continence.

The mainstay of management is accurate urodynamic assessment to assess bladder emptying, incontinence and the risks to the upper tract. The upper tracts should be assessed with regular ultrasound scanning, and assessment of the patient's mobility, intelligence and motivation is vital. The important factors to assess urodynamically are:

- Bladder emptying;
- Bladder capacity and bladder pressure during filling;
- Continence.

1

SURGERY

Small bladder capacity☛ The capacity of the bladder may be considerably diminished in several conditions. This can cause crippling urinary frequency and incontinence. It may follow tuberculosis, radiotherapy or interstitial cystitis. Radiotherapy for pelvic cancer can also cause this problem.
Drug-induced incontinence ☛ The detrusor muscle is basically under postganglionic parasympathetic control and the main neurotransmitter system is cholinergic. A number of drugs can induce urinary retention **(anticholinergic agents, tricyclic antidepressants, lithium and some antihypertensives).**
Constant dribbling of urine coupled with normal micturition ☛ This occurs when there is a ureteric fistula or an ectopic ureter associated with a duplex system opening into the urethra beyond the urethral sphincter in females, or into the vagina. The history is diagnostic, and intravenous pyelography or ultrasound scanning may reveal the upper pole segment which is often poorly functioning. These segments are very liable to infection. Treatment is by excision of the aberrant ureter and portion of kidney which needs it. A ureteric fistula can be difficult to diagnose and may require retrograde ureterography and a high degree of suspicion to demonstrate.

⇨ Rupture of the Bladder

This may be **intraperitoneal (20 Percent)** or **extraperitoneal (80 Percent)**

Intraperitoneal rupture may be secondary to a blow, kick or fall on a fully distended bladder and it is more common in the male than in the female, and usually follows a bout of beer drinking. More rarely, it is due to surgical damage. Extraperitoneal rupture is usually caused by a fractured pelvis or is secondary to major trauma or surgical damage.
➠ **Sudden, agonising pain in the hypogastrium, often accompanied by syncope**
➠ **The shock later subsides and the abdomen commences to distend** ☛
➠ **No desire to micturate** ☛
➠ **Varying degrees of abdominal rigidity and abdominal distension are present on examination** ☛
➠ **No suprapubic dullness, but there is tenderness** ☛
➠ **There may be shifting dullness**
➠ **If the urine is sterile, symptoms and signs of peritonitis are delayed**
Extraperitoneal Rupture
In many cases of pelvic trauma, this is difficult to distinguish from rupture of the membranous urethra.
Confirming a suspected diagnosis of intraperitoneal rupture
✓ Plain X-ray in the erect position may show the ground-glass appearance of fluid in the lower abdomen
✓ Intravenous urography (IVU) may confirm a leak from the bladder
✓ A peritoneal 'tap' may be of value if facilities for radiological examination are not available
✓ If doubt still exists and if there is no sign of fracture then retrograde cystography can be performed safely. With careful asepsis a small [14 French gauge (FG)] catheter is passed. Usually some blood-stained urine will drain. A solution made from 60 ml of 35 percent Hypaque® or Conray® with 120 ml of sterile isotonic saline is injected into the bladder and radiographs are taken.

Ectopia Vesicae (Syn. exstrophy of the bladder) ☛
Caused by the incomplete development of the infra-umbilical part of the anterior abdominal wall, associated with incomplete development of the anterior wall of the bladder owing to delayed rupture of the cloacal membrane.
Clinical features of ectopia vesicae
➠ One in 50 000 births (four male: one female)
➠ **Characteristic appearance because of the pressure of the viscera behind it**
➠ **Edges of abdominal wall can be felt**
➠ **Umbilicus is absent**

➲ Urethral Stricture: High Yield for AIPGMEE, AIIMS, PGI 2012/2013

Urethral Stricture ☛	
The causes of urethral stricture are:	
➠ Congenital;	
➠ Traumatic; MC Cause.	AI 2003
➠ Inflammatory:	
– **Postgonorrheal;**	
– **Post urethral chancre;**	
– **Tuberculous;**	
➠ Instrumental:	
– **Indwelling catheter;**	
– **Urethral endoscopy;**	
➠ Postoperative:	
– **Open prostatectomy;**	
– **Amputation of penis.**	

⇨ Extravasation of Urine

Superficial extravasation is likely with **complete rupture of the bulbar urethra** and in ruptured urethral abscess.
➠ The extravasated urine is **confined in front of the midperineal point** by the attachment of Colles fascia to the triangular ligament, and by the attachment of Scarpa's fascia just below the inguinal ligament. The external spermatic fascia stops it getting into the inguinal canals. ➠ Extravasated urine **collects in the scrotum and penis and beneath the deep layer of superficial fascia in the abdominal wall.**
Treatment is by **urgent operation** to drain the bladder by suprapubic cystostomy. This prevents further extravasation.

1

SURGERY

Deep extravasation occurs with **extraperitoneal rupture of the bladder or intrapelvic rupture of the urethra.**
➡ It can also occur if the ureter is damaged or if there is perforation of the prostatic capsule or bladder during transurethral resection.
➡ Urine extravasates in the layers of the **pelvic fascia and the retroperitoneal tissues.**
Treatment is by **suprapubic cytostomy** and drainage of the retropubic space.

▶ Urethral injury associated with #pelvis: membranous urethral injury☛	MAHE 2007
▶ Urethral injury associated with High flying prostate: membranous urethral injury☛	
▶ Bladder injury associated with #pelvis: extraperitoneal rupture.☛	

⇨ Injuries to the Male Urethra

Rupture of the Bulbar Urethra ☛	
Rupture of the bulbar urethra is the **most common urethral injury**.	
There is a **history of a blow to the perineum** usually due to a fall astride a projecting object. Cycling accidents, loose manhole covers and gymnasium accidents astride the beam account for a number of cases.	MAHE 2007
Clinical Features	
The triad of signs of a ruptured bulbar urethra is	
✓ **Retention of urine,**	AIIMS 2006
✓ **Perineal hematoma and**	MAHE 2007
✓ **Bleeding from the external urinary meatus.**	AI 2007
Rupture of the membranous urethra ☛	
Extra peritoneal rupture of the urethra	
Intrapelvic rupture of the membranous urethra occurs near the apex of the prostate Like extraperitoneal rupture of the bladder, it may be due to penetrating wounds but in civilian life it is most usually a result of **pelvic fracture.**	
Fracture of the pubic and ischial rami is most likely to result when sudden force is applied to one lower limb in a car accident or in landing on one leg after falling from a height. There is an associated disruption of the sacroiliac joint so that one half of the pelvis and ischiopubic ramus is pushed up above the other. This applies a traction force on the prostate which is firmly bound by ligaments to the back of the symphysis pubis. The torn ends of the urethra may be widely displaced by this type of injury.	
Catheterization is best avoided.	AIIMS 2001

Congenital valves of the posterior urethra	
➡ These are symmetrical folds of urothelium which can cause obstruction to the urethra of boys.	
➡ They are **usually found just distal to the verumontanum** but they may be within the prostatic urethra. They behave as flap valves so, although urine does not flow normally, a urethral catheter can be passed without difficulty.	DELHI 1993

- In some instances, the valves are incomplete and the patient remains without symptoms until adolescence or adulthood.
- In such cases the prostatic urethra is grossly dilated and saccules and diverticula are present within it.

⇨ Other Important Points about Posterior Urethral Valves: AIIMS 2003

- Symmetrical folds of **urothelium**
- Common **distal to verumontanum**
- Occur in **males** only. AIIMS 1984
- MC cause of urinary obstruction in male infant. AI 2001
- Cause **obstruction to passage of urine and catheter.**
- Diagnosis is by **VCUG**. And Endoscopy. PGI 2002
- Associated with **VURD syndrome**. (Urethral valves, unilateral reflux, Renal Dysplasia)

➲ Overactive Bladder: HIGH Yield for 2011-2012

Includes Symptoms of

- **Urgency,**
- **Frequency and**
- **Urge incontinence.**

The prime effector of continence is the **synergic relaxation of the bladder wall muscle (detrusor) and contraction of bladder neck and pelvic floor muscles.**

The sympathetic nerve fibres originating from the T11 to L 2 segments of the spinal cord, which innervate smooth-muscle fibres around the bladder neck and proximal urethra, cause these fibres to contract, allowing the bladder to fill.

As the bladder fills, sensory stretch receptors in the bladder wall trigger a central nervous system (CNS) response. **The parasympathetic nervous system** causes **contraction of the detrusor, while the muscles of the pelvic floor and external sphincter relax.**

The PNS fibres, as well as those responsible for somatic (voluntary) control of micturition, originate from the sacral plexus from the S 2 to S 4 segment of the spinal cord.

Causes:

- **Idiopathic**: The majority of cases
- **Neurological Injuries**: spinal cord injury or CVA.
- **Neurological Diseases**: As multiple sclerosis, dementia, Parkinson"s disease, medullary lesions.
- **Non-neurogenic Causes**: Such as UTI, Ca bladder, bladder calculi, bladder inflammation, or bladder outlet obstruction (BOO).
- **Drug Therapy**: Diuretics can lead to symptoms of urge incontinence as result of increasing filling of the bladder, stimulating the detrusor.

Types of Urinary Incontinence:

Urge Incontinence: Involves a strong, sudden need to urinate, immediately followed by a bladder contraction, resulting in an involuntary loss of urine.

Stress Incontinence: Is characterised by an involuntary loss of urine when the intra-abdominal pressure is suddenly increased, for example, during coughing, sneezing and laughing or during physical activity.
Overflow Incontinence: Is the involuntary loss of urine associated with an overdistended bladder. It occurs when bladder filling exceeds the bladder functional capacity.

Functional Incontinence: Occurs in patients who would otherwise be continent but for whom physical and/or cognitive impairments interfere with the ability to reach a toilet in time.

Mixed Incontinence: Involves a combination of different type of incontinence, typically stress and urge incontinence occurring simultaneously.

Treatment:

- **Antichloinergics:** Since acetylcholine is the neurotransmitter that mediates detrusor contractions, medicationwith anticholinergics is used to inhibit the premature detrusor muscle contraction. Consequently, the most frequently used drugs to treat this condition aim to reduce the involuntary contraction of the detrusor muscles by blocking the muscarinic receptors.
- **Oxybutynin:** Is used to treat detrusor overactivity and its efficacy in treating OAB is well documented. However, the effects of oxybutynin are not tissue specific
- **Tolterodine:** Has a greater inhibitory effect on bladder contraction. Therefore it has fewer side effects such as dryness of mouth, but with comparable efficacy.
- **Tricyclic antidepressants: Imipramine or doxepin** have also been used to treat OAB.
- **Bladder Training:** Management of urge incontinence usually begins with a program of bladder retraining. Occasionally, electrical stimulation and biofeedback therapy may be used in conjunction with bladder retraining.

  Pelvic Floor Exercises: Known as pelvic muscle training exercises or Kegel exercises are primarily used to treat people with stress incontinence. However, these exercises may also be beneficial in relieving the symptoms of urge incontinence.
- **Surgery:** Is rarely used to treat OAB. It is reserved for patients who are severely debilitated by their incontinence and who have an unstable bladder (severe inappropriate contraction) and poor ability to store urine.
- **Augmentation cystoplasty** is the most frequently performed surgical procedure for severe urge incontinence.

  In this reconstructive surgery a segment of the bowel is removed and used to replace a portion of the bladder.

  Neuromodulation: It requires the surgical implantation of a small device at the base of the spinal cord. It electrically or magnetically stimulates the sacral nerves that inhibit detrusor muscle contraction.

➲ High Yield for AIPGMEE, AIIMS, PGI 2012/2013

⇨ Hypospadias

Hypospadias	DNB 2011
▶ Hypospadias occurs in one in 350 male births	
▶ Is the most common congenital malformation of the urethra.	
▶ The external meatus opens on the underside of the penis or the perineum, and the inferior aspect of the prepuce is poorly developed **(Hooded Prepuce).**	**PGI 1999**
▶ **Meatal stenosis** also occurs	**PGI 1999**
▶ **Bifid scrotum.**	**PGI 2001**
Hypospadias is classified according to position of the meatus.	
Glandular hypospadias ☛this is the **most common type** and does not usually require treatment. The normal site of the external meatus is marked by a blind pit, although it occasionally connects by a channel to the ectopic opening on the underside of the glans.	**MAH 2012**
Coronal Hypospadias – The meatus is placed at the junction of the underside of the glans and the body of the penis.	
Penile and Penoscrotal Hypospadias – The opening is on the **underside of the penile shaft**	
Perineal Hypospadias – This is the **most severe abnormality.** The scrotum is split and the urethra opens between its two halves. There may be testicular maldescent which may make it difficult to determine the sex of the child.	
The more severe varieties of hypospadias represent an absence of the urethra and corpus spongiosum distal to the ectopic opening. The absent structures are represented by a fibrous cord which deforms the penis in a downward. Direction **(chordee).** The more distant the opening from its normal position, the more pronounced the bowing.	
6-10 months of age is the best time for surgery.	**AI 2003**

⇨ The Tunica Vaginalis **DNB 2011**

Is derived from the peritoneum as the **processus vaginalis** at the time of testicular descent, is a secretory membrane. Fluid is generated by the serous surface of the tunica vaginalis, with fluid formation being enhanced by inflammation or trauma. Fluid within the tunica vaginalis is resorbed at a constant rate through the extensive venous and lymphatic systems of the spermatic cord. **Hydrocele,** the excessive accumulation of this serous fluid, results when there is increased production or decreased resorption, the latter condition usually being idiopathic.

⇨ Cryptorchidism

The term cryptorchidism (Greek cryptos = hidden, orchis = testis) should be reserved for impalpable, usually abdominal, testes.

- There is a higher incidence of undescended testes in **premature** than in full-term babies.
- Two-thirds of undescended testes in newborn infants will descend, usually by 6 weeks in term and 3 months in preterm babies.
- There is an increased incidence of cryptorchidism in **anencephalics** and other cerebral anomalies.

1

SURGERY

- **Cryptorchism** is the **absence of one or both testes from scrotum**, usually represent failure of testes to move or descend during fetal development from abdominal position through inguinal canal into the ipsilateral scrotum.
- Most testes descend by the first year of life (the majority within three months). About 2/3 of cases are unilateral 1/3involve' both testes.
- In 90% testes can be palpated in the inguinal canal. Complication include
  - **Reduce fertility,**
  - **Increased risk of testicular germ line tumors,**
  - **Torsion,**
  - **Infarction,**
  - **Atrophy and inguinal hernia.**
- **Investigation: Pelvic USG** is usually the first investigation. **MRI is the investigation of choice.**
- **Treatment: Orchiopexy** usually performed in infancy and the **best time is 6 months.** **AIPGME 2010**

⇨ Syndromes Associated with Undesceded Testis

- Microcephaly
- Arthrogryposis
- Multiplexa congenital
- Prune belly syndrome
- Posterior urethral valve
- Exomphalos
- Ectopia vesicae
- Gastroshisis
- Neural tube defects

⇨ Ectopic Testes

These have descended as far as the external inguinal ring and then become deviated into the

- **Superficial inguinal,** **AIIMS 1987**
- **Perineal,** **AIIMS 1987**
- **Suprapubic or**
- **Femoral ectopic sites.**
- The commonest by far is the superficial inguinal pouch, above and lateral to the external inguinal ring.

⇨ Retractile Testes

The cremasteric reflex in young children will draw the testes into the region of the superficial inguinal pouch very readily but they can be manipulated back down to the bottom of the scrotum. The testis would normally reside in the scrotum if such a child is in a warm bath or relaxed in bed.

⇨ Ascending Testis

Some boys with recorded testicular descent at routine clinic checks in infancy may be found later at preschool or school medicals to have an undescended testis. This phenomenon of the 'Ascending Testis' was noted first by Atwell. It has been suggested that this is caused by failure of elongation of the spermatic cord during differential body growth, so that the testis is drawn up by absorption of the processus vaginalis.

Anorchia

Anorchia may be on one or both sides. If on one side alone there may be ipsilateral renal agenesis. If the baby is fully masculinized but both testes are absent it must be assumed that they have atrophied subsequent to torsion or infarction during development. **Absence of testicular tissue** and therefore lack of müllerian inhibitory hormone during early gestation can lead to müllerian development along female lines. The lack of androgenic stimulation (testosterone) from the testes leads to failure of wolffian duct development.

⇨ Predisposing Factors for Torsion of Testis are

- **Inversion of testis**
- **Long Mesorchium**
- **Undescended/ectopic testis**
- **High investment of tunica vaginalis**
- **Initiating factors: Spasm of cremaster**
- **Torsion of spinal cord involves twisting of spermatic cord along its long axis. Left testis rotates anticlockwise and Right testis rotates clockwise. i.e. away from midline.**
- **"De torsion" is the initial treatment.**

➲ Remember: High Yield for AIPGMEE, AIIMS, PGI 2012/2013

- Torsion of the testicle should be corrected as soon as possible after the diagnosis is entertained. **AIIMS 2004**
- Incomplete torsion can cause partial strangulation, the effects of which may be overcome if surgical intervention is accomplished within 12 hours, whereas severe torsion with complete compromise of the blood supply results in loss of the testis unless surgical intervention occurs within approximately 4 hours.
- The contralateral scrotum should also be explored at the time of the operation, since the primary anatomic defect—insufficient attachment of the testicle to the scrotal sidewall—most often is a bilateral phenomenon.
- If the contralateral scrotum is not explored, the patient runs a very high risk of undergoing torsion on the other side and the possible complication of loss of both testes **AIIMS 2001**

⇨ Hazards of Incomplete Descent are

- Sterility in bilateral cases;
- Pain due to trauma;
- An associated indirect inguinal hernia that is often present and, in older patients, it is frequently the hernia which causes symptoms;

1

SURGERY

- Torsion;
- Epididymo-orchitis that, in an incompletely descended testis, is extremely rare but of interest because, on the right side, it mimics appendicitis;
- Atrophy of an inguinal testis that can occur even before puberty, possibly due to recurrent minor trauma;
- Increased liability to malignant disease. All types of malignant testicular tumour are more common in incompletely descended testes even if they have been brought down surgically. **AIIMS 1999**
- **Operate at between 9-15 months of age. AI 2004**

Testicular torsion	Epididymitis
▶ Usually <30 yrs age	▶ Usually >30 yrs age
▶ Pain stays same/ worsen with testicular elevation (Prehns test) **DNB 2011**	▶ Pain ↓with testicular elevation
▶ Immediate exploration needed	▶ Immediate exploration NOT needed

⇨ Remember Normal Values for Semen Analysis

World Health Organization Reference Values for Semen Analysis Testing 2009 **PGI**

- **Volume > 2 ml**
- **Sperm concentration > 20 million/ml**
- **Sperm number > 40 million per ejaculate**
- **Sperm motility > 50% progressive or> 25% rapidly progressive**
- **Morphology (Strict Criteria) > 15% normal forms**
- **White blood cells < 1 million/ml**
- **Immunobead or mixed < 10% coated**
- **Antiglobulin reaction test***
- **Vitality ≥ 75% living**
- **pH ≥ 7.2**
- **Liquification time < 60 minutes**

- Motility (ability to swim) - More than 50% should be actively motile (moving).
- More than 14% nomal forms - The heads and tails are properly shaped.
- Less than 5 white blood cells per high power microscope filed.
- **Normozoospermia:** Semen parameters fall within the WHO reference values (i.e. >20 million sperm/ml of semen and no morphological or genetic defects in the sperm);
- **Oligozoospermia:** Refers to seminal fluid in which the concentration of sperm is lower than the WHO reference values.

Remember:

Aspermia: No ejaculate
Oligospermia: Sperm count less than 20 million /ml
Polyzoospermia: Count>350 million/ml
Azoospermia: No spermatozoa in semen
Asthenozoospermia: Reduced sperm motility
Necrozoospermia: Spermatozoa are dead
Teratozoospermia: >70% Spermatozoa with abnormal morphology

⇨ **Oligospermia**

Oligospermia, by definition, indicates a sperm count of less than 20 million per ml. and under such circumstances fertility is difficult.
The principal causes of defective spermatogenesis include:
❐ **Congenital inadequacy of the seminiferous tubules;**
❐ **Testicular damage as a consequence of infection, trauma, or infarction;**
❐ **Klinefelter's syndrome;**
❐ **Hypopituitarism;**
❐ **Varicocele; and**
❐ **Cryptorchidism.**
❐ Other causes of oligospermia may relate to the transport of spermatozoa. Chronic prostatitis and seminal vesiculitis may result in fibrosis and impede transport and delivery of sperm. Infection spreading into the vas deferens may induce fibrosis and stricture even to the point of total occlusion.

Azoospermia, complete absence of spermatozoa in the ejaculate, may be caused by:
➠ Total occlusion of the sperm transport system, vasa, seminal vesicles, or ejaculatory ducts. Congenital absence of the vas and seminal vesicles may occur as an isolated anatomic defect, and congenital absence of the vas is the rule in males with cystic fibrosis.
➠ Gonococcal epididymitis and vasitis may cause complete stenosis and azoospermia.
➠ Complete nonresponsiveness of the germinal epithelium as in primary gonadal failure may also produce a picture of azoospermia despite elevated follicle-stimulating hormone levels.
➠ Trauma to the vasa in the course of an inguinal hernia operation or orchidopexy.

⇨ Testicular Cancer:

Classification of Germ Cell Tumors

Benign: Mature Teratomas, Dermoid Cysts

Malignant:

- Seminomas
- Non-seminomatous germ cell tumors
- Immature teratoma
- Teratoma with malignant components
- Choriocarcinoma
- Endodermal cell (yolk sac) tumors
- Mixed germ cell tumors

Germ Cell Tumors have the Following Subtypes and Frequencies:

- Seminoma (40%)
- Embryonal tumors (25%)
- Teratocarcinoma (25%), teratomata (5%)
- Choriocarcinoma (1%)
- Other (5%)

❒ **Primary germ cell tumors (GCTs) of the testis**, constitute 95□ of all testicular neoplasms. ☛Infrequently, GCTs arise from an extragonadal site, including the **mediastinum**, retroperitoneum and, very rarely, the pineal gland.	
❒ **Yuvraj singh (Cricketer) suffered from Mediastinal Seminoma.**	
❒ **Bilateral in 10% cases.**	AI 2006
❒ **Cryptorchidism** is associated with a several fold higher risk of GCT. ☛	
❒ **Abdominal cryptorchid testes** are at a **higher risk** than inguinal cryptorchid testes.☛	PGI 2003
❒ Orchiopexy should be performed before puberty, if possible. ☛	
❒ **Testicular feminization syndromes** increase the risk of testicular GCT, and ☛	PGI 2003
❒ **Klinefelter's syndrome** is associated with mediastinal GCT.	PGI 2003
❒ An isochromosome of the short arm of **chromosome 12** is pathognomonic for GCT ☛	
❒ **A painless testicular mass** is pathognomonic for a testicular malignancy.	
❒ **Mc tumor of testis in younger age group: seminoma**	JK BOPEE 2011
❒ **Mc histological subtype: mixed**	
❒ **Mc tumor in infants: yolk sac tumor**	AIIMS 2008
❒ **Mc tumor in aged elderly: lymphoma**	AI 2001

Commonest testicular malignancy is: Seminoma
Most malignant testicular cancer is: Choriocarcinoma

⇨ Seminoma

Seminoma	
❑ Has a median age in the fourth decade,	
❑ Generally follows a more indolent clinical course.	
❑ Seminomas are radiosensitive.	PGI 2005
❑ **But Surgery is the TOC.**	PGI 2005
❑ Seminomas metastasize by lymphatics.	
❑ Seminomas correspond to dysgerminomas of ovary.	PGI 99

⇨ Spermatocele

➠ Spermatocele is a **unilocular retention cyst.**	
➠ It **almost always** lies in relation to the head of the epididymis.	
➠ The fluid **contains spermatozoa and resembles" barley fluid".**	JK 2009
➠ Treatment for small spermatoceles is conservative followup while as larger ones should be aspirated or excised.	
➠ A spermatocele is a diverticulum of the epididymis that contains cloudy fluid with spermatozoa. It is unilocular or multilocular and often confused with hydrocele because both a spermatocele and a hydrocele can be transilluminated. Differential diagnosis of spermatocele and hydrocele is aided by the localization of the mass: hydrocele generally surrounds the testis, while the spermatocele is more eccentric, can often be palpated in direct conjunction with the epididymis, and is often tender.	
"Transillumination" is also seen in:	**AIPGME 2012**
➠ **Cystic hygroma**	
➠ **Newborn hydrocele**	
➠ **Spinal meningocele**	

⇨ Cysts Connected with the Epididymis

Epididymal Cysts

These are filled with a **crystal-clear fluid** (as opposed to the barley-water fluid of a spermatocele or the amber fluid of a hydrocele). They are very common, usually multiple and vary greatly in size at presentation. They represent cystic degeneration of the epididymis.

Cyst of a Testicular Appendage

Cyst of a testicular appendage is usually unilateral and is felt as a small globular swelling at the superior pole. Such cysts are liable to torsion and should be removed if they cause symptoms.

⇨ Hydrocele

The tunica vaginalis, derived from the peritoneum as the processus vaginalis at the time of testicular descent, is a secretory membrane. Fluid is generated by the serous surface of the tunica vaginalis

- Congenital hydrocele may follow **failure of obliteration of the processus vaginalis**, and fluid formed within the peritoneal cavity may gravitate into the tunica vaginalis.
- There may sometimes be an **associated palpable inguinal hernia**
- In older persons, hydrocele is frequently the result of **epididymo-orchitis or trauma.**
- **Lords plication is used for hydrocele** AI 2010

➲ Types of Hydrocele: High Yield for AIPGMEE, AIIMS, PGI 2012/2013

Infantile Hydrocele

Infantile hydrocele does not necessarily appear in infants. The tunica and processus vaginalis ate distended to the inguinal ring but there is no connection with the peritoneal cavity.

Congenital Hydrocele

The processus vaginalis is patent and connects with the general peritoneal cavity. The communication is usually too small to allow herniation of intra-abdominal contents. Digital pressure on the hydrocele does not usually empty it but the hydrocele fluid may drain into the peritoneal cavity when the child is lying down. Ascites or even ascitic tuberculous peritonitis should be considered if the swellings are bilateral. **Herniotomy is the procedure of choice.** MAH 2012

Encysted Hydrocele of the Cord

There is a smooth oval swelling near the spermatic cord which is liable to be mistaken for an inguinal hernia. The swelling moves downwards and becomes less mobile if the testis is pulled gently downwards.

Hydrocele of the canal of Nuck is a similar condition. It occurs in females and the cyst lies in relation to the round ligament. Unlike a hydrocele of the cord, a hydrocele of the canal of Nuck is always at least partially within the inguinal canal.

Postherniorrhaphy Hydrocele

Postherniorrhaphy hydrocele is a relatively rare complication of inguinal hernia repair. It is possibly due to interruption to the lymphatics draining the scrotal contents.

Hydrocele of a Hernial Sac

Hydrocele of a hernial sac occurs when the neck is plugged with omentum or occluded by adhesions.

Filarial Hydroceles and Chyloceles

Filarial hydroceles and chyloceles account for up to 80 percent of hydroceles in some tropical countries where the parasite is endemic. Filarial hydroceles follow repeated attacks of filarial epididymo-orchitis. They vary in size and may develop slowly or very rapidly. Occasionally the fluid contains liquid fat which is rich in cholesterol. This is due to rupture of a lymphatic varix with discharge of chyle into the hydrocele. Adult worms of the Wuchereria bancrofti have been found in the epididymis removed at operation or at necropsy. In long-standing chyloceles, there are dense adhesions between the scrotum and its contents. Filarial elephantiasis supervenes in a small number of cases.

⇨ Epididymitis

Acute tuberculous epididymitis should come to mind when the **vas is thickened** and there is little response to the usual antibiotics.

Acute Epididymo-Orchitis of Mumps

- Develops in about 18 percent of males suffering from mumps, usually as the parotid swelling is waning.
- The main complication is **testicular atrophy** which may cause infertility if the condition is bilateral (which is not usual). Partial atrophy is associated with persistent testicular pain. The epididymitis of mumps sometimes occurs in the absence of parotitis, especially in infants. The epididymis and testis may be involved by infection with other enteroviruses and in brucellosis and lymphogranuloma venereum.

➲ Idiopathic Scrotal Gangrene

Idiopathic scrotal gangrene **(Syn. Fournier's gangrene)** is an uncommon and nasty condition It is a vascular disaster of infective origin which is characterized by: ☛

- Sudden appearance of scrotal inflammation;
- Rapid onset of gangrene leading to exposure of the scrotal contents;
- Absence of any obvious cause in over half the cases.

It has been known to follow minor injuries or procedures in the perineal area, such as a bruise, scratch, urethral dilatation, injection of hemorrhoids or opening of a periurethral abscess.

The **hemolytic streptococcus** ☛(sometimes microaerophilic) is associated with other organisms (staphylococcus, E. coli, Clostridium welchii) in a fulminating inflammation of the subcutaneous tissues which results in an obliterative arteritis of the arterioles to the scrotal skin.

⇨ Varicocele

Is an **abnormal enlargement of the veins in the scrotum draining the testicles**. Defective valves, or compression of the vein by a nearby structure, can cause dilatation of the veins near the testis, leading to the formation of a varicocele.

Symptoms of a Varicocele May Include:

- **Dragging-like or aching pain within scrotum**
- **Feeling of heaviness in the testicle**
- **Atrophy (shrinking) of the testicle**
- **Visible or palpable enlarged vein, likened to feeling a bag of worms.**

— 98% of idiopathic varicoceles occur on **the left side**, apparently because the left testicular vein runs vertically up to the renal vein, while the right testicular vein drains directly into the inferior vena cava. **AIIMS 2011**

— Isolated right sided varicoceles are rare, and should prompt evaluation for an abdominal or pelvic mass.

— A **secondary varicocele** is due to compression of the venous drainage of the testicle. A pelvic or abdominal malignancy is a definite concern when a right-sided varicocele is newly diagnosed in a patient older than 40 years of age.

1

SURGERY

- Later development of a varicocele may be an indicator of left renal tumor because the left spermatic vein system drains into the renal vein and obstruction at that point could produce dilatation of the veins of the left cord. Most varicoceles are idiopathic, although there may be a defect in the valve system of the spermatic vein, particularly on the left where the vein takes a longer course. Varicocele rarely causes symptoms, but there may be a heavy, dragging, aching sensation in the scrotal compartment.
- In Left sided Varicocele, a thorogh investigation should be done to rule out Renal cell carcinoma. AIPGME 2012
- One non-malignant cause of a secondary varicocele is the so-called **"Nutcracker syndrome"**, a condition in which the superior mesenteric artery compresses the left renal vein, causing increased pressures there to be transmitted retrograde into the left pampiniform plexus.
- The most common cause is renal cell carcinoma followed by retroperitoneal fibrosis or adhesions.

- The pampiniform plexus is a network of many small veins found in the human male spermatic cord. It is formed by the union of multiple spermatic veins from the back of the testis and tributaries from the epididymis.
- The veins of the plexus ascend along the cord in front of the ductus deferens. Below the superficial inguinal ring they unite to form three or four veins, which pass along the inguinal canal, and, entering the abdomen through the deep inguinal ring, coalesce to form two veins. These again unite to form a single vein, the testicular vein, which opens on the right side into the inferior vena cava, at an acute angle, and on the left side into the left renal vein, at a right angle.The pampiniform plexus forms the chief mass of the cord.

- Dilatation and tortuosity of the veins of the **pampiniform plexus**
- Most commonly observed on the **left.** MP 1997
- Development of a varicocele may be an **indicator of left renal tumor** because the left spermatic vein system drains into the renal vein and obstruction at that point could produce dilatation of the veins of the left cord.
- There may be a **heavy, dragging, aching sensation** in the scrotal compartment.

BAG OF WORMS AI 1998

- May be a feature of renal cancer.
- Negative transillumination test MP 1997
- Reducible
- Cough impulse+
- MC cause of surgically treated male infertility. MAHE 1998

⇨ Prostate Gland:

- Shape: Chest nut shaped
- Type: Fibro musculo glangular organ
- Corresponding female orga: Paraurethral glands of Skene

▶ Volume: 8-12 ml.	
▶ Carcinoma arises from: Peripheral zone	AIIMS 2000
▶ BHP arises from: Periurethral Zone	AIIMS 2000
▶ Fracture of the bony pelvis may often result in laceration and transection of the **membranous urethra** just distal to the prostate, and urinary extravasation as well as bleeding may displace the prostate and bladder superiorly.	
MC site of urethral cancer is also membranous urethra	AI 2010

⇨ Urethral Cancer

- Most common site of urethral tumor in males is **Membranous urethra** followed by penile and prostatic urethra.
- Most common type of primary urethral cancer is **Transitional cell carcinoma**
- Urethral cancer are **extremely rare lesion**, comprising <1% of total malignancies.
- In females the most common site of tumor invasion are **labia, vagina, and bladder neck.**

Symptoms

- Diminished stream, straining to void, and other **obstructive** voiding symptoms
- Frequency, nocturia, itching, dysuria, and other **irritative** voiding symptoms
- Incontinence , Hematuria, urethral or vaginal spotting
- May produce no symptoms except a hard nodular area in the perineum, labia, or along the course of the penis
- Purulent, foul-smelling, or watery discharge, Hematospermia
- Perineal, suprapubic, or urethral pain
- Dyspareunia,Swelling, Tenesmus, Priapism

Surgery is indicated to confirm a diagnosis of clinically suspected urethral cancer.

More extensive surgery is indicated for local control ofa primary urethral neoplasm and depends on the size, location, and extent of the tumor and the overall condition of the patient.

⇨ Benign Prostatic Hypertrophy (BPH, BHP):

Fibro musculo glandular hyperplasia. (All 3 elements involved in varying proportion)☛

Is the **most common cause of bladder outlet obstruction** in men older than 50 years of age.☛

Mechanical pressure phenomena cause:

- **Upward displacement of the base of the bladder,**
- **Fishhooking of the lower ureters due to trigonal displacement,**
- **Hypertrophy of the bladder wall with trabeculation,**
- **Cellule formation,**
- **Diverticula of the bladder.**
- **Complete bladder outlet obstruction may result in decompensation of the detrusor muscle and total urinary retention.**

- ✓ In the early stages the patient complains of **diminished size and force of the urinary stream.**
- ✓ **Hematuria** may be caused by prostatic enlargement with engorgement of the small mucosal vessels covering the adenomatous gland, ruptured as a consequence of straining to urinate.
- ✓ Rectal examination shows most often **symmetric enlarged prostate and rubbery.**
- ✓ As enlargement progresses, the gland protrudes posteriorly, compressing the anterior rectal wall and sometimes producing symptoms of **constipation.**
- ✓ The size of the gland **bears little relationship** to the degree of symptomatic difficulty
- ✓ **Anticholinergic drugs and antihistamines should be avoided** because they may precipitate urinary retention.

Indications for a surgical procedure include:

- **Residual urine of more than 100 ml.**, particularly when there is associated azotemia of any degree;
- **Persistent or recurrent urinary infection** refractory to usual therapeutic methods; gross hematuria on more than one occasion;
- **Acute urinary retention**
- **Chronic urinary retention** with overflow dribbling.

Conservative therapy is by drugs.

Surgical procedures are:

- **TURP**
- **Transvesical Prostatectomy**
- **Retropubic prostatyectomy**
- **Perineal prostatectomy**

Ho YAG LASER is used **AI 2003**

- **MC complication of TURP: Retrograde ejaculation.** **COMED 2007**
- **Irrigation fluid used now in TURP: 1.5% Glycine** **COMED 2008**
- **Altered sensorium with drowsiness after TURP might indicate: Hyponatremia** **AIIMS 2007**

⇨ Indications of TURP

- Recurrent UTIs
- Refractory urinary retention
- Bladder stones and bladder diverticuli
- Upper tract changes (hydroureteronephrosis)
- Deranged renal function
- Recurrent hematuria

⇨ Complications of Prostatectomy

- ✓ Hemorrhage
- ✓ Bladder perforation
- ✓ Retrograde ejaculation / impotence
- ✓ Incontinence

- ✓ Urethral stricture
- ✓ Hyponatemia
- ✓ Sepsis
- ✓ Osteitis pubis

⇨ Minimally Invasive Procedures

- ▶ **Trans urethral needle ablation of Prostate. (TUNA)**
- ▶ **Trans urethral micro wave operation (TUMT)**
- ▶ **Trans urethral US guided laser induced prostatectomy (TULIP)**
- ▶ **Trans urethral vapourization of Prostate (TUVP)**
- ▶ **Trans urethral incision of prostate. (TUIP)**

➲ Carcinoma of the Prostate: High Yield for AIPGMEE, AIIMS, PGI 2012/2013

- ❒ **Adenocarcinoma** of the prostate is the most common
- ❒ Most often has its origin in **glandular acini of the peripheral group of glands** located in the **posterior and posterolateral regions** of the prostate.
- ▶ **Mc Neals Zone is referred to as cancer zone.** KAR 2006
- ▶ **Peripheral zone is the commonest site.** AIIMS 2001
- ▶ **PSA is the initial screening test marker.** PGI 1999
- ❒ Unique qualities of prostatic carcinoma is that many tumors produce an enzyme, **acid phosphatase,** which can be detected in the serum of patients **with metastatic disease** or at least a very large local lesion.
- ❒ **Prostate-specific antigen density (PSAD)** is calculated by dividing the serum PSA level by the estimated prostate weight calculated from transrectal ultrasonography (TRUS). **Values >0.15** suggest the presence of cancer. PSAD levels also increase with age.
- ❒ **PSA velocity** is derived from calculations of the rate of change in PSA before the diagnosis of cancer was established. Increases of >0.75 ng/mL per year are suggestive of cancer.
- ❒ The noninvasive proliferation of epithelial cells within ducts is termed **"Prostatic intraepithelial neoplasia" (PIN).** It is considered the precursor of cancer, but not all PIN lesions develop into invasive cancers
- ❒ Histologic grade is based most commonly on the **"Gleason system"** MAH 2012
- ❒ **Direct spread** is most common to seminal vesicles
- ❒ **Blood borne** metastasis is most common to: bones
- ❒ **Lymphatic spread** is most common to obturator nodes. PGI 1999
- ❒ Secondaries are **osteoblastic.**
- ❒ Metastasis to vertebrae is through **Batesons vertebral venous plexus.** AI 2001
- ❒ Carcinoma characteristically is **hard, nodular, and irregular.**
- ❒ **Digital rectal examination plus PSA levels** are used for **screening.** PGI 2006
- ❒ **Gleasons staging is used for Ca prostate.** PGI 2000

1

SURGERY

⇨ The Penile Structure

Phimosis ☛

Ahesions between the foreskin and the glans penis may persist until the boy is 6 years of age or more, giving the false impression that the prepuce will not retract. Rolling back the prepuce causes its inner lining to pout and the meatus comes into view. This condition should not be confused with true phimosis in small boys where there is scarring of the prepuce which will not retract without fissuring. In these cases, the aperture in the prepuce may be so tight as to cause urinary obstruction.

Paraphimosis ☛

- When the tight foreskin is retracted, it may sometimes be difficult to return and a paraphimosis results.
- In this condition, the venous and lymphatic return from the glans and distal foreskin is obstructed and these structures swell alarmingly causing even more pressure within the obstructing ring of prepuce. Gangrene may occur. **AIIMS 1998**
- Ice bags, gentle manual compression and injection of a solution of hyaluronidase in normal saline may help to reduce the swelling.
- Such patients can be treated by **circumcision** if careful manipulation fails. **AIIMS 1998**
- A dorsal slit of the prepuce under local anaesthetic may be enough in an emergency

Balanoposthitis ☛ Inflammation of the prepuce is known as posthitis; inflammation of the glans is balanitis. The opposing surfaces of the two structures are often involved – hence the term balanoposthitis.

Chordee ☛Chordee (French = corded) is a fixed bowing of the penis due to hypospadias or, more rarely, chronic urethritis. Erection is deformed and sexual intercourse may be impossible. Treatment is usually surgical.

Peyronie's Disease.

- Peyronie's disease is a relatively common cause of deformity of the erect penis.
- On examination, hard plaques of fibrosis can be palpated in the tunica of one or both corpora cavernosa. The plaques may be calcified the presence of the unyielding plaque tissue within the normally elastic wall of the corpus cavernosum causes the erect penis to bend, often dramatically, towards the side of the plaque.
- The aetiology is uncertain, but it may be a result of past trauma – there is an association with Dupuytren's contracture **UP 2007**
- Usually self limiting **UP 2006**

Paget's disease of the Penis (Syn. Erythroplasia of Querat)☛ Is 'a persistent rawness of the glans like a long-standing balanitis followed by cancer of the substance of the penis' (Sir James Pager). Treatment is by circumcision, observation and excision if the lesion does not resolve. **AIIMS 2001**

Buschke–Lowenstein tumour☛ Is uncommon. It has the histological pattern of a verrucous carcinoma. It is locally destructive and invasive, but appears not to spread to lymph nodes or to metastasise. Treatment is by surgical excision.

⇨ Cancer of the Penis

- Is a rare tumor
- Has a much higher proportion in populations where **circumcision and personal hygiene are not well established.**
- The most common form of cancer of the penis is **squamous cell carcinoma**☛
- Seen associated with **chronic balanoposthitis** from lack of circumcision
- Lymphadenopathy common. **AIIMS 2001**

Premalignant Lesions:

- **Buschke lownstein tumor**☛
- **Erythroplasia of Querat / Pagets disease of penis**☛
- **Bowens disease**☛
- **Leukoplakia**
- **Balanitis xerotica obliterans**☛
- Diagnosis is established by **biopsy.**
- Treatment consists of **partial or total penectomy**; a proximal margin-free tumor of at least 1.5 cm is desirable.
- Inguinal node dissection with excision of both superficial and deep inguinal nodes is advocated when clinically palpable nodes persist after amputation.
- Lymphadenopathy may occur from secondary infection seen in most cases of advanced penile carcinoma.

⇨ Peyronie's Disease (Details) AIIMS 2002

- A **localized induration of the fibrous investments of the penile shaft**, first described by the French surgeon Peyronie.☛
- After age 40 years usually
- **Penile Fibromatosis**☛
  - A **firm fibrotic thickening of the "Fascia of the Corpora Cavernosa"** is observed, usually involving the dorsolateral aspects of the penile shaft or the intracavernous septum between the corpora cavernosa,
  - Histologically similar to **Keloid or Dupuytren's contracture.** ☛ **UP 2006**
  - The fibrous plaques themselves **may be painless**
  - Often **compromise of erectile capacity of the penis** with **"deviation of the penis on erection"** and pain **as a consequence** of this derangement.☛
  - Deviation of the penis that **interferes with intromission and coitus.** ☛
  - Progression is slow, and spontaneous remissions are observed
  - **Nesbitts operation** is done☛

⇨ Priapism

- Prolonged
- Pathologic ☛
- Painful erection of the penis ☛
- In recognition of the Greek god of sexual excess, Priapus.

- Pelvic venous thrombosis predisposes to priapism, **metastatic malignant diseases, leukemia, pelvic trauma, sickle cell disease or trait, trauma to the corpora, or spinal cord injury.** ☛
- Prompt recognition and therapy are essential because prolonged unrelieved priapism almost inevitably leads to subsequent Permanent impotence from fibrosis of the corpora cavernosa.

➲ Brain Tumors Adults: High Yield for AIPGMEE, AIIMS, PGI 2012/2013

Glioblastoma

- Most Common primary bone tumor☛
- Prognosis: grave
- Pseudopallisading pattern of tumor cells☛

Meningoma

- Psammoma bodies☛
- Arises from Arachnoid cells☛
- Second most common brain tumor in adults

Oligodendroglioma

- Most common in Frontal Lobes
- Fried egg appearance of tumor cells☛

Schwanommas

- Origin from Schwann cells☛
- Bilateral scwannomas found in NF2☛
- Two Patterns: ANTONI A and Antoni B☛

Pituitary Tumors

- Secrete Prolactin
- Derived from Rathkes Pouch☛

⇨ CNS Tumors

- **MC site of CNS lipoma☛ Corpus Callosum**
- **MC site of Germinoma☛ Pineal Gland**
- **MC site of Chordoma Clivus**
- **MC source of Metastasis to Brain (Females)☛ Breast**
- **MC source of Metastasis to Brain (Males)☛ Lung**
- **Imaging of choice is: ☛ Contrast enhanced MRI**
- **Most specific test: ☛ Stereotaxic needle biopsy**
- **Bleeding brain tumors:☛ Glioblastoma multiforme,**

➲ Calcification in Brain: High Yield for AIPGMEE, AIIMS, PGI 2012/2013

▶ Calcification of cerebral cortex (Railroad Calcification)	❒ Sturge Weber Syndrome☛
▶ Diffuse Nodular calcification	❒ Toxoplasmosis
▶ Amorphous Supracelluler Calcification	❒ Craniopharyngioma ☛
▶ Basal ganglia calcification	❒ Hypoparathyroidism (Commonest)
▶ Rice grain Calcification	❒ Cysticerosis☛
▶ Periventricular Calcification	❒ CMV Infection☛
▶ Sunray Calfication with spicules of brain	❒ Meningioma☛
▶ Bone thickening at site of brain tumor	❒ Meningioma
▶ Punched out Rarefication	❒ Multiple myeloma, sarcoidosis, Gout☛
▶ Pepper pot or Salt and pepper app	❒ Hyperparathyroidism☛
▶ Beaten silver app	❒ Raised intracranial pressure☛
▶ Post clenoid erosion	❒ Raised intracranial pressure☛
▶ Candle grease dripping or trouser leg appearance	❒ Intramedullary tumors in myelography

⇨ Waterhouse-Friderichsen Syndrome

Waterhouse-Friderichsen Syndrome. ☛

- **Massive bilateral adrenal cortical hemorrhage** occurs in eases of fulminating **meningococcal septicemia** and in some cases of streptococcal, staphylococcal or pneumococcal septicemia.
- Most cases occur in infants and young children, but it can happen in adults with severe hemorrhage or burns. The onset is catastrophic, with rigors, hyperpyrexia, cyanosis and vomiting.
- Petechial hemorrhages into the skin which coalesce rapidly into purpuric blotches are a constant feature. Profound shock follows, and before long the patient passes into coma.
- The condition is one of overwhelming sepsis that pursues a galloping course, death occurring in most eases within 48 hours of the onset of symptoms unless correct treatment is given without delay.

⇨ Conditions Involving Pituitary Gland

Craniopharyngioma. ☛

- Craniopharyngiomas represent 3 to 5% of intracranial neoplasms and arise from either sellar or extrasellar remnants of **Rathke's pouch**.
- These tumors **usually affect children** and produce symptoms of increased **intracranial pressure** (headache, vomiting, somnolence) as well as visual disturbances.
- **Calcification within the tumor** is readily seen on CT.☛
- **Transfrontal resection** is the treatment of choice for craniopharyngioma.☛
- Craniopharyngiomas are **generally resistant to radiation therapy.** ☛

1

SURGERY

Pituitary Apoplexy.
— Pituitary apoplexy follows **sudden hemorrhage into or infarction** of a pituitary tumor. Symptoms occur suddenly due to **expansion of blood within the sella** and include severe headache, **stiff neck, loss of vision, and extraocular nerve palsies.**
— Secondary adrenal insufficiency may lead to hypotension and shock.
— Pituitary apoplexy most often occurs in an undiagnosed pituitary tumor but can appear during radiation therapy for pituitary tumors, during anticoagulation, or after closed-head trauma.
— Acute pituitary apoplexy is a neurosurgical emergency that requires acute transsphenoidal decompression of the sella.

⇨ Sites of Origin of Brain Tumors

— Craniopharyngiomas occur in the **suprasellar region** and produce endocrine symptoms.
— Ependymomas arise in the floor of the **fourth ventricle**, and grow to occupy its lumen.
— Medulloblastomas arise in the **cerebellar vermis** and grow down into the fourth ventricle.
— Meningiomas are extrinsic tumors that arise from the **arachnoid cap cells**. They are very common in adults, but are rare in children.

➲ High Yield for AIPGMEE, AIIMS, PGI 2012/2013

Sheehan's Syndrome.

Pituitary necrosis may occur rarely after **postpartum hemorrhage and hypovolemia**. The degree of subsequent hypopituitarism reflects the extent of pituitary necrosis and may include adrenal insufficiency hypothyroidism, and amenorrhea. An inability to breastfeed postpartum due to destruction of oxytocin containing neurons of the posterior pituitary is an early clue to this diagnosis.

Empty Sella Syndrome.

Results from **arachnoid herniation through an incomplete diaphragma sellae.** This syndrome may occur in the absence of a recognized pituitary tumor and is either primary due to a congenital diaphragmatic defect or secondary due to an injury to the diaphragm by pituitary surgery, radiation, or infarction.

Primary empty sella syndrome occurs in **obese, multiparous, hypertensive women who experience headaches but have no underlying neurologic disorders**. Pituitary function is usually normal, but occasionally PRL is increased and GH reserve is reduced. Secondary empty sella syndrome is observed in patients with otherwise benign CSF hypertension and in patients with a loss of pituitary function due to apoplexy or surgical therapy.

➲ Herniation Syndromes:

⇨ The Classic Presentation

Foramen Magnum Herniation

Clinical Findings	Imaging Findings	Complications
✓ Bilateral arm dysesthesia ✓ Obtundation	✓ Cerebellar tonsils at the level of the dens on axial images ✓ Cerebellar tonsils on sagittal images 5 mm below foramen magnum in adults; 7 mm below in children	✓ Obtundation and Death

⇨ Ascending Transtentorial Herniation

Clinical Findings	Imaging Findings	Complications
Nausea Vomiting Obtundation	Spinning top appearance of midbrain Narrowing of bilateral ambient cisterns Filling of the quadrigeminal plate cistern	Hydrocephalus Rapid onset of obtundation and possibility of death

⇨ Descending Transtentorial Herniation

Clinical Findings	Imaging Findings	Complications
✓ Ipsilateral dilated pupil ✓ Contralateral hemiparesis ✓ Ipsilateral hemiparesis if Kernohan's Notch is present (false localizer)	✓ Contralateral temporal horn widening ✓ Ipsilateral ambient cistern widening ✓ Ipsilateral prepontine cistern widening ✓ Uncus extending into the suprasellar ✓ Cistern	✓ Occipital infarct from posterior cerebral artery compression

⇨ Subfalcine Herniation

Clinical Findings	Imaging Findings	Complications
✓ Headache ✓ Contralateral leg weakness	✓ Amputation of the ipsilateral aspect of the frontal horn ✓ Asymmetric anterior falx ✓ Obliteration of the ipsilateral atrium of the lateral ventricle ✓ Septum pellucidum shift	✓ Ipsilateral anterior cerebral artery (ACA) infarction as ACA is entrapped under the falx ✓ Other associated herniations

⇨ Caroticocavernous Fistulas

- ✓ Can be caused by **trauma.**
- ✓ Blunt and penetrating head injuries can result in a caroticocavernous fistula.
- ✓ They also can occur spontaneously.
- ✓ Most caroticocavernous fistulas are of spontaneous origin and unknown etiology.
- ✓ Penetrating head injury can lead to fistula formation by direct laceration of intracavernous vessels.

Spontaneous fistula formation has been associated with:

- **Ruptured intracavernous aneurysm,**
- **Fibromuscular dysplasia,**
- **Ehlers-Danlos syndrome and other collagen vascular diseases,**
- **Atherosclerotic vascular disease,**
- **Pregnancy, and**
- **Straining.**

- The onset is usually sudden.
- Ocular manifestations can include **ophthalmic venous hypertension and orbital venous congestion, proptosis, corneal exposure, chemosis, and arterialization of episcleral veins.**
- Other ocular manifestations may include **diplopia, visual loss, cranial nerve palsy (III, IV, V, VI), central retinal vein occlusion, retinopathy, and glaucoma.**
- **Bruit and headache** also may be present upon clinical presentation.

1

SURGERY

⇨ Intra Spinal Tumors

Can be divided into: Extradural, Intradural extramedullary, and Intramedullary

Extradural neoplasms

- Are usually malignant.
- Metastasis, lymphoma and myeloma.
- Typically, such a tumor begins within the vertebral bone and extends into the epidural space or begins within the epidural space.
- In either case, the tumor gradually compresses the spinal cord or cauda equina and interferes with the blood supply to this neural tissue.
- The most common location for an extradural neoplasm is in the thoracic area of the spine.

Intradural Extramedullary Neoplasms

- Tumors that occur within the spinal subarachnoid space are of two types:
- **Benign neoplasms that arise from the meninges (meningiomas) or the nerve roots (neurofibromas, schwannomas),** or
- **Meningiomas present as subdural masses.** **AIIMS 2011**
- **Malignant tumors that have spread through the spinal subarachnoid space from a primary intracranial location (e.g., medulloblastoma, ependymoma, certain pineal region tumors) or from a malignancy elsewhere in the body (meningeal carcinomatosis).**
- A nerve root tumor occasionally extends along the nerve, with one end within the dural sac, an isthmus extending through the intervertebral foramen (and enlarging it), and the other end outside the spine; a tumor with this configuration is called a **dumbbell tumor.**

Intramedullary Neoplasms

- Intramedullary tumors develop within the spinal cord, enlarging it in a fusiform manner.
- The patient experiences a **progressive myelopathy,** and the radiographic studies demonstrate evidence of spinal cord expansion. Although plain X-ray films and CT scans may show enlargement of the spinal canal, MRI with gadolinium enhancement is the most useful test for demonstrating the tumor and any associated syrinx.

⇨ Surgical Conditions Related to Hand:

- **Acute paronychia** subcuticular infection caused by **staph aureus**
- **Chronic Paronychia** chronic nail infection caused by **Candida**
- **Felon** Terminal pulp space infection
- Deep Palmar abscess abscess beneath flexor tendons (Frog Hand)
- Dupuyntern's contracture, Thickening of Palmar/Plantar Fascia

➲ Accessory Surgical Conditions of Limbs/Trunk

High Yield for AIPGMEE, AIIMS, PGI 2012/2013

Klippel–Feil syndrome. This comprises multiple congenital abnormalities in the cervical spine leading to a characteristic **short, stiff neck and a low hairline.** Torticollis, facial asymmetry and webbing of the neck may be apparent.

Sprengel shoulder.☛ This is due to a failure of normal descent of the scapula which **remains high and small** There may be a bony tether, the omovertebral bar, between scapula and spine, which is also prone to anomalies.

Polydactyly Extra digits can be an isolated abnormality, part of a pattern of limb malformation (e.g. tibial deficiency with diplopodia) or syndromic, as in chondroectodermal dysplasia **(Ellis—van Creveld syndrome)** which consists of short-limbed dwarfism, dysplastic nails, hair and teeth, polydactyly and congenital heart disease.

Hereditary multiple exostoses (diaphyseal aclasis)☛ This is a relatively common, **autosomal dominant dysplasia**. Cartilaginous-capped exostoses occur at the metaphysis and the **osteochondromas** grow with the child and stop growing at maturity.

Achondroplasia: This is the commonest cause of **short-limbed dwarfism** The inheritance trait is **autosomal dominant**, although many cases arise as new mutations. The limbs are short with wide metaphyses, there is lumbar lordosis, the forearm bulges and the nasal bridge is low. Trunk height is maintained but spinal stenosis is common.

Cleidocranial dysostosis: ☛This generalised dysplasia includes partial or complete absence of clavicles, ossification defects in the skull, abnormal dentition and a wide symphysis pubis. The absence of clavicles allows the shoulders to be brought together in front of the chest.

Carpal tunnel syndrome: Median Nerve Involvement The typical patient awakens with painful tingling over the radial side of the hand; there is often loss of fine dexterity because of weakness of the abductor pollicis brevis muscle and altered sensation over the thumb, index and middle fingertips. On examination, **Tinel's percussion sign is positive** over the carpal tunnel and **Phalen's test may be positive** (tingling in the hand when the wrist is fully flexed). In advanced cases, the **thenar eminence is wasted**. The diagnosis, if not certain clinically, is confirmed with electrophysiology. Treatment includes splinting the wrist in extension at night, injecting steroid into the carpal canal and surgical release of the transverse carpal ligament.

De Quervain's disease☛ The **extensor pollicis brevis tendon and abductor pollicis longus** tendon run in a compartment beneath the extensor retinaculum. This compartment can constrict the tendons, causing pain at the base of the thumb. Usually occurring spontaneously in middle-aged women, it is also associated with late pregnancy and overuse. **Finkelstein's test** is positive there is pain over the radial side of the wrist when the patient's thumb is grasped and the hand is quickly abducted ulnarward.

Dupuytren's contracture ☛The condition is inherited as an **autosomal dominant** trait and is more common in males, with age, smoking, pulmonary tuberculosis, epilepsy, acquired immunodeficiency syndrome (AIDS) and alcoholic cirrhosis. **Myofibroblasts in the palmar fascia proliferate and contract**. Initially, there is a nodular swelling in the palm. The overlying skin then puckers. Cords running into the fingers contract causing a flexion deformity of the metacarpophalangeal and proximal interphalangeal joints. The skin over the back of the proximal interphalangeal joints may thicken **(Garrod's knuckle pads)** and a few patients may have thickening in the penis **(Peyronie's disease)** or on the sole of the foot **(Ledderhose's disease)**.

1

SURGERY

⇨ Intravascular Catheter Related Infectious

- ❐ Indwelling vascular catheters are a leading source of bloodstream infections.
- ❐ Amongst indwelling vascular catheters, **central venous catheters are the most common culprits.**

Pathogenesis

Potential sources for catheter related infections-

- **The skin insertion site**
- **The catheter hub**
- **Hematogenous seeding from a distant infection**
- **Contaminated infusate**

- The skin insertion site and the catheter hub are by for the two most important sources.
- Approximately **65%** of catheter related infections originate from the skin flora, 30% from the contaminated hub and 5% from other pathways.
- For **short term catheters**, skin contamination is the most likely mechanism of pathogenesis.
- On the other hand, for **long term catheters,** hub contamination is more frequent because such catheters often have to be intercepted and manipulated.
- **Skin organisms** migrate from the skin insertion site along the external surface of catheter, colonizing the distal intravascular tip of the catheter I and ultimately causing blood-stream infection. On the other hand, in hub. Related infections, organisms are usually introduced into the hub from the hands of medical personnel and the organisms migrate along the internal surface of the catheter, where they can cause a bloodstream j infection.

Microbiology

- ✓ Most of the micro-organisms implicated in CRIs arise from the skin flora.
- ✓ **Staphylococci are the most frequently isolated pathogens, paricularly coagulase-negative staphylococci.**

⇨ Commonly asked and used Scoring Parameters

BLS has three components:	**JK BOPEE 08**
A Airway B Breathing C Circulation	
ATLS is advanced trauma Life Support	
GCS is Glasgow Coma Scale	
ABCDE is Airway, Breathing, Circulation, Disability assessment, Exposure	
TRISS includes (RR, BP, GCS)	**AI 2010**
APACHE (Acute Physiology and Chronic Health Evaluation)	
HESS and HUNT scale is used for SAH	**AI 2010**

⇨ ICU Management: A to J

A: Asepsis/Airway
B: Bedsore/encourage Breathing/Blood pressure
C: Circulation/encourage Coughing/Consciousness
D: Drains
E: ECG
F: Fluid status
G: GI losses/Gag reflex
H: Head positioning/Height
I: Insensible losses
J: Jugular venous pulse

⇨ Important Surgical Points in Diabetes

The most common site of infection in diabetics is the urinary tract.

- **Pyelonephritis,**
- **Papillary necrosis,**
- **Emphysematous pyelonephritis, and**
- **Perinephric abscesses** are all more common in diabetics.

Unusual infections are also seen, including

- **Rhinocerebral mucormycosis**, an invasive fungal infection of the nose and sinuses
- **Malignant external otitis**, an invasive bacterial infection of the auditory canal usually caused by Pseudomonas aeruginosa.
- **Necrotizing cellulitis and** especially in the perineal region of male diabetics who have recently had urethral catheterization. Known as **Fournier's gangrene**
- Impaired Wound Healing
- Cholelithiasis
- **Gangrene of the gallbladder**

- ✓ **A peripheral, symmetric sensorimotor neuropathy** with
- ✓ The most common manifestation is **peripheral neuropathy of the feet** and distal lower extremity, with loss of protective sensation in the foot.
- ✓ Minor trauma may develop into a serious necrotizing infection with tissue loss.
- ✓ Normal adjustments of the foot in weight bearing do not occur, and **heavy calluses** form over pressure points, adding to the pressure and causing necrosis under the callus.
- ✓ **Foot problems are the most common indication for hospital admission in diabetics. Necrobiosis lipoidica diabeticorum.**

The **most common site of infection in diabetics is the urinary tract.** **DNB 2011**

Pyelonephritis, papillary necrosis, emphysematous pyelonephritis, and perinephric abscesses are all more common in diabetics.

Pulmonary infections with common bacterial organisms such as Streptococcus pneumoniae, Escherichia coli, and Staphylococcus aureus also occur frequently and are associated with high mortality rates. Unusual infections are also seen, including rhinocerebral mucormycosis, an invasive fungal infection of the nose and sinuses, and **malignant external otitis**, an invasive bacterial infection of the auditory canal usually caused by Pseudomonas aeruginosa. **AIPGME 2012**

Necrotizing cellulitis and fasciitis can occur, especially in the perineal region of male diabetics who have recently had urethral catheterization. Known as Fournier's gangrene, this polymicrobial infection with aerobic and anaerobic organisms must be treated with prompt aggressive surgical débridement, colostomy, and systemic antibiotics.

⇨ Interesting Facts in Relation to Fruits and Vegetables, etc.

▶ **Potato Nodes:** Sarcoidosis☛
▶ **Potato Tumor:** Chemodectoma☛
▶ **Potato/oyster ovary:** PCOD☛
▶ **Straw berry Gallbladder** Cholesterosis
▶ **Straw Berry Tongue** Scarlet Fever
▶ **Straw Berry Cervix** Trichomonas Vaginalis
▶ **Strawberry hemangioma:** Nevus vasculosus
▶ **Barley coloured fluid cyst:** Spermatocele☛
▶ **Aple jelly nodules:** Lupus Vulgaris☛
▶ **Apple core lesion:** Ca Colon☛
▶ **Raspberry tumor:** Umbilical adenoma☛
▶ **Raspberry thorn sign:** Crohns disease

➲ Surgical Oncology: High Yield for AIPGMEE, AIIMS, PGI 2012/2013

⇨ Latest Tumor Markers

▶ **Alpha feto protein**	Hepatocellular carcinoma
▶ **CEA☛**	Adenocarcinoma colon, pancreas, lung, ovary
▶ **PSA**	Prostate cancer
▶ **Neuron Speciic enolase☛**	Small cell lung cancer, Neuroblastoma
▶ **LDH**	Lymphoma
▶ **Cathecolamines**	Pheochromocytoma
▶ **Beta 2 microglobulin☛**	Multiple Myeloma Lymphoma
▶ **Bladder Tumor Antigen☛**	Bladder Tumor, UTI, Renal Calculi

▶ CA27.29	Breast Cancer
▶ CA 72.4	Ovarian and Pancreatic Cancer
▶ LASA -P (Lipid Associated Sialic Acid)	Ovarian Cancer
▶ NMP 22	Bladder Cancer
▶ HCG	Gestational Trophoblastic Disorders
▶ CA 125	Ovarian Cancer
▶ Placental Alkaline Phosphatase	Seminoma
▶ S100	Melanoma, Neural Tumors

Serum Thyroglobulin. MARKER OF THYROID CANCER. KCET 2012

Thyroglobulin is produced **only by thyroid tissue**. Normal persons have low but detectable thyroglobulin levels. Total surgical removal of thyroid tissue for cancer should result in undetectable thyroglobulin levels. **Determination of thyroglobulin levels by immunoassays has its most useful application following thyroid cancer surgery**. The upper normal limit of thyroglobulin is 20 to 25 ng per deciliter, and levels above that range may indicate a return of thyroid cancer. Thyroglobulin levels also increase when patients become hypothyroid, as occurs, for example, in preparation for radioactive iodine scanning and treatment.

⇨ Also Remember

▶ Intermediate Filament	▶ Tumor
▶ Keratin	▶ Carcinoma
▶ Vimentin	▶ Sarcoma
▶ Desmin	▶ Muscle
▶ Neurofilaments	▶ Phechromocytoma, Neuroblastoma
▶ Glial Fibrillary Acidic Protein (GFAP)	▶ Astrocytomas, Ependymomas

⇨ Types of Secondaries

Osteo lytic secondaries	Osteoblastic Secondaries
▶ Kidney	▶ Prostate, Seminoma
▶ Lung	▶ Breast, Uterus, Ovary
▶ Thyroid	▶ Carcinoid
▶ GIT	▶ Osteosarcoma

⇨ Spontaneous Regression is Seen in:

- ▶ Renal cell carcinoma
- ▶ Retinoblastoma
- ▶ Choriocarcinoma
- ▶ Neuroblastoma
- ▶ Malignant Melanoma

⇨ Radiation Induced Tumors/Cancers

- Acute Leukemia (MC)
- Pappilary ca of thyroid
- Breast vca
- Lung ca (Radon)
- Angisarcoma of liver (Thorotrast)
- Skin cancers (BCC, SQ CALL, Malig Melanoma)
- Brain Tumor
- Osteosarcoma

⇨ Sentinel Node Biopsy is done in

- Ca Breast
- Melanoma
- Ca penis

⇨ Immunotherapy is done in: High Yield for AIPGMEE, AIIMS, PGI 2012/2013

- BCG: Bladder ca☚
- Levamisole: Colorectal ca
- IFN α: Melanoma, Lymphoma
- Cytokines: RCC, Melanoma☚
- Corynebacterium Parvum: Ovarian Cancer☚

➲ Pulsating Tumors: High Yield for AIPGMEE, AIIMS, PGI 2012/2013

- RCC Secondaries☚
- Osteosarcoma☚
- Osteoclastoma☚
- Sec from Follucular Ca Thyroid☚

Cancer Type Environmental Risk Factor

- Lung: Smoking, Asbestos, Nickel, Radon, Coal, Arsenic , Chromium,
- Mesothilioma: Asbestos
- Bladder Ca Smoking, Aniline dyes, Schistomiasis
- Skin Ca: UV light exposure, coal, Tar, Arsenic
- Liver: Alcohol, Vinyl chloride, Aflatoxins
- Pancreas: Smoking
- Renal Cell Carcinoma: Smoking
- Stomach: Alcohol, Nitrosamines

⇨ Screening and Tumors: PGI 2009

- Breast Cancer: Self examination +mammography
- Cervical Cancer: Pap smear examination
- Colorectal Cancer: Fecal occult blood test, digital rectal examination , Sigmoidoscopy and colonoscopy in high-risk group particularly.
- Prostate: Digital rectal examination and PSA level

⇨ Extent of Minimal Access surgery

Laparoscopy

A rigid endoscope is introduced through a metal sleeve into the peritoneal cavity which has been previously inflated with carbon dioxide to produce a pneumoperitoneum.

Thoracoscopy

A rigid endoscope is introduced through an incision in the chest to gain access to the thoracic contents.

Endoluminal Endoscopy

Flexible or rigid endoscopes are introduced into hollow organs or systems, such as the urinary tract, upper or lower gastrointestinal tract, and respiratory and vascular systems.

Perivisceral Endoscopy

Body planes can be accessed even in the absence of a natural cavity. Examples are mediastinoscopy, retroperitoneoscopy and retroperitoneal approaches to the kidney, aorta and lumbar sympathetic chain.

ORGAN	MAXIMUM COLD STORAGE TIME
❒ Kidney	48 hrs ☛
❒ Liver	24 hrs
❒ Pancreas	24 hrs
❒ Small intestine	8 hrs
❒ Heart	6 hrs
❒ Lung	8 hrs

➲ "Important Surgeries" (Frequently Asked)☛:

High Yield for AIPGMEE, AIIMS, PGI 2012/2013

- Nissens Fundoplication Hiatus Hernia ☛
- Ramsteads Pyloromyotomy Hypertrophic Pyloric Stenosis ☛ ☛
- Whipples Pancreaticoduodenectomy ☛
- Hellers Operation Achlasia Cardia ☛ ☛

1

SURGERY

Prolapse Rectum	
➨ Thierischs Surgery	
➨ Ripsteins Surgery ☚	
➨ Delormes Surgery ☚	AI 2010
➨ Wells Surgery	
➨ Lauhats Surgery	
Hydronephrosis	
➨ Anderson Hynes Pyeloplasty ☚	AI 2010
Inguinal Hernia Repair	
➨ Bassini Repair ☚	
➨ Shouldice Repair	
➨ Lytle Plication	
Femoral Hernia	
➨ Mc Eveddy ☚	
➨ Losenthein	
➨ Lockwood	
Varicose veins	
➨ Tredlenburgs ☚ ☚	
➨ Coccket and Dodd	
Hirschsprungs Disease	
➨ Modiofied Duhamel ☚	
➨ Swensons	
➨ Soaves	
Meconium Ileus	
➨ **The Bishop-Koop enterostomy or double-barrel enterostomy**, which were popular methods of treatment in the past, are rarely necessary in the present era. Avoidance of an enterostomy facilitates early discharge from the hospital and reduces the risk of hospital-acquired cross-infection. In instances of meconium ileus complicated by atresia, volvulus, perforation, or gangrenous bowel, bowel resection and anastomosis or temporary enterostomy is required.	KCET 2012

⇨ Surgical Shunts for Praipism

- A transglanular to corpus cavernosal scalpel or needle-core biopsy (**Ebbehoj or Winter technique**) is the first reasonable approach for refractory cases. A unilateral shunt is often effective. Bilateralshunts are used only if necessary.
- **Quackel shunts** are cavernosal-spongiosum shunts (unilateral or bilateral) and are performed via a perineal approach.
- **Gray hack shunt** is a cavernosal-saphenous vein shunt (rarely necessary or indicated).

The operations done in morbid obese patients are as follows Classification of surgical procedures:

Predominantly Malabsorptive Procedures
1. Biliopancreatic diversion
2. Jejunoileal bypass
3. Endoluminal sleeve
Predominantly Restrictive Procedures
1. Vertical Band Gastroplasty
2. Adjustable gastric band
3. Sleeve gastrectomy
4. Intragastric balloon
Mixed Procedures
1. Gastric Bypass Surgery
2. Sleeve gastrectomy with duodenal switch
3. Implantable Gastric Stimulation   AIPGME 2010

➲ Obesity

- ❐ **Is a state of excess adipose tissue mass.**
- ❐ **Body mass index (BMI), which is equal to weight/height^2 (in kg/m^2)**
- ❐ Specifically, **intraabdominal and abdominal subcutaneous fat have more significance** than subcutaneous fat present in the buttocks and lower extremities.
- ❐ **Appetite** is influenced by many factors that are integrated by the brain, most importantly within the hypothalamus Hormonal signals include leptin, insulin, cortisol, and gut peptides such as cholecystokinin, which signals to the brain through the vagus nerve.
- ❐ These diverse hormonal, metabolic, and neural signals act by influencing the expression and release of various hypothalamic peptides e.g., **neuropeptide Y (NPY), Agouti-related peptide (AgRP), a melanocyte-stimulating hormone (MSH), and melanin concentrating hormone (MCH)** that are integrated with serotonergic, catecholaminergic, and opioid signaling pathways.
- ❐ Mutations in the gene encoding **proopiomelanocortin (POMC)** cause severe obesity through failure to synthesize a-MSH, a key neuropeptide that inhibits appetite in the hypothalamus.

Specific Syndromes Associated with Obesity:

- **Cushing's Syndrome**
- **Hypothyroidism**
- **Insulinoma**
- **Craniopharyngioma**

⇨ Pathologic Consequences of Obesity

- **Insulin Resistance and Type 2 Diabetes Mellitus**
- **Reproductive Disorders** Male hypogonadism, menstrual abnormalities in women
- **Cardiovascular Disease**
- **Pulmonary Disease**
- **Gallstones**
- **Cancer** cancer of the gallbladder, bile ducts, breasts, endometrium, cervix, and ovaries
- **Bone, Joint, and Cutaneous Disease** increased risk of osteoarthritis.

⇨ Treatment

- ✓ **Behavior Modification** The principles of behavior modification provide the underpinnings for
- ✓ **Diet** Reduced caloric intake is the cornerstone of obesity treatment.
- ✓ **Exercise** Exercise is an important component of the overall approach to treating obesity.
- ✓ **Drugs**
  - **Phentermine** is an amphetamine-like drug
  - **Sibutramine** is a central reuptake inhibitor of both norepinephrine and serotonin
  - **Recombinant human leptin**
  - New drugs are also being developed based on insights into central pathways that regulate body weight. These include antagonists for **NPY receptors (subtypes Y1, Y5) and agonists for melanocortin 4 receptors.**
- ✓ Surgery for Morbid obesity
- ✓ **Morbid obesity is a serious and increasingly common disease that represents a severe handicap and is associated with major health problems, including diabetes, hypertension, biliary disease, arthritis, and a number of other disorders. Because diets rarely produce sustained weight loss in these patients, operation has become the treatment of choice. Three operations are done:**
  - **The gastric bypass,**
  - **The vertical banded gastroplasty,** **DNB 2011**
  - **Kuzmak's Silastic banding**

➲ Important Pouches in Surgery

High Yield for AIPGMEE, AIIMS, PGI 2012/2013

- **Morrisons Pouch: Hepatorenal pouch** is a potential space, the hepatorenal recess is not normally filled with fluid. However, this space becomes **significant in conditions in which fluid collects within the abdomen** (most commonly **ascites** and **hemoperitoneum**). As little as 30 or 40 ml of fluid in the abdominal cavity may be visualized in this space. Early visualization of fluid in the hepatorenal recess on **FAST scan** may be an indication for urgent laparotomy.
- **Rectouterine pouch (Pouch of Douglas)**: Is the extension of the peritoneal cavity between the **rectum** and **back wall of the uterus in the female human body**. The rectouterine pouch is used in the treatment of end-stage renal failure in patients who are treated by peritoneal dialysis. The tip of the dialysis catheter is placed into the deepest point of the pouch.

- **Rectovesical Pouch** Between the **rectum and the bladder**, the peritoneal cavity forms, in the male, a pouch or **rectovesical pouch** about 7.5 cm. from the orifice of the anus. A membranous partition called the Rectoprostatic fascia (Denonvillier's fascia) is located at the lowest part of the rectovesical pouch.
- **Rathke's pouch** is a **depression in the roof of the developing mouth in front of the buccopharyngeal membrane**. It gives **rise to the anterior pituitary (adenohypophysis)**, a part of the endocrine system. The pouch eventually loses its connection with the pharynx giving rise to the anterior pituitary. The anterior wall of Rathke's pouch proliferates, filling most of the pouch to form pars distalis and pars tuberalis. The posterior wall forms pars intermedia. **Rathke's pouch may develop benign cysts. (Craniopharyngioma)** is a neoplasm which can arise from the epithelium within the cleft.
- The **Ileoanal pouch** is a **surgical treatment option for chronic ulcerative colitis, colon cancer and familial polyposis patients who need to have their large intestine (colon) removed.** An ileoanal reservoir (or pouch) is an internal pouch formed of small intestine. This pouch provides a storage place for stool in the absence of the large intestine. Anal sphincter muscles assist in holding in the stool. Several times a day, stool is passed through the anus. Ileoanal reservoir surgery is a widely accepted surgical treatment for ulcerative colitis or familial polyposis because it eliminates the disease, gives the patient control of bowel movements and does not require a permanent ileostomy. Each patient considering this surgery is carefully evaluated to determine if this procedure is appropriate for them. This procedure is performed in one, two or three stages, but is most often done in two stages, usually 2-3 months apart.
- **Hartmann's pouch** is an **out-pouching of the wall of the gallbladder at the junction of the neck of the gallbladder** and the cystic duct. Its identification is useful in delineating biliary anatomy when performing a cholecystectomy.

Graft-Versus-Host Disease

- GVHD is the result of **allogeneic T cells that were either transferred with the donor's stem cell inoculum or develop from it, reacting with antigenic targets on host cells.**
- GVHD developing within the first 3 months posttransplant is termed **acute GVHD,**
- GVHD developing or persisting beyond 3 months posttransplant is termed **chronic GVHD.**
- Acute GVHD most often first becomes apparent between 2 and 4 weeks posttransplant and is characterized by an erythematous maculopapular rash; persistent anorexia or diarrhea, or both; and by liver disease with increased serum levels of bilirubin, alanine and aspartate aminotransferase, and alkaline phosphatase.
- **Diagnosis usually requires skin, liver, or endoscopic biopsy** for confirmation. In all these organs, endothelial damage and lymphocytic infiltrates are seen.
- **Grade I acute GVHD is of little clinical significance**, does not affect the likelihood of survival, and does not require treatment.
- In contrast, **grades II to IV GVHD are associated with significant symptoms and a poorer probability of survival and require aggressive therapy.**
- One general approach to the prevention of GVHD is the **administration of immunosuppressive drugs early after transplant.** **HIGH Yield for 2011-2012**

➲ Surgical Oncology:

High Yield for AIPGMEE, AIIMS, PGI 2012/2013

- MC Cancer in Gynecology: Endometrial Carcinoma
- MC Cancer in Infancy: Hemangioma
- MC Cancer in Kids: Leukemia
- MC Cancer in Men: Prostate CA
- MC Cancer in Women: Leiomyoma (fibroids)
- MC Cancer of the Adrenal Medulla- **adults** -Pheochromocytoma
- MC Cancer of the Adrenal Medulla- **kids**- Neuroblastoma
- MC Cancer of the Appendix: **Carcinoid**
- MC Cancer of the Bone Metastases from **Breast & Prostate**
- MC Cancer of the Bone - **primary** - adults -Multiple Myeloma
- MC Cancer of the Brain- Child- **Medulloblastoma** (cerebellum)
- MC Cancer of the Breast -Infiltrating ductal adenocarcinoma
- MC Cancer of the Connective Tissue -Benign Lipoma
- MC Cancer of the Esophagus: Leiomyoma
- MC Cancer of the Esophagus - Malignant SCC (60%) > adenocarcinoma (40%)
- MC Cancer of the Heart - adults -Metastases
- MC Cancer of the Heart - **Primary**- **adults** -Myxoma
- MC Cancer of the Heart - **Primary**- **kids**- Rhabdomyoma
- MC Cancer of the Liver Metastasis; Lung > GI
- MC Cancer of the Liver - Benign Cavernous hemangioma
- MC Cancer of the liver - Primary Hepatocellular CA

- ❒ MC Cancer of the Mouth - SCC or Mucoepidermoid CA
- ❒ MC Cancer of the Mouth - Upper lip Basal Cell CA
- ❒ MC Cancer of the Nasal cavities: SCC
- ❒ MC Cancer of the Ovary - **Benign** -Serous cystadenoma
- ❒ MC Cancer of the Ovary - **Malignant** - Serous cystadenocarcinoma
- ❒ MC Cancer of the Pancreas- Adenocarcinoma (usually in the head)
- ❒ MC Cancer of the Pituitary Prolactinoma
- ❒ MC Cancer of the Placenta - benign Cavernous hemangioma
- ❒ MC Cancer of the Salivary Glands: Pleimorphic Adenoma
- ❒ MC Cancer of the Skin: Basal Cell Carcinoma
- ❒ MC Cancer of the Small Bowel Carcinoid - frequent metastasis from **ileum**

- ❐ MC Cancer of the Spleen - Benign Cavernous hemangiomas
- ❐ MC Cancer of the Stomach Gastric Adenocarcinoma
- ❐ MC Cancer of the Testicles: Seminoma
- ❐ MC Cancer of the Thyroid: Papillary Carcinoma
- ❐ MC Cancer that invades the Female GU tract Endometrial Adenocarcinoma
- ❐ MC Cancer; Site of metastasis **Regional Lymph Nodes (2nd most common)** Liver

Esophagus:	
— **MC type** of esophageal cancer: squamous cell ca	**AI 91**
— **Mc site** of esophageal cancer: lower end	**AIIMS 97**
— Mc site of Adeno carcinoma: lower end	**AIIMS 2000**
— Most common site of squamous cell ca: middle 1/3	**AI 2001**
Pancreas	
— **Most common is:** Ductal adenocarcinomas,	
— **Most common in:** Pancreatic head (70% of cases)	**PGI 2000**
— **Most common symptom is:** Pain and weight loss.	**PGI 2000**
— **Most common physical sign is:** Jaundice.	
GallBladder	
— Adenocarcinoma **most common type.**	
— Fundus is the **most common site.**	
— Biliary colic is the **most common presentation.**	
— Gallstones are the **most common predisposition.**	
— **Adeno carcinoma** is the most common type of **Rectal cancer**	**PGI 2005**
— **Epidermoid cancer** is the most common type of **Anal cancer**	**PGI 2007**

⇨ Thyroid:

— Thyroid tumor associated with MEN II: Medullary carcinoma	
— Thyroid tumor in **Throglossal cyst:** Papillary carcinoma	
— Thyroid tumor in **Hashimotos Thyroioditis:** Papillary carcinoma	
— Thyroid tumor with **best prognosis:** Papillary carcinoma	
— Thyroid tumor **least malignant:** Papillary carcinoma	**AIIMS 2003**
— Thyroid tumor associated with worst prognosis: Anaplastic cancer	
— Thyroid tumor rarest : Anaplastic	

- ❐ MC **anterior** mediastinal mass: Thymoma
- ❐ MC **middle** mediastinal mass: Bronchogenic cyst
- ❐ MC **Posterior** mediastinal mass: Neurogenic tumor
- ❐ MC **malignant** mass of Mediastinum: Lymphomas

1

SURGERY

➲ Commonest Site of Intestinal Lesions:

High Yield for AIPGMEE, AIIMS, PGI 2012/2013

Lesion	Area
✓ Lipoma	— Cecum
✓ Lymphoma(Non hodgkins)	— Stomach (Least : Rectum)
✓ Adenomatous polypi	— Sigmoid, rectum
✓ Polypi in Puetzjeghers syndrome	— Always Jejunum is involved
✓ Familial Polyposis and Gardener's syndrome	— Colon
✓ ZES gastrinoma	— Pancreas
✓ Carcinoma small intestine	— Jejunum
✓ Carcinoma Colon	— Sigmoid colon and ectosigmoid,
✓ Tuberculosis Ulcer	— Small Intestine **(Transverse)**
✓ Typhoid Ulcer	— Small Intestine **(Longitudinal)**
✓ Crohn's disease	— Starts at or near Ileo cecal Valve
✓ Ulcerative Colitis	— Starts at rectum
✓ Diverticulosis	— 90% in sigmoid (Rectum is never involved)
✓ Perforation in Typhoid	— Small intestine near Ileo cecal Junction
✓ Pneumatosis Cystoides	— Small Intestine
✓ Commonest Type of Intussesception	— Ileo cecal
✓ Volvulus Neonatorum	— Midgut (Whole small intestine and Cecum)
✓ Volvulus Small intestine	— ileum
✓ Ischemic Colitis	— Splenic flexure
✓ Dilatation of Gut in Chaga's disease	— Esophagus and Colon
✓ in Blast Injury	— Pelvic Colon

➲ Clinical Wrap UP: High Yield Questions Repeated

⇨ Important Clinical Scenarios: High Yield for AIPGMEE, AIIMS, PGI 2012/2013

▶ **Sixth post operative day, salmon colored fluid on dressing**	▶ **Wound Dehiscence**
▶ **Burning retrosternal pain aggreviated by bending,** lying flat	▶ **GERD**
▶ A 35 year old with **dysphagia for liquids more than solids** regurgitating undigested food	▶ **Achlasia cardia** ▶
▶ An **elderly man** who is a smoker and drinks as well has **progressive dysphagia** and loses weight	▶ **Gastric Ca**

▶ After a heavy drink and violent episode of vomiting, a patient feels **severe epigastric pain** and is diaphoretic	▶ **Boorhavees rupture**
▶ After a heavy drink patient **vomits bright red blood repeatedly**	▶ **Mallory Weiss Tear**
▶ An elderly man who is a heavy drinker faints during his job. His examination shows **occult blood in stools**	▶ **Colonic cancer**
▶ A patient of **Ulcerative colitis has severe abdominal pain,** leukocytosis and high temperature with **massively distended colon on X-ray**	▶ **Toxic Megacolon**
▶ A patient postoperatively **on clindamycin** complains of **watery diarrhea, crampy abdominal pain**	▶ **Pseudomembranous colitis**
▶ A patient with **perianal pain, cant sit down with fever and chills with tender, fluctuant mass** between anus and ischial tuberosity	▶ **Ischiorectal abscess**
▶ A **six year old boy** passes a **bloody bowel movement**	▶ **Meckels diverticulitis**
▶ A young boy complains of **right flank colicky pain radiating to inner thigh or scrotum**	▶ **Ureteric colic**
▶ A 45 years female complains of Colicky right hypochondriac pain with **radiation to rt scapula**	▶ **Acute Cholecystitis**
▶ A 75 year old male with nausea, vomiting, colicky abdominal pain. ▶ X-rays show distended loops of bowel with large air shadow like **parrots beak.**	▶ **Sigmoid volvolus**

▶ A cirrhotic develops malaise, right hypochondric pain with weight loss and **AFP levels**	▶ **Hepatoma**
▶ A person with colonic ca shows nodularities in liver with **CEA levels**	▶ **Metastatic tumor**
▶ A 30 year old female **on OCPS develops sudden onset abdominal pain** with tachycardia and hypotension. No history of trauma.	▶ **Bleeding from ruptured hepatic adenoma**
▶ A 55 year old has **progressive jaundice with weight loss, ↑alkaline phosphatase, nagging epigastric** and back pain USG reveals **dilated intra and extra hepatic ducts** with **thin walled GB**	▶ **Pancreatic Ca**
▶ After treatment of **acute pancreatitis**, the patient comes after 7 weeks with **ill defined epigastric mass**	▶ **Pancreatic pseudo cyst**
▶ After an **automobile accident**, the patient comes after 7 weeks with ill **defined epigastric mass**	▶ **Pancreatic pseudo cyst**

▶ A patient with **recurrent** peptic ulcer disease. H. pylori was **not detected.** There are **multiple ulcers** on First and second portions of duodenum	▶ Gastrinoma
▶ A 44 years old female has **migratory necrolytic dermatitis.** She is **diabetic** and thin	▶ Glucagonoma
▶ A 33 year old male with **pounding headache, palpitations, perspirations and increased VMA levels**	▶ Pheochromocytoma
▶ A 55 years old female with flushing, **non healing diarrheas and bronchospasm with increased 5HIAA levels**	▶ Carcinoid Tumor
▶ A 20 years old female with **hypertension not responding to antihypertensives** with **bruit over renal area**	▶ Fibromuscular Dysplasia
▶ A 75 years old with **hypertension not responding to antihypertensives** with bruit over renal area	▶ Renal artery Stenosis

- ❒ 30 years of women comes with dysphagia for both solid and liquids and barium swallow shows Parrot beak appearance. On esophageal manometry. Increased LES pressure is: **Achalasia cardia**
- ❒ Increasing difficulty in swallowing both for solids and liquids in a woman with **bird's beak** appearance in X-ray seen in: **Achalasia cardia.** Management includes: **PGI June 2008, MAH 2012**

❒ A 67 year old male presents with **adenomatous polyposis; osteomas of the mandible, skull, and long bones; and a sebaceous cysts.** Most likely diagnosis is:	Gardeners syndrome High Yield for 2011-2012
❒ A 65 year old has **Tuberculous involvement of Spine** with **paraspinal abscess extending beneath the paraspinal muscle and extending down the psoas muscle** and presents as a mass in the medial thigh. On incision, this **mass produces caseous necrotic material** without any associated erythema. This clinical presentation is known as:	Cold abscess
❒ The type of **lymphedema most commonly involving the dorsum of the foot** and lower extremity up to the level of the knee with a **familial history** is	Milroys disease High Yield for 2011-2012
❒ A 34 year old **has Frontal osteomyelitis with marked overlying soft tissue swelling** that is secondary to frontal sinusitis is referred to as:	Potts puffy tumor High Yield for 2011-2012
❒ An **elderly patient** who usually takes high fibre diet presents with **acute onset of severe colicky pain, nausea, vomiting, and obstipation.** On abdominal examination a **compressible mass extending from the right lower quadrant to the midabdominal region is felt.** Plain abdominal roentgenograms reveals **marked distention of the cecum as well as small bowel dilatation.** Barium enema classically reveals the narrowing accompanying the twisting of the colon **(so-called bird's neck deformity).** Most likely cause is:	Cecal volvolus

❒ A 25 year old medical student has **enlarged hair follicles in otherwise normal skin**. The follicle holds a single hair shaft surrounded by rings of keratin. The **cavity contains pus under pressure** and a wall of edematous fat; polymorphonuclear cells predominate. The cavity has a wall of **fibrous tissue lined by granulation tissue of capillaries, lymphocytes, and giant cells.** The cavity is laden with Staphylococcus aureus and other organisms, including anaerobes. Most likely diagnosis is:	**Pilonidal sinus** **High Yield for 2011-2012**
❒ **A prematurely borne** infant fails to tolerate attempted feeding. **Bilious vomiting** is observed and initiates a diagnostic evaluation. Plain x-ray of the abdomen demonstrates **one air bubble in the stomach and the second in the duodenum proximal** to the obstruction. Most Likely diagnosis is:	**Duodenal atresia** **High Yield for 2011-2012**
❒ An infant appears **dyspneic, tachypneic, and cyanotic** and has severe retractions with an increased chest diameter. **Bowel sounds are heard on auscultation of the affected chest**. An anteroposterior chest X-ray demonstrates **air-filled viscera in the chest.** Compression of ipsilateral lung which is **hypoplastic** is also noted. Most likely diagnosis is:	**Congenital Diaphragmatic Hernia** **High Yield for 2011-2012**
❒ A 34 year old female presents with **abdominal mass accompanied by pain, nausea, and vomiting.** The mass is diagnosed on physical examination. It displays a **characteristic lateral mobility and is associated with the bowel mesentery.** The most likely diagnosis is:	**Mesentric cyst**
❒ An **Infant** presents with **abdominal distention and failure to pass meconium in the first 24 hours** of life. Plain abdominal radiographs demonstrate **loops of distended bowel** with air-fluid levels. Barium enema shows a **microcolon extending up to the descending at which point the colon becomes dilated and copious intraluminal material (thick meconium plug)** is observed. Following instillation of the contrast material, large pieces of inspissated meconium is passed and the obstruction is completely relieved. Most likely cause is:	**Meconium plug syndrome** **High Yield for 2011-2012**
❒ A 44 year old has **findings of bilateral hydronephrosis and hydroureter** proximal to the site of **extrinsic compression of the ureters.** The ureters are seen to be **fibrosed over a substantial distance, starting inferiorly and progressing superiorly.** The ureters are **deviated medially** toward the midline. Most likely diagnosis is:	**Ormonds disease** **High Yield for 2011-2012**
❒ A 55 year old patient presents with **seeing double, periorbital edema and headache.** He has BP 130/80 mm Hg. On evaluation he was found to have fever. Ophthalmologist finds **lateral gaze palsy with ptosis and dilated pupil.** Most likely cause is:	**Cavernous sinus thrombosis** **High Yield for 2011-2012**
❒ A 45 year old female has developed a small **nodule at a site of previous** injury with granulation tissue formation. The lesion is neither **non bacterial nor a true granuloma.** Microscopically, **proliferating blood vessels in an immature fibrous stroma are seen.** Most likely the lesion is a:	**Pyogenic granuloma** **High Yield for 2011-2012**

1

SURGERY

❒ A **6 to month-old** brought by his mother presents with **episodes of distress and crying** interspersed with quiet periods of normal behavior and playing. His mother says that **he passes stool mixed with mucus and blood, the jelly stool.** The abdomen is soft and non tender. **A sausage-like mass** may be palpable in the upper abdomen. Most Likely diagnosis is:	Intussesception
❒ A young **girl** presents with **Polyostotic fibrous dysplasia, precocious puberty, café au lait spots, short stature.** Most likely the diagnosis is:	Albrights syndrome High Yield for 2011-2012
❒ A **nonsuppurative inflammatory process** of the retroperitoneum that causes problems by **extrinsic compression of retroperitoneal structures such as the ureters, aorta, and inferior vena** with ureteral obstruction as one of the most common presentation of this disease process is:	Idiopathic retroperitoneal fibrosis High Yield for 2011-2012
❒ A 42 year old non alcoholic presents to Gastroenterologist with multiple episodes of **chest pain, regurgitation of saliva and undigested food.** The characteristic appearance of the esophagram shows a tapered **"bird's beak"** deformity at the level of the esophagogastric junction. Further Manometry yields high resting pressures of the lower esophageal sphincter, which fails to relax. Most likely the disease is:	Achlasia High Yield for 2011-2012 MAH 2012
❒ An 81-year-old man with Alzheimer disease who lives in a nursing home undergoes surgery. For a fractured femoral neck. On the 5th postoperative day, it is noted that his **abdomen is grossly distended and tense, but not tender.** He has occasional bowel sounds. The **rectal vault is empty on digital examination, and there is no evidence of occult blood.** X-ray films show a few **distended loops of small bowel** and a very distended colon. The **cecum measures 9 cm in diameter, and the gas pattern of distention** extends throughout the entire large bowel, including the sigmoid and rectum. No stool is seen in the films. Other than the abdominal distention, and the ravages of his mental disease, he does not appear to be ill. **Vital signs are normal** for his age. The most likely diagnosis is:	Ogilives disease High Yield for 2011-2012
❒ A **29-year-old man** comes to the **clinic with a 2-day history of severe left-sided scrotal pain and swelling.** He **is sexually active and has multiple sexual partners.** He has no history of sexually transmitted diseases. **His temperature is 38.2 C (100.8 F), blood pressure is 120/70 mm Hg, and pulse is 80/min.** Examination shows **unilateral intrascrotal tenderness and swelling. Testicular support makes the pain less intense.** The most likely diagnosis is:	Epididymitis
❒ **A syndrome of Congenital AV fistulas+ Hemangiomas+ Varicose veins + Hypertrophy of limbs is most likely**	Klippel Trenauny syndrome

❑ A 67-year-old man comes to the clinic complaining of **steady, dull back pain** over the past 3 weeks. He states that he has recently moved after retiring from a career in banking and is searching for a new primary care physician. His past medical history is significant for diverticulosis, prior smoking, and hypertension. He says that he has run out of his blood pressure medication. He denies trauma to his back and otherwise feels well. **On physical examination his blood pressure is 170/93 mm Hg with a pulse of 88/min.** He has no tenderness over the spinal processes or paraspinal areas. His abdomen is obese but there is a **suggestion of a non-tender, pulsatile mass in the epigastric region**. The remainder of the physical examination is normal. Most likely diagnosis is:	**Abdominal aortic aneurysm (AAA)** **High Yield for 2011-2012**
❑ A 40 -year-old woman comes to a physician after four months **of intermittent abdominal cramps and diarrhea accompanied by skin flushing** that is most pronounced in the head and neck area. Physical examination **reveals a murmur heard over the tricuspid valve.** Urine special studies for **5-hydroxyindoleacetic acid show excretion of 99mg/day** [reference range 0.5-9.0 mg/day]. **CT scan of the liver demonstrates a 2-cm lesion.** Most likely diagnosis is:	**Carcinoid** **High Yield for 2011-2012**
❑ A developmental abnormality in which the **roof of the fourth ventricle fails to perforate** to form the foramen of Magendie. The resultant **cystic dilatation of the fourth ventricle** expands the posterior fossa, elevating the tentorium and causing **hydrocephalus** because of obstruction of the aqueduct of Sylvius, with concomitant hypoplasia of the cerebellar vermis. Most likely diagnosis is:	**Dandy-Walker malformation** **High Yield for 2011-2012**
❑ A 75 years old presents with symptoms of nonpleuritic chest pain, dyspnea secondary to pleural effusion, Weight loss, fever, and cough also occur with high frequency. Physical examination is notable for dullness to percussion and diminished breath sounds. They **stain positive for keratin.** The chest X-ray shows **pleural plaques, pleural effusion** .Computed tomography demonstrates extrapleural soft tissue invasion and diaphragmatic involvement. The most likely diagnosis is:	**Mesothelioma** **High Yield for 2011-2012**
❑ A 55 year old man presents with **severe hemoptysis.** An organism is isolated and found that it has a tendency to **invade pre-existing pulmonary cavities** and form a **rounded necrotic mass of matted hyphae, fibrin, and inflammatory cells.** This mass usually lies free in the cavity and can change its location as the patient moves from an upright to a recumbent position. On the chest X-ray, **a crescentic radiolucency adjacent to a rounded mass within a cavitary lesion is seen.** A filamentous organism with coarse, septate, fragmented hyphae is isolated.Most likely diagnosis is:	**Aspergillosis**

❐ A young child presents with fever, generalized malaise, and localized **pain in the left lower extremity**. Laboratory examination reveals a leukocytosis> 17,000 cells per ml, **mild to moderate anemia, and a markedly elevated erythrocyte sedimentation rate.** The patient appears toxic and irritable, and any manipulation of the extremity produces paroxysms of pain. The child refuses to **move the involved limb, mimicking a neurologic deficit.** The condition is called:	**Reflex dystrophy** **High Yield for 2011-2012**
❐ A **benign growth of hyaline cartilage** lying in the medullary cavity of a bone arising from **ectopic cartilaginous rests in the phalanges** and metacarpals and Radiographically, producing a **lucent defect with well-defined margins and surrounding sclerotic reactive bone** are most likely:	**Enchondroma** **High Yield for 2011-2012**
❐ **A 55 year old male has diabetes mellitus, weight loss and skin rash.** Rash is prominent on buttocks. Dermatologist refers it to as **necrolytic migratory erythema.** Most likely diagnosis is:	**Glucagonoma**

❐ A **16 year old** female **has firm, rubbery mass** in right breast **moving with palpation**	**Fibroadenoma**
❐ A 16 year old female has firm, rubbery mass in right breast is **8 cms in** diameter	**Giant Fibroadenoma**
❐ A 30 year old female has history of **bilateral breast tenderness related to menstrual cycle** with lumps coming and going.	**Fibrocystic disease**
❐ A 30 year old female has **bloody discharge** from nipple. **No other palpable masses** are seen.	**Intraductal Pappiloma**
❐ A 30 year old **lactating mother has red, hot, tender mass** with **fever and** leucocytosis	**Breast abscess**
❐ A **55 year old woman has 3.5 cms hard mass** in her left breast **with ill defined borders** and **not mobile.** The skin overlying has orange peel appearance	**Breast ca**
❐ A 60 year old has **headaches not responding** to medications. She had **undergone Modified radical Mastectomy** 1 year back	**Brain metastasis from Breast ca**

❐ A 50 year old notices **coldness and tingling in his left hand and forearm** pain while doing **heavy work** along with **vertigo, blurred vision**	**Subclavian Steal Syndrome**
❐ A 50 year old has **a 6 cms pulsatile mass deep in abdomen**	**AAA (Abdominal Aortic Aneurysm)**
❐ A 65 year old has **sudden onset, tearing chest pain radiating to back** with BP 220/120 with **unequal arm pressures** and normal cardiac enzynes	**Dissecting aneurysm of Thoraxic Aorta**
❐ A 20 year old with **BP 195/120 in upper limb** with **normal BP in lower limbs and rib notching**	**Coarctation of Aorta**

❒ A 10 year old girl with round 1 cm mass in **midline of neck** moving with **movement of tongue**	❒ Throglossal duct Cyst
❒ A 15 year old girl with round 1 cm on side of **neck beneath and in front of sternocleidomastoid.**	❒ Branchial cyst
❒ A 6 year old with **fluid filled translucent mass** in supraclavicular area	❒ Cystic hygroma
❒ A 35 year old with **enlarged lymph nodes in cervical region** with **night sweats and pruritis plus axillary lymphadenopathy**	❒ Lymphoma

❒ **Critical pH** in Mendelsons syndrome is **2.5**	ORISSA 2004
❒ **Best site** for TPN is **Subclavian vein**	MAH 2002
❒ **IV fluid monitoring** in trauma is judged by: **Urine output**	PGI 2006
❒ **Cryoprecipitate** is stored at **-40°C**	UPSC 2006
❒ **Period of onset of tetanus** refers to **time between is symptom to spasm.**	PGMEE 2006
❒ **Triple therapy** immunosupppresion for renal transplant is: **Cyclosporine, Azathioprine, Prednisolone**	AI 2006
❒ Organ for which **HLA Matching is not necessary: Liver**	JIPMER 2002
❒ Commonest pattern of **basal cell cancer** is : **Nodular**	COMED 2008
❒ **Marjolins ulcer** is **Squamous cell carcinoma**	PGI 2007, AI 2006
❒ **Wolfes graft** is **Full thickness graft**	UP 2007
❒ **Basal cell carcinoma** spreads by **Direct route**	MAHE 2007
❒ Chronic **Burrowing ulcer** is caused by **Microaerophilic streptococci**	AI 2007
❒ **Most important** aspect of management of Burn injury in first 24 hours is **Fluid Management**	UPSC 2007
❒ **IV Rule** for burns is: **%BSA X Wt in Kg X4=Volume in ml**	
❒ Indications for **referral to BURN UNIT:** ✓ 10% burns in infants ✓ 10% deep burns in adults ✓ Scalds on head and face ✓ Burns on palm ✓ >20% superficial burns	PGI 2004

❒ **Pseudoaneurysms** in IV drug abusers is most commonly seen in **femoral artery**	PGI 2007
❒ **Patchy meningitis hemorrhagica interna** is manifested by **Subdural hemmorhage**	MANIPAL 2006
❒ **Cleft lip** is due to nan failure of **maxillary process with medial nasal process**	PGI 2001
❒ **Cleft lip** is repaired by **Tennisons Method, Millards Method, Le Mesuriers Method.**	AIIMS
❒ **Unilateral clefts** are common on **left side**	PGI 88
❒ **Pierre Robinsons Syndrome** is Cleft palate +Mandibular hypoplasia+ Respiratory obstruction	

- ❐ **Most frequent tooth** to be impacted is : **Lower Third Molar** — UPSC 2007
- ❐ **Floating teeth** are seen in **Histiocytosis X** — Kar 2002
- ❐ **Epulis** arises from **Gingiva** — PGI
- ❐ **Ranula is retention cyst of sub lingual gland**

- ❐ **Most common cause** of **anorectal abscess** is **inflammation of anal gland** — MAHE 2007
- ❐ **External haemmoroids** are painful **below dentate line** — AI 2007
- ❐ Treatment of choice for **squamous cell carcinoma anus** is **Chemoradiation** — AI 2006
- ❐ **Adeno carcinoma** is the most common type of **Rectal cancer** — PGI 2005
- ❐ **Epidermoid cancer** is the most common type of **Anal cancer** — PGI 07
- ❐ **Rotation of sigmoid volvolus** occurs **Anticlockwise** — UP 2007
- ❐ **Rotation of cecal volvolus** occurs **clockwise**
- ❐ **Acute pseudo obstruction** of colon is called **Ogilives Syndrome** — UP 2007
- ❐ **Borcharts triad** of epigastric pain, inabiltity to pass catheter, violent retching is seen in **Acute Gastric Volvolus** — JK 2005
- ❐ **Gallstone ileus** is impaction at **Distal ileum** — JK BOPEE 2009
- ❐ **Oliguria**: excretion of less than **300 ml in 24 hours.** — JIPMER 87
- ❐ **Normal capacity** of renal pelvis: **7 ml** — AIIMS 86
- ❐ Commonest cause of **UTI**: **E. coli** — AP 85
- ❐ Commonest organism isolated in **emphysematous pyelonephritis: E. coli** — COMED 2008
- ❐ **Spider leg deformity** in excretory urogram is seen in **Polycystic kidney.** — UP 2007
- ❐ **Canberry juice** helps in **prevention of UTI.** — AIIMS 2007
- ❐ **Stone resistant** to lithotripsy: **Cysteine stone** — AIIMS 2007
- ❐ **Ethylene glycol poisoning** is characterized by **Oxalate stones.**

- ❐ Irrigation solution used in **TURP** is: **1. 5 % Glycine** — COMED 2008
- ❐ The most common complication of **TURP** is: **Retrograde ejaculation** — COMED 2007
- ❐ **Carcinoma prostate** arises from: **Peripheral zone** — UP 2007
- ❐ **Altered sensitiveness and drowsiness** after TURP is because of : **Hyponatremia** — AIIMS 2007
- ❐ **Most sensitive screening** of Prostate cancer is by: **DRE+PSA** — AI 2007
- ❐ **Mc Neals** peripheral zone of prostate is seat of: **Cancer** — PGMEE 2006
- ❐ **In fourniers gangrene** testis are usually **spared** — MAHE 2007
- ❐ Ideal age for **orchiopexy** for cryptorchidism is **<1 year** — AIIMS 2007
- ❐ **Orchidopexy** for undescended Testis is recommended best at 2 years — KAR 2006
- ❐ **Testicular cancer** most sensitive to radiation is **Seminoma** — UPSC 2005

❒ **Optical urethroplasty** is done for: Congenital urtethral stricture	UP 2007
❒ **Peyroines disease** is seklf limiting associated with **Dupynterns contracture**	UP 2007
❒ **Prostatitis** is accompanied by **seminal vesculitis**	AIIMS 07
❒ **Tear drop bladder** is seen in **Pelvic hematoma**	KAR 98
❒ **Secondary vesical calculus** refers to stones formed after **UTI**	PGMEE 2006
❒ **Suprapubic aspiration** is the **most reliable** method of urine collection	UPSC 2005
❒ Management in case of **strangulated hernia is: Immediate surgery**	PGI 2006
❒ **Spigelian Hernia** is **Infra umbilical hernia**	JK BOPEE 2009
❒ **Scrambled egg appearance** is seen in: **Carcinoma Pancreas**	COMED 2007
❒ **Gases** used for pneumoperitoneum: **CO_2, O_2, N_2O**	PGI 2007
❒ **Cushings reflex** is: **↑Mean Arterial pressure with ICP**	UP 2007
❒ **Shoulder pain** in laproscopy indicates **Co_2 Narcosis**	AIIMS 2007
❒ **Best way** of Preventing DVT in postoperative period is: **Prophylactic Heparin**	AIIMS 2006
❒ **Lambert sutures** in abdominal surgery refer to **Sero muscular sutures**	KAR 2006
❒ Commonest site for **Lymphomas** of GIT IS: **Stomach**	COMED 2007
❒ **Dukes classification** is used for: **Colorectal Ca**	UP 2007
❒ **FNAC** is not useful in: **Follicular ca Thyroid, Aneurysmal Bone Cyst**	AI 2006
❒ **Soft tissue sarcoma** that metastasizes to **lymph nodes** mostly is: **Embryonal Rhabdomyosarcoma**	AI 05
❒ **Buschke Lownstein Tumor** is **Giant copndyloma acuminata**	TN 2003
❒ **Gleasons staging** is done for **Cancer prostate**	MAH 2012

❒ **Double bubble sign** is seen in **duodenal atresia.**	AIIMS 2009
❒ **Dye used in chromoendoscopy** for detection of GIT cancer is: **methlyene blue.**	AIIMS 2009
❒ **Most common cause** of esophagitis is **reflux.**	AIIMS 2009
❒ **Sister mary josephs nodule** is seen in **stomach cancer.**	AIIMS 2009
❒ Most common **cause of death** in Crohns disease is : **malignancy** (Although rare)	AIIMS 2009
❒ **Skip lesions** are seen in **crohns disease.**	AIIMS 2009
❒ **MC site of curlings ulcer** is **duodenum**	AIIMS 2008
❒ **Best test** to diagnose **GERD** and quantify acid out put is: **24 hour p H monitoring.**	AIIMS 2008
❒ **Hunteraian ligature operation** is done for: **Aneurysms**	AIIMS 2008
❒ **Glomus tumor** is seen in **fingers** (digits)	AIIMS 2008
❒ **Ductal ectasia** is treated by surgery: **Hadfeld operation.**	AIIMS 2008
❒ **Nicolodoni sign** is also called as **Branhams sign.**	AIIMS 2008

1

SURGERY

NOTES

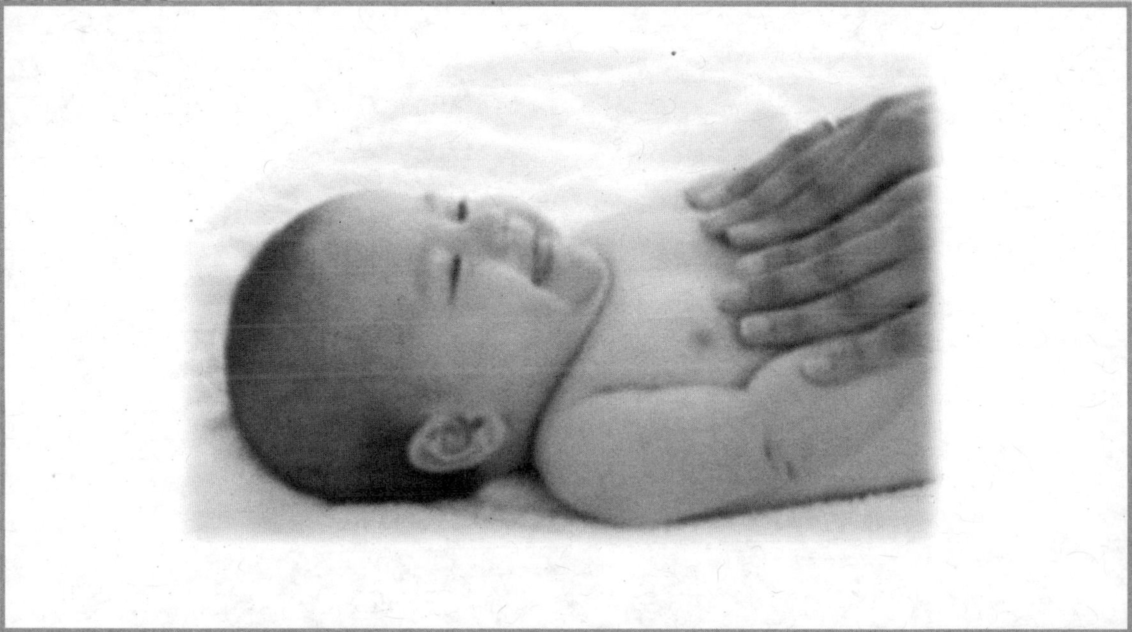

OBSTETRICS AND GYNECOLOGY

Remember:

❒ Fertilization occurs in "Ampulla" of fallopian tubes. ☛
❒ Sperm binds with "Secondary" oocyte.
❒ "Zona pellucida" must degenerate before implantation occurs. ☛
❒ "Implantation" occurs in posterosuperior wall of uterus. ☛
❒ Endometrium of pregnant uterus is called "Decidua".
❒ Deciduas basalis is part of deciduas in contact with blastocyst. ☛
❒ Deciduas capsularis is part of deciduas covering the ovum. ☛
❒ Deciduas parietalis is the rest of deciduas outside the implantation area. ☛

➲ Important Events Following Fertilization

▶ 0 hour	➦ Fertilization☛☛
▶ 30 hours	➦ 2 cell stage (Blastomeres)
▶ 40-50 hours	➦ 4 cell stage
▶ 72 hours	➦ 12 cell stage☛☛
▶ 96 hours	➦ 16 cell stage. (Morula) enters the uterine cavity
▶ 5th day	➦ Blastocyst
▶ 6-7th day	➦ Zona pellucida disappears, Interstitial implantation occurs ☛
▶ 9th day	➦ Lacunar period; Endometrial vessels tapped☛
▶ 10-11th day	➦ Implantation completed
▶ 13th day	➦ "Primary" villi☛
▶ 16th day	➦ "Secondary" villi
▶ 21st day	➦ "Tertiary" villi
▶ 21st-22nd day	➦ Fetal heart. Feto-placental circulation

➲ Placenta: Frequently asked Questions (High Yield for 2011/2012)

❒ Biscoidal placenta:	➦ Placenta has two disks. ☛☛
❒ Lobed placenta:	➦ Placenta divides into lobes. ☛
❒ Diffuse placenta:	➦ Chorionic villi persist all around the blastocyst. ☛
❒ Placenta succenturaita:	➦ Small part of placenta separated from the rest.
❒ Fenestrated:	➦ Placenta has hole in center. ☛
❒ Circumvallate:	➦ Edge of placenta is covered by circular fold of deciduas. ☛

⇨ According to "Umbilical Cord" Attachment:

- **Marginal:** Marginal as well as battle dore placenta refers to placenta with cord attached to margins. ☛
- **Furcate:** Blood vessels divide before reaching the placenta. ☛
- **Velemantous insertion:** blood vessels are attached to amnion where they ramify before reaching the placenta. ☛

➲ Placentation in Humans is an Important PG Topic

► In humans implantation is **Interstitial.** ☛	
► Human placenta is **Hemochorial**☛	
► Human placenta is **6 -8 inches** in diameter. ☛	
► Human placenta weighs about **500 gms.**	
► Human placenta has a surface area of **14 m^2.**	
► Human placenta has **60-100 fetal cotlydens**☛	
► Human placenta has **15-20 maternal cotlydens.** ☛	
► Zone of fibrinoid degeneration where trophoblast and decidua meet is called **Nitbauchs layer.**	AIIMS 04

► Oogonia are derived from: **yolk sac**	JIPMER 1992
► Zygote reaches uterine cavity as **16 celled stage**	KERALA 2003
► Commonest site of fertilization is: **ampulla**	DNB 2004
► Placental circulation is established on **17th day of fertilization**	UPSC 2006
► Placenta has **2 areteries, one vein.**	DNB 1999
► **Folds of Hoboken** are a feature of umblical cord	DNB 1999

- ❒ **Placenta accerta:** placenta directly anchored to Myometrium without intervening deciduas
- ❒ **Placenta incerta :** placenta invades muscle bundle☛
- ❒ **Placenta percerta:** placenta invades serosa. Treated by hysterectomy. ☛☛
- ► **Absence of deciduas basalis** is seen.
- ► **Absence of nitbauchs fibrinoid layer** is seen. ☛

⇨ Hormones of Placenta:

Protein Hormones☛☛☛

- ► **Human Chorionic Gonadotrophin (HCG)**
- ► **Human Placental Lactogen (HPL)**
- ► **Human Chorionic Thyrotrophin (HCT)**
- ► **Human Chorionic Corticotrophin (HCC)**
- ► **Pregnancy specific Beta-1 Glycoprotein**

Steroid Hormones☛
➨ Estrogens: Estriol, Estradiol and Estrone
➨ Progesterone

➲ Human Chorionic Gonadotrophin (hCG): (High Yield for 2011/2012)

- "Glycoprotein"
- 2 subunits
- **Alpha Subunit____"Hormone nonspecific"** ☛☛
- **Beta Subunit______Hormone "specific"**☛☛
- Alpha Subunit is **chemically similar to LH, FSH and TSH**☛
- **Beta Subunit** is relatively **unique** to HCG☛☛
- Synthesised by the **syncytiotrophoblast**☛
- Secreted into the blood of both mother and fetus.
- Half-life is about **1.5** day
- By RIA, it can be detected in the maternal serum or urine as early as **8-9** days following Ovulation.
- The **doubling time** of hCG in plasma is **about 2** days. ☛
- The blood and urine levels reach maximum ranging **100 IU and 200 IU/ml** ☛
- hCG **disappears** from the circulation within **2 weeks** following delivery. ☛

⇨ Human Placental Lactogen (HPL)

- Also known as **human chorionic somatotrophin**☛
- Synthesized by **Syncytiotrophoblast**☛ Promotes **growth hormone (GH) release** and **insulin** Secretion but **decreases** insulins peripheral effects, Liberates maternal fatty acids so sparing maternal glucose use. (**i.e; Insulin resistance** (Seen during pregnancy) ☛
- Stimulates mammary growth and maternal **casein, lactalbumin andlactoglobulin** production.
- Values of **HPL<5mg/ml after the 35 weeks** indicate the possibility of **fetal distress.**

⇨ Pregnancy Specific β-1 Glycoprotein

- Produced by the **trophoblast**☛
- Detected in maternal serum as early as **7 day after ovulation.** ☛
- Used as a **specific test** of pregnancy.

⇨ Estrogen

- ❒ Produced by the **Syncytiotrophoblast**☛☛
- ❒ Its synthesis depends much on the precursor derived mainly from the fetus.
- ❒ In late pregnancy, **estriol** is the most important estrogen.

- Estrogen increases the secretion and ciliary beating in fallopian tubes.
- Estrogen changes the cuboidal lining of vagina to stratified.
- Estrogen changes the break down of glycogen into lactate in vagina.
- Estrogen initiates **breast development.**
- Estrogen causes **early epiphyseal closure.**
- Estrogen causes **water retention.**

Progesterone

- Produced by **Syncytiotrophoblast**
- Chief hormone of **Corpus luteum**
- After delivery, its level decreases rapidly and is **not** detectable **after 24 hours.**

Amniotic Fluid

50 ml at 12 weeks.	**DNB 2005**
400 ml at 20 weeks	
1000ml at 36 weeks	
600-800ml at term.	**UPSC 2004**
Replaced every 3 hours	**Delhi 2000**

Green colored:	Fetal distress	AP 96
Golden colored:	Rh Incompatibility	
Saffron colored:	Post maturity	
Dark brown:	IUD	

Amnoicentesis: (High Yield for 2011/2012)

Done in:

- ✓ Pregnancy above the age of **35 years** (Chance of **Downs Syndrome**)
- ✓ A **previous** child with chromosomal abnormalities (e.g; **Autosomal Trisomy**)
- ✓ **X-linked** genetic recessive disorders
- ✓ To detect **inborn errors** of metabolism

Investigation to be done

- **Culture of the desquamated foetal cells in the amniotic fluid**
- **Chromosomal study of the desquamated foetal cells in the amniotic fluid**
- **Fetal sex is determined by karyotyping of cultured amniotic cells.**

Other Related **points to be remembered**

- Fetal serum also contains AFP in a concentration **150 times** that of maternal serum.
- **Acetyl cholinesterase levels** in amniotic fluid is **more specific** than AFP in predicting Neural tube defects

⇨ Therapeutic Indications

FIRST HALF OF PREGNANCY

- Induction of **abortion** (Instillation of chemicals e.g; **hypertonic saline, urea, prostaglandin**)
- Repeated **decompression** of the uterus in **acute hydramnios.**

SECOND HALF OF PREGNANCY

- **Decompression** of uterus in unresponsive cases of **chronic hydramnios**
- To give intrauterine foetal **transfusion** in severe hemolysis following Rh-isoimmunisation.

⇨ Preferred Sites for Amniocentesis

EARLY MONTHS: 1/3rd of the way up the **uterus from symphysis pubis**

Later months:

- **Trans-isthmic suprapubic** approach after lifting the presenting part **OR**
- Through **the flanks** in between the foetal limbs **OR**
- Below **the umbilicus** behind the neck of the fetus.

Other points to be remembered

- ✓ A **20-22** gauze **spinal needle** is used.
- ✓ **Length** of needle **is 4''(inches or 10 cm)**
- ✓ Amount to be collected for diagnostic purposes is **10 ml.**

Precautions for amniocentesis

- **Prior USG localization** of placenta to prevent feto-maternal bleeding.
- Prophylactic administration of **100 microgram of anti-D Ig** in Rh-negative non- immunised mother.

Hazards of amniocentesis

MATERNAL COMPLICATIONS

- Infection
- Hemorrhage(placental or uterine injury)
- Premature rupture of the membranes
- Premature labor

FETAL COMPLICATIONS

- Trauma
- Feto-maternal Hemorrhage

⇨ Causes of Maternofetal Hemorrhage

a. Early pregnancy loss

b. Miss carriage

c. Missed abortion

d.	Elective abortion
e.	Ectopic pregnancy
f.	Chorione villus sampling
g.	Aminocentesis
h.	Fetal blood sampling

⇨ ↑Maternal Serum Alpha Fetoprotein Levels

Maternal Conditions ☛☛		Fetal Conditions ☛☛
❒ Neural tube defects	AIIMS 87, DNB 2002	❒ Low Weight☛
❒ Gastrochisis, Exomphalos	UP 2000	❒ Hepatocellular Ca☛
❒ Renal agenesis, Posterior urethral valves☛		❒ SLE☛
❒ Amniotic band disruption		
❒ IUGR		
❒ Osteogenesis imperfecta		
❒ Placental tumors		
❒ Umblical cord tumors		
❒ Sacrococcygeal teratoma		
❒ Cystic hygroma		
❒ Twins	AI 1996	

⇨ Maternal Serum Alpha Fetoprotein Levels

❒ Downs syndrome☛
❒ Cystic fibrosis☛
❒ Hydrocephalus☛
❒ Increased maternal weight☛
❒ Overestimated gestational age☛

⇨ Triple Test

It Includes:

- HCG☛☛
- Estriol☛☛
- Alpha feto protein (Maternal). ☛

In Downs Syndrome: ☛

HCG↑	AFP↓	Estriol ↓

In Edwards syndrome:

HCG↓	AFP↓	Estriol ↓

➲ Quadrple Test is done for Downs Syndrome

It involves Triple Test Plus Inhibin.
1. Alpha fetoprotein
2. HCG
3. Estriol
4. Inhibin

⇨ Chorionic Villus Sampling

▶ 10-12 weeks preferebally	AIIMS 2005, Orissa, AI 1996
▶ Done transcervically: 10-12 weeks	
▶ Done transabdominally: 10 weeks to term	AIIMS 2009
▶ Done before 10 weeks results in oromandibular limb defects	AIIMS 2002
▶ Slightly higher risk of fetal loss.	

▶ Chorionic villus sampling: 10-12 weeks	AIIMS 2005, Orissa, AI 1996
▶ Done before 10 weeks results in oromandibular limb defects	AIIMS 2002
▶ Amniocentesis: 14-16 weeks	
▶ Percutaneous umblical blood sampling: 18 weeks	
▶ Fetoscopy: 16-20 weeks	

⇨ Screening Methods Chromosomal Abnormalities AIIMS 2010

First Trimester
➡ Maternal age.
➡ NT
➡ NB (nasal bone)
➡ Free beta+free-h CG+Papp-A
➡ NT+ NB + free beta - hCG + Papp - A.
Second trimester
➡ Triple test
➡ Quadrple test
➡ Genetic sonogram
➡ Quadrple test+Genetic sonogram.

AIIMS 07, UPSC 07, PGI 2000, 2001, JIPMER 91

Oligohydramnios DNB 2003, DNB 2004, UP 2000	Polyhydramnios UP 2005, Kar 2003, Delhi 2004
➡ Renal agenesis	➡ Esophageal atresia
➡ Multicystic dysplastic kidneys.	➡ Duodenal atresia
➡ Amnion nodosum	➡ Diabetes **mellitus** not Insipidus

➡ IUGR☛	➡ Multiple pregnancy☛
➡ Post maturity	➡ Open neural tube defects☛
➡ Premature rupture of membranes	➡ Chorioangioma placenta☛
➡ Post urethral valves	
➡ AF index<5	

⇨ Doppler Flow

- ✓ Peak velocity of blood flow occurs **during systole**
- ✓ Small amount of blood flow occurs in diastole.
- ✓ S/D ratio assessments are used.

Abnormal Flows:

- ❐ **Absence of blood flow**
- ❐ **Reverse flow**
- ❐ **Notching of wave form at end of systole**

Abnormal Flows Cause:

- ✓ IUGR
- ✓ Fetal distress

Remember:

► Cardiac activity of fetus seen by USG at: **6 weeks.**	**TN 1999**
► **Anencephaly is the earliest** fetal anomaly detected by USG.	
► External genitalia earliest diagnosed by USG at: **10 weeks.**	
► Fetal respiratory movements occur at: **12 weeks**	**JIPMER 1991**
► Fetal bradycardia is **less than 120 bpm for 15 minutes** period of continuous monitoring	**TN 1999**
► Fetal scalp p H **<7.2 is abnormal.**	**AMC 2000**

⇨ Crown Rump Length

- ➡ Crown Rump Length is an accurate parameter used to calculate gestational age in the first trimester **especially during 5-15 weeks.** ☛☛
- ➡ CRL is **linear measure of longest axis.** ☛
- ➡ Usually three images are taken on USG and maximum length is used as the final CRL. ☛
- ➡ Other parameters such as BPD, Femur length, Abdominal or head circumference are less accurate initially.

CRL at I month : 5 mm

CRL at 2 month: 30 mm

CRL at full term: 300 mm

► **HCG is a glycoprotein.**☛☛	**PGI 2002**
► **HCG has 2 subunits.** ☛	**PGI 2002**
► **HCG is Secreted by trophoblasts.** ☛	**AIIMS 2006**

⇨ Selective and Nonselective Genetic Screening

In pregnant women is achieved by fetal sonography, chorionic villus biopsy, or amniocentesis coupled with biochemical, chromosomal, or molecular analyses of cultured fetal cells. Maternal blood is a useful screening source for the fetal disorders Down syndrome and spina bifida. If maternal blood concentrations of a-fetoprotein, chorionic gonadotropin, or estriol vary above or below mean values of normal at a specific age of gestation, further fetal studies by sonography and amniocentesis are indicated.

➲ Normal Pregnancy:

⇨ Total Duration: 280 days

▶ Gravidity:	➠ Total number of previous pregnancies (normal or abnormal)
▶ Parity:	➠ State of having given birth to an infant or infant weighing 500 gms or more dead or alive.
▶ Immature infant :	➠ Weighing <1000 gms and completed <28 weeks
▶ Premature infant	➠ Weighing >1000 gms and completed >28 weeks
▶ Low birth weight:	➠ Live born infant weighing 2500 gms or less.
▶ Mature infant:	➠ Live born infant completed 38 weeks of gestation and weighing more than 2500 gm.
▶ Postmature infant:	➠ Live born infant completed 42 weeks of gestation or more

⇨ "Presumptive" Manifestations of Pregnancy:

- ▶ Amenorrhea☛
- ▶ Nausea and vomiting☛
- ▶ Breast tenderness☛
- ▶ Quickening (first Perception of fetal movements) at 18-20 weeks in primi, 14-16 weeks in multigravida.
- ▶ Bladder irritability, frequency and nocturia☛☛

⇨ "Changes" in Pregnancy are

Hemodynamic Changes ☛☛☛

❒ Increased cardiac output.	PGI 2003
❒ Increased blood volume.	AIIMS 2006
❒ Increased plasma volume.	AIIMS 2006
❒ Increased pulse rate.	
❒ Compression of sup vena cava (supine hypotension syndrome) in 3rd trimester	
❒ Decreased Peripheral vascular resistance.	AIIMS 2006
❒ Decreased pulmonary vascular resistance. ☛	
❒ Decreased arterial BP.	

Integumentary System:

- ↑Pigmentation of aerola ☛☛
- Cholasma ☛
- Linea Nigra (On Abdomen in midline) ☛
- Spider angioma
- Palmar erythema
- Stria gravidarum

Respiratory:

- ↓TLC, FRC, RV☛
- ↑Tidal volume☛
- ↑Minute ventilation☛
- ↑O_2requirements

Genitourinary:

- ↑Urinary frequency☛☛
- ↑UTI, Pyelonephiritis☛
- Glycosuria ☛

Others:

- ↑Incidence of **Carpal Tunnel Syndrome**
- ↑Total Thyroxine and ↑Thyroxine binding globulin levels. **Normal TSH**
- ↑Incidence of **Gallstones, GERD (Reflux)** ☛
- ↑Renal blood flow, ↑GFR☛

⇨ Pregnancy Causes Increase in Concentrations of — PGI 2001

- ↑ **Glogulin**
- ↑ **Fibrinogen**
- ↑ **Transferrin**
- ↑ **Leukotrienes**

⇨ Fetal Growth is Predominantly by — AI 99

- ✓ IGF 1,
- ✓ Insulin,
- ✓ Growth factors.

⇨ Signs of Pregnancy

- **Chadwicks Sign: Congestion of pelvis causes bluish/purplish hue of vagina/cervix** — K CET 2012
- **Leucorrhea: Non fern pattern of cervical mucus**

▶ Goodells Sign: Cyanosis and softening of cervix	UPSC 2007, PGI 2000
▶ Ladins Sign: Softening of uterus in anterior midline	
▶ Hegars Sign: Compressibility of isthmus on bimanual examination	PGI 2000, PGI 97
▶ Mc Donalds Sign: Uterus becomes flexible at utero cervical junction.	
▶ Von Frendwals sign: Irregular softening of fundus at site of implantation.	
▶ Piskaceks sign: Softening of cervix with lateral implantation	UP 07, Manipal 2006
▶ Osianders sign: Pulsations in lateral vaginal fornix	JIPMER 2000
▶ Palmers sign rythmic contractions of uterus	PGI 2000, KAR 1999
▶ Weinberg sign: Abdominal pregnancy	DNB 2005

⇨ Probable Manifestations of Pregnancy:

- Abdominal enlargement
- Uterine contractions (painless uterine contractions: Braxton Hicks contractions)
- Uterine ballotment
- Uterine soufflé

⇨ Pseudocyesis: PGI 2001

- ✓ Patient having an intense desire for pregnancy and develops symptoms of pregnancy.
- ✓ No FHS
- ✓ No USG documentation of gestational sac
- ✓ Refer to pshyciatrist

⇨ X-ray Evidence of Fetal Death:

✓ Overlapping ofskull bones -Spadling sign	
✓ Gas in Aorta-Roberts sign	KCET 2012
✓ ↑Curvature of fetal spine	
✓ Angulation of spine	

True Labor	False Labor
Regular uterine contractions	Irregular uterine contractions
Effacement and dilatation of cervix occur	Effacement and dilatation of cervix don't occur

✓ Ideal number of antenatal visits: 12-14	MAHE 2007
✓ Minimum number of antenatal visits: 3	MAHE 2007

- ❒ Total duration: 280 days
- ❒ Quickening occurs at 20 weeks in primi, 18 weeks in multi

❒ Earliest detection of pregnancy by USG is by: gestational sac ☛☛	PGI 2000
❒ Pregnancy is confirmed by:	PGI 2004
✓ FHR,	AI 1995, DNB 2000
✓ FM,	
✓ Fetal sac on USG	
❒ TVS detects gestational sac at 14 days after ovulation. ☛☛	PGI 2000
❒ Fetal parts can be detected by x ray at: 16 weeks. ☛☛	

Important Terms Frequently Asked

- **Fetal presentation:** ☛☛ **Designates fetal parts which lie over the inlet.**
- **Fetal lie:** ☛☛ **Refers to relation of long Axis of fetus to long axis of mother.**
- **Fetal position: relationship of point of direction of presenting part to one of the four quadrants of maternal pelvis.**

The Pelvis

▶ Normal female pelvis is **Gynaecoid pelvis**	
▶ Most common type of pelvis is **Gynaecoid pelvis** ☛☛	DNB 2004
▶ Transverse diameter is more than AP Diameter in **Gynecoid pelvis.**	

▶ Transverse diameter is more than AP Diameter in **Platypelloid pelvis.** ☛☛	PGI 88
▶ Flat type of pelvis is **Platypelloid pelvis.**	KAR 1989
▶ Least common type of pelvis is **Platypelloid pelvis.**	UPSC 85
▶ Engagement occurs by asyncitilism in **Platypelloid pelvis** ☛☛	

▶ Male type/Wedge shaped pelvis is **Android pelvis** ☛☛	
▶ All diameters are reduced in **Android pelvis** ☛☛	
▶ Engagement is delayed in **Android pelvis** ☛☛	
▶ Deep transverse arrest/Persistent occipito posterior position is common in **Android pelvis**	AI 1995

▶ Ape like pelvis is **Anthropoid pelvis** ☛☛	
▶ Non rotation/Face to pubis delvery is common in **Anthropoid pelvis** ☛☛	
▶ Only pelvis with AP diameter >transverse diameter is **Anthropoid pelvis**	PGI 1988
▶ Face to pubis delivery is common in **Anthropoid pelvis**	DELHI 2003

▶ **Shortest diameter of pelvic inlet** is obstretic conjugate.	DNB 2004
▶ **Most important diameter during labor is** interspinal diameter of outlet. ☛☛	
▶ **Shortest diameter of fetal skull is Bitemporal.**	UP 2005, DELHI 2005, KERALA 94
▶ **Largest diameter of fetal skull is submento vertical**	DNB 2004, BHU 97

ENGAGING DIAMETER	PRESENTATION	
❐ Suboccipitobregmatic	Vertex☛☛	
❐ Suboccipitofrontal	Vertex☛☛	
❐ Occipitofrontal	Vertex	
❐ Mentovertical	Brow	
❐ Submentovertical	Face ☛☛	AI 88
❐ Submentobregmatic	Face ☛☛	AI 88

➠ Inlet contraction:	➠ If AP diameter is 10cms or less. ☛☛
➠ Mid pelvic contraction:	➠ If inter ishial diameter is <9.5 cms☛☛
➠ Mid pelvic contraction :	➠ Prominent ischial spines, converging pelvic walls☛☛
➠ Outlet contraction:	➠ Intertuberous diameter is 8 cms or less. ☛☛

- When sagittal suture is midway between pubic and sacrum: synclitism☛☛
- When sagittal suture deviates from midline: asynclitism☛☛
- Sub pubic angle : 85° ☛☛
- Commonest type of vertex presentation: LOA (left occipito anterior) AIIMS 87
- Commonest presentation: cephalic☛☛
- Commonest presenting part: vertex☛☛

⇨ Bishops Scoring

AI 2007, PGI 1998, PGI 1997

Is used for labor.

Bishops scoring includes:

- ❐ Dilatation of cervix, ☛☛
- ❐ Effacement of cervix, ☛☛
- ❐ Consistency of cervix☛☛
- ❐ Position of cervix ☛☛
- ❐ Station of head, ☛☛

Bishops score >6 indicates beginning of labor.

➲ Labor

- Graphical representation of stages of labor is **partogram.** DNB 2000
- Assessment of labor is **best done** by Partogram. COMED 2008, PGI 1997
- **Graph showing relationship between cervical dilatation and labor is cervicograph** KERALA 2003
- Cervical ripening is **mainly due to** PGE_2. ☛☛
- **Sensitivity of uterine musculature is ↑ by: estrogen.** ☛☛ AIIMS 2006
- Cervical ripening is done by PGE_2, **oxytocin, misoprostol.** ☛☛

⇨ Stages of Labor

	Primi	Multi
I st stage labor☚☚ ✓ onset of labor-dilatation of cervix KERALA 1994 ✓ 8-10 hours in primi ✓ 6-8 hours in multi gravida	6-20 hours☚☚	2-10 hours☚☚
2nd stage labor☚☚ ✓ From full dilatation of cervix -complete birth of baby ✓ Not more than 2 hours	30 minutes-3 hours ☚☚	5-30 minutes
3 rd stage labor☚☚ ✓ Birth of infant to delivery of placenta	0-30 minutes☚☚	0-30 minutes

Third stage of labor is managed by:

- Early cord clamp — PGI 2011
- Oxytocin injection — PGI 2011
- Controlled cord traction
- Uterine massage and
- Methergin after delivery of anterior shoulder. — PGI 2011

⇨ Signs of Placental Separation: ☚☚

- Gush of blood☚☚
- Lengthening of cord. ☚☚
- Uterus becomes globular
- Fundal height increases

⇨ Cardinal Movements of Labor are: PGI 2008, PGI 2000

- Engagement (in relation to BPD) ☚☚ — KAR 2006
- Descent ☚☚
- Flexion☚☚
- Internal rotation☚☚
- Extension☚☚
- Restitution
- External rotation
- Expulsion

⇨ Trial of Labor

UPSC 2007, PGI, KAR

Indications: Minor CPD

Contraindications:

- ✓ Elderly primi
- ✓ Major CPD (disproportion)
- ✓ Severe PET
- ✓ Previous cesarean
- ✓ Malpresentation
- ✓ Outlet contraction

⇨ Postdecidual Secretions: Lochia

AI 1997

Lochia rubra:	1-4 days usually	Reddish
Lochia serosa:	5-9 days	Yellowish
Lochia alba:	10-15 days	Pale white

▶ Puerpurium is 6 weeks period after delivery.	UP 2006 , TN 97
▶ Uterus becomes a pelvic organ 2 weeks after delivery.	UPSC 2007
▶ Involution of uterus is complete by: 6 weeks.	UPSC 85

✓ Mc site of purpureal infection:	✓ Placental site.	
✓ Mc manifestation of purpureal infection:	✓ Endometritis.	
✓ Mc cause of purpureal infection:	✓ Streptocococcus	DNB 1998
✓ Mc route of purpureal infection spread:	✓ Direct spread	AIIMS 1995

✓ Mammogenesis:	➙ Preparation of breast for feeding	
✓ Lactopoesis:	➙ Synthesis of milk	
✓ Galactokinesis:	➙ Ejection of milk	JIPMER 2004
✓ Galactopoesis:	➙ Maintanence of lactation	
✓ Galactorrhea:	➙ Excessive and inappropriate milk secretion.	

➲ Band's Ring

Retraction ring

Seen in CPD, malpresentation

- ▶ **Average pressure** of uterine contractions during first stage of labor: **30 mm Hg** immediately following delivery, height of uterus corresponds to 20 weeks.
- ▶ Graph showing relationship **between cervical dilatation and duration of labor** is called **cervicograph.** Kerala 2003
- ▶ **Assessment of labor** is best done by **Partogram** PGI 97, COMED 2008
- ▶ Pressure inside uterus during **second stage of labor is 100-120 mm Hg** MAHE 2007
- ▶ **Precipitate labor** is labor occurring in less than 2 hours.

⇨ Preterm Labor

Is defined as labor occurring before 37 completed weeks of gestation.

Differentiate from premature baby: < 38 weeks.

Prediction of Preterm Labor:

- ✓ Symptoms of preterm labor.
- ✓ Uterine contraction greater than 4 per hour.
- ✓ Cervical length less than 2.5 cm — AI 2005, AI 2003
- ✓ **U-shaped cervix is indicative** — AI 2007
- ✓ Presence of fibronectin in vaginal discharge between 24-36 weeks
- ✓ Bishops score greater than 4
- ✓ Cervical dilatation greater than 2cm and effacement 80%.
- ✓ Vaginal bleeding
- ✓ Prior preterm

Causes of Preterm Labor are:

Chorioamnionitis

- **Bacterial Vaginosis**
- Previous history
- Recurrent UTI
- Smoking
- Low Socioeconomic and nutritional status
- **Uterine anomalies**
- Medical and surgical illnesses
- **Cervical incompetence**
- Increased amniotic fluid **IL-6 levels** and **Neoptrin** are considered as markers of preterm labor.

⇨ Tocolytics

Are drugs used to **arrest premature labor.**

Important Tocolytics are:

- ❐ Beta mimetics: **Ritodrine, Salbutamol, Isoxsuprine** — MAH 2012 AI 2008
- ❐ Oxytocin antagonists: Atosiban
- ❐ Magnesium Sulfate — AI 1999
- ❐ Nifedepine
- ❐ Glyceryl Trinitrate
- ❐ Progesterone,
- ❐ Diazoxide, — AI 1999
- ❐ Ethyl Alchohol,
- ❐ Atropine
- ❐ PG inhibitors: Indomethacin, Sulindac

Abortion:

❒ Threatened abortion	Os closed
❒ Inevitable abortion	Os open
❒ Incomplete abortion	Patulous os
❒ Complete abortion	Os closed with expulsion of gestational sac

Septic Abortion

- ✓ Any abortion with clinical evidence of infection of uterus or its contents.
- ✓ Rise of temp at least 100^0 F for at least 24 hours
- ✓ Presence of offensive/ purulent vaginal discharge
- ✓ Presence of evidence of pelvic infection.
- ✓ Most commonly follows illegal abortion.
- ✓ Infection is polymicrobial.

Tests Done for Recurrent Abortions

- ✓ Complete blood counts
- ✓ Lupus anticoagulant
- ✓ Anticardiolipin antibody level.
- ✓ TSH level
- ✓ Luteal phase endometrial biopsy
- ✓ Hysterosalpingography
- ✓ Karyotyping (most important) PGI 2006
- ✓ Not TORCH Infections AI 2008, PGI 2003, JK

- ► Abortion is expulsion of **fetus less than 500 gms./before 20 weeks** MAHE 2005, KERALA 2000
- ► MTP is **legal up to 20 weeks.**
- ► **First trimester abortions** are mainly due to (SAME)
  - ✓ **Chromosomal aberrations.** AI 2003
  - ✓ **(Embryonic) defect** PGI 1997
  - ✓ **Germ cell defect** AIIMS 1995
  - ✓ Ovofetal factor HPU 85
- ► **Commonest cause of first trimester abortions is trisomy.** PGI 99
- ► **Among trisomies commonest to cause abortion is Trisomy 16** DELHI 1997
- ► **Blighted ovum is avascular villi.** UP 2002
- ► **Second trimester abortions** are mainly due to **incompetent cervix.**
- ► **Cervical incompetence** is treated by: **Shirodkars procedure, Mc Donalds procedure, Wurms procedure.** PGI 2006, PGI 2003

- Induction of mid trimester abortions is usually done by: **Intraamniotic saline, intraamniotic**
- **prostaglandins, hysterotomy**
- **Best method** of Induction of **mid trimester abortions** is by: **Intraamniotic prostaglandins,**
- **Female with recurrent abortions and ↑APTT** is most likely having: **Antiphospholipid antibody syndrome** MAHE 2007, AIIMS 2007
- Dose of anti D following first trimester abortion is: **50μg.** COMED 2008

Ectopic Pregnancy: (High Yield for 2011/2012)

- A young girl with 8 weeks ammenorrhea comes in shock. Likely diagnosis is: Ectopic AI 2000
- A young girl with 6 weeks ammenorrhea presents with mass abdomen, USG shows empty uterus. Likely diagnosis is: ectopic AI 2001
- A young girl with 6 weeks ammenorrhea comeswith pain abdomen USG shows fluid in pouch of douglas. Aspiration yields dark colored fluid failing to clot. Likely diagnosis is: ruptured ectopic. AI 2001

Is associated with:

- Tubal diseases (Commonest) UPSC 2007 Kerala, AIIMS 96, DNB 98, AI 96
- Endometriosis PGI 2007
- PID UPSC 2007
- Tuberculosis
- IUCD
- Following Tubal procedures
- Congenital tubal anomalies
- Progastasert PGI 99

- **Ectopic pregnancies are characterized by fairly normal early development of the embryo, with the formation of placental tissue, the amniotic sac, and decidual changes.** An abdominal pregnancy is occasionally carried to term. With tubal pregnancies, however, the invading placenta eventually burrows through the wall of the oviduct, **causing intratubal hematoma (hematosalpinx), intraperitoneal hemorrhage, or both**. The tube is usually locally distended as much as 3 to 4 cm by a contained mass of freshly clotted blood in which may be seen bits of gray placental tissue and fetal parts.
- **The histologic diagnosis depends on the visualization of placental villi or, rarely, of the embryo.**

- **Most common feature** of ectopic is **abdominal pain.** PGI 1998
- Most reliable indicator of ectopic gestation is **no gestational sac in USG.**
- Expelled products in ectopic originate from: **Decidua vera.** JIPMER 99
- Medical treatment of ectopic pregnancy is by: **Methotrexate, actinomycin-D, mifepristone, prostaglandins** AI 2005, MAHE 2005
- **STUDOFORD CRITERION** is for primary abdominal pregnancy

- **Laproscopy** is the best investigation for diagnosis.
- **Commonest type which ruptures is: Isthimic** AI 94, AIIMS 1995
- **Trans vaginal USG** and **HCG** levels are also used

Bagel sign: It is a sign of ectopic pregnancy in Ultrasonography. JK BOPEE

It is a hyperechoic ring around gestational sac in adenexal region.

Blob sign is inhomogeneous mass adjacent to ovary or moving separate from ovary.It is a gestational sac without cardiac activity.

SALPINGOSTOMY for unruptured tubal pregnancy **(Tubes to be preserved)** PGI 2000

SALPINGECTOMY for ruptured tubal pregnancy with no desire for future pregnancy.

⇨ Indications of Medical Management of ECTOPIC PREGNANCY PGI 2007

- ✓ Hemodynamic stability
- ✓ Gestational sac not more than 4 cm
- ✓ Serum hCG level not more than 10000 miu/L
- ✓ Willing for follow-up
- ✓ No evidence for acute intraabdominal Hemorrhage
- ✓ Preferably absent fetal cardiac activity

⇨ Arias Stella Reaction

Is typical adenomatous change of endometrial glands.

- Loss of polarity of cells
- Hyperchromatic nuclei
- Vacuolated cytoplasm
- Occasional mitosis
- It occurs in 10-15% cases of ectopic pregnancy
- It is because of progesterone influence

⇨ Post-term Pregnancy:

Post term pregnancy is characterized by:

- **Wrinkled skin appearance.**
- **Overgrown nails**
- **Absence of Vernix caseosa.**
- **"Scanty saffron colored meconium and subsequent oligohydraminos".**
- **Placental calcification.**
- **Hypoxia and RDS.**
- **Polycythemia**
- **Hypoglycemia.**

- **Golden colored meconium: Rh incompatibility**
- **Saffron colored meconium: Post maturity**
- **Dark brown meconium: IUD.**

⇨ Rh Incompatibility

The manifestations in such condition are:

Fetal and neonatal:

- **Hydrops fetalis** (severe anemia, tissue anoxemia and metabolic acidosis)
- **Intrauterine fetal death**
- **Sonography**: real time with pulse Doppler detects edema in the skin, scalp and pleural or percardial effusion and echogenic bowel.
- Straight X-ray abdomen showing **"Buddha" position of the fetus"** with a halo around the head due to edematious scalp.
- **Enlargement of liver and spleen**
- Placenta is large, pale and edematous with fluid oozing from it.
- **Icterus gravis neonatorum**: baby born alive without evidences of jaundice but soon develops it within 24 hrs of birth.
- **Congenital anemia** of the newborn

Maternal:

Mainly affects the baby, but may also affect the mother, There is increased incidence of:

- **Pre-eclampsia,**
- **Polyhydramnios**
- **Big baby with its hazards**
- **Hypofibrinogenemia due to prolonged retention of dead fetus in uterus**
- **Postpartum Hemorrhage due to big placenta and blood coagulapathy**
- **Maternal syndrome: generalized edema, proteinuria and pruritus due to cholestasis. These features are ominous indicating imminent detal death in-utero.**

(a) Number of living children (Ref: Dutta, Platinum notes)

Risk of GTT is associated with:

- **Blood group AB**
- **High HCG titers**
- **Multiparity**

⇨ Hydatid Mole

- Molar pregnancy is an abnormal form of pregnancy, characterized by the presence of a hydatidiform mole **(or hydatid mole, mola hytadidosa).**
- Molar pregnancy comprises two distinct entities, **partial and complete moles.**
- **Complete moles** have no identifiable embryonic or fetal tissues and arise when an empty egg with no nucleus is fertilized by a normal sperm.
- **Partial mole** occurs when a normal egg is fertilized by two spermatozoa. Hydatidiform moles may develop into choriocarcinoma,

Caused by triploidy	**AI 2010**
Causes persistent GTD	**AI 2010**
Choriocarcinoma. Fortunately, pure choriocarcinomas account for only a small number of the germinal cell tumors. The tumor is **extremely rapidly invasive, with trophoblasts invading the venous system early** in the course of the disease. **Metastasis may be both blood-borne and through lymphatics** and **has usually occurred by the time of diagnosis.** Unlike choriocarcinoma in the female, which responds well to methotrexate, choriocarcinoma in the male is best treated with other agents such as cisplatin, bleomycin, and additional agents. **The prognosis for these patients is usually far worse than for other patients because of the advanced stage at time of diagnosis.**	**DNB 2011**

- A hydatidiform mole is a pregnancy/conceptus in which the placenta contains **grapelike vesicles** that are usually visible with the naked eye. The vesicles arise by distention of the chorionic villi by fluid. When inspected in the microscope, **hyperplasia of the trophoblastic tissue** is noted. If left untreated, a hydatidiform mole will almost always end as a **spontaneous abortion.**
- Hydatidiform moles are a common complication of pregnancy, occurring once in every 1000 pregnancies in the US, with much higher rates in **Asia**
- Blood tests will show **very high levels of human chorionic gonadotropin (hCG).**
- The diagnosis is strongly suggested by ultrasound (sonogram), but **definitive diagnosis requires histopathological examination**. The mole grossly resembles a bunch of **grapes ("cluster of grapes" or "honeycombed uterus" or "snow-storm")**
- There is **increased trophoblast proliferation** and enlarging of the chorionic villi. Angiogenesis in the trophoblasts is impared as well.
- **Sometimes symptoms of hyperthyroidism** are seen, due to the extremely high levels of hCG, which can mimic the normal Thyroid-stimulating hormone (TSH).
- Hydatidiform moles should be treated by **evacuating the uterus by uterine suction or by surgical curettage** as soon as possible after diagnosis, in order to avoid the risks of choriocarcinoma. Patients are followed up until their serum human chorionic gonadotrophin (hCG) level has fallen to an undetectable level.
- Invasive or metastatic moles (cancer) may require chemotherapy and often respond well to **methotrexate.** The response to treatment is nearly 100%.

⇨ Complications of H. Mole

- Hemorrhage and shock due to separation of vesicles from its attachment to deciduas.
- Massive intraperitoneal hemorrhage
- Sepsis
- Perforation of uterus
- Preeclampsia with convulsions
- Acute pulmonary insufficency due to Pulmonary embolism
- Thyroid storm
- Development of choriocarcinoma.

➲ Nutshell: (High Yield for 2011/2012)

- ❒ Large for date uterus☛☛
- ❒ Chromosome configuration is: 46XX☛☛
- ❒ Excessive nausea/ vomiting☛☛
- ❒ Early onset PET. ☛☛
- ❒ Absent fetal heart☛☛
- ❒ Grape like vesicles per vaginum☛☛
- ❒ Bilateral theca leutin cysts associated☛☛
- ❒ High HCG☛☛
- ❒ Snow storm appearance on USG☛☛
- ❒ Investigation of choice to diagnose H mole is USG — UPSC 07
- ❒ Confirmation of diagnosis is by vaginal eamination. ☛☛
- ❒ Evacuate by suction evacuation. ☛☛
- ❒ Immediate complication of evacuation of H mole is bleeding.

Associations: UPSC 07

- ✓ PIH
- ✓ Thyrotoxicosis
- ✓ Hyperemesis

- ► Commonest complication of H mole is sepsis. ☛☛
- ► Imaging technique of choice for diagnosing H. mole is USG — UPSC 2007
- ► Chromosomal configuration in H. mole is 46 XX. ☛☛
- ► Treatment of choice in H. mole is suction evacuation. ☛☛ — KERALA
- ► In a female of age 40 and above with h. mole and completed family treatment of choice is total hysterectomy☛☛
- ► Immediate complication of H. mole is bleeding. ☛☛
- ► Hydropic degeneration of villi is histological characteristic of H.mole. — UP 2007

  The typical hydatidiform mole is a voluminous mass of swollen, sometimes cystically dilated, chorionic villi, appearing grossly as grapelike structures. The swollen villi are covered by varying amounts of normal to highly atypical chorionic epithelium.

- ► Most common gestational trophoblastic disease following H. mole is: invasive mole. — AI 2007
- ► Molar pregnancy is usually diagnosed in First trimester. — MANIPAL 2006

➲ Gestational Trophoblastic Tumor (High Yield for 2011/2012)

Signs and Symptoms:

- **Irregular vaginal bleeding**
- **Offensive, purulent discharge**
- Persistent ill health
- Continued amenorrhea due to very high levels of **HCG secreted by the metastatic growth outside the uterus.**
- Symptoms of **lung metastasis** cough, dyspnea hemoptysis and chest pain.
- Headache, convulsions, paralysis coma due to **brain metastasis.**
- Irregular and brisk bleeding due to **vaginal metastasis.**
- Epigastric pain and jaundice due to **liver metastasis.**
- **Uterine enlargement.**
- Purple hemorrhagic projections within vagina due to retrograde spread along venous channels of vaginal plexus.
- **PV examination** reveals subinvolution of uterus, purplish red nodule, U/L or B/L enlarged ovaries.

Vesicular mole is a premalignant condition and can develop into choriocarcinoma.

In case of transformation of a molar pregnancy to choriocarcinoma the following features are seen:

- **Subinvolution of the uterus. The uterus remains enlarged and does not return back to normal size**
- **Rising levels of HCG**
- **Theca leutin cysts will persist**
- **Sites of metastasis**

- In cases of ovarian failure and menopause the **FSH is very high.**
- In pituitary failure the **FSH will be very low.**
- In pregnancy, **FSH is suppressed** due to high levels of prolactin.
- **Normal FSH and amenorrhea** point towards uterine pathology.

⇨ Sarcoma Botyrides☛☛☛☛

- ❐ Sarcoma botyrides is an **embryonal rhabdomyosarcoma**
- ❐ **Mesenchymal in origin.** ☛☛
- ❐ **Readily bleeds on touching**☛☛
- ❐ Tumor cells resemble **Tennis racket**☛☛
- ❐ Presents as **grape like mass buldging through vaginal orifice**
- ❐ **Locally invasive**
- ❐ **Chemoradiation** is treatment of choice

2

OBSTETRICS AND GYNECOLOGY

⇨ Twinning: ☛☛☛

▶ **Negroes** have the highest rate of twinning.	
▶ **Hellins law** indicates chances of twinning.	PGI 2000
▶ **Most common** types of twins are **both vertex.**	PGI 1997
▶ **Superfecundation** is fertilization of two ova released at same time by sperms released at two different occasions of sexual intercourse.	
▶ **Siamese twins** have **highest mortality**	JIPMER 1993
▶ **Thoracophagus** is the most common type of **conjoined twins.**	UPSC 2007
▶ **A double headed monoster** is called **dicephalous**	SGPI 2004
▶ **Twin peak sign is seen in diamniiotic dichorionic twins**	PGI 2005
▶ **In multiple fetal pregnancy fetal reduction is done by: potassium chloride**	AIIMS 1998
▶ **Most common cause of perinatal mortaslity in twins is prematurity**	CMC 1998
▶ **Twin pick sign is seen in dichorionicity**	AI 2010

Siamese/conjoined twins: Twins fused to each other
✓ **Thoracophagus: fused in region of thorax**☛☛
✓ **Ischiophagus: fused in region of pelvis**☛☛
✓ **Pyophagus: fused in region of back**☛☛
✓ **Craniophagus: fused in region of head**☛☛
Superfecundation: Fertilization of two different ova released in same cycle. ☛☛
Superfetation: Fertilization of two ova released in two different cycles☛☛

⇨ Anencephaly

❐ Associated with: Face presentation, hydraminos, post maturity, prematurity.
❐ Best diagnosed by USG at 10-12 weeks.

➲ Malpresentations

⇨ Breech:

▶ Most common cause of breech is **prematurity.**
▶ Most common type of breech is **frank breech.**
▶ **Engagement occurs earliest** in frank breech.
▶ Mortality in breech is mainly due to **intracranial hemorrhage.**
▶ Commonest position is **left sacroanterior.**
▶ Engaging diameter is **bitrochanteric.**
▶ Head is borne by **flexion.**

Delivery of head is by: UP 2007

- **Burns Marshall Method**
- **Maureciau-smeille-veit method**
- **Pipers forceps**

Extended legs: **Pinards Maneuver.**

Extended arm: **Lovests Maneuver.**

Prematurity, congenital anomilies and birth asphyxia are the main causes of perinatal mortality.

Most unfavorable presentation is Mento posterior.

⇨ Shoulder Dystocia

AIIMS 2009

- Impaction of anterior shoulder of fetus against symphysis pubis after fetal head has been delivered.
- Occurs when breadth of shoulders is greater than BPD.

Risk factors are:

- ✓ Diabetes
- ✓ Obesity
- ✓ Post term baby
- ✓ Excessive weight gain in pregnancy.

Approach is:

- **Apply suprapubic pressure.** **AI 2010**
- **Legs in flexion (Mc Roberts Maneuver)** **AI 2010**
- **Woods procedure** **AI 2010**
- **Release posterior shoulder**
- **Manual corckscrew**
- **Episiotomy**
- **Rollover**

Turtle sign positive: Head delivers but retracts against symphisis pubis.

Complications: Erbs palsy, klumpkes palsy# clavicle, humerus, spine, PPH (Injury to perineum), Fetal hypoxia.

Treatment

- ❐ **Cleidotomy**
- ❐ **Zanavelli maneuver: replacement of fetus to uterine cavity and cesarean section**
- ❐ **Symphisiotomy**

⇨ Management of Shoulder Dystocia

- **Never give fundal pressure**
- Moderate suprapubic pressure can be applied
- If it is **bilateral shoulder dystocia** directly proceed to perform **LSCS** after doing the Zavanelli maneuver
- The rest of the maneuvers can be tried for unilateral shoulder dystocia

- **The McRobert's maneuver:** The maneuver consists of removing the legs from the stirrups and sharply flexing them up onto the abdomen.
- **Woods corkscrew maneuver.**
- Delivery of the posterior shoulder.
- **Rubin maneuver.**

⇨ Rh Incompatibility

- **Immune hydrops** — **JIPMER 2003**
- **Father Rh+, mother Rh–, fetus Rh+**
- **Ist child escapes usually.**

Can have adverse effects on baby as well as mother such as:

- Preeclampsia
- Polyhydraminos
- Big baby
- Hypofibrinogenemia
- PPH
- Maternal syndrome: Generalised edema, proteinuria, pruritis.

- **Immune Hydrops in fetus** — **MP 2000**
  - ✓ **Pericardial effusion**
  - ✓ **Large placentas**
  - ✓ **Skin edema Earliest sign on USG** — **UPSC 1996**
  - ✓ **Ascites**
- **Icterus neonatorum gravis in fetus**
- **Hemolytic anemias in fetus.**

- Anti D immunoglobulin should be given within 72 hours of delivery. — **JIPMER 1986**
- **300 μg following delivery**
- **50 μg following abortion**
- **Prognosis depends on serum bilirubin.** — **AI 1996**
- **Immediate cord ligation is done.** — **UP 2003**
- **Feto maternal transfusion is detected by: Kleihauer-Betke test** — **UPSC 2008**

Diabetes and Pregnancy

Gestational Diabetes:

- Is defined as **glucose intolerance** that either has its onset or its first recognition during pregnancy.
- Gestational diabetes is usually diagnosed by means of oral glucose tolerance testing. Patients with gestational diabetes and normal fasting glucose levels have two major risks. **The first is fetal macrosomia.** Women with gestational diabetes are known to have largerbabies, and this creates an **increased risk of complications of delivery including shoulder dystocia and cesarean delivery.** The second risk is of the eventual **development of overt diabetes.**
- Patients with gestational diabetes and abnormal fasting glucose levels do have an **increased risk of stillbirth.**
- Overt diabetes and gestational diabetes with abnormal fasting glucose levels are associated with stillbirth.

- The metabolic changes are accompanied by maternal insulin resistance, caused in part by placental production of steroids, a growth hormone variant, and placental lactogen.
- Pregnancy complicated by diabetes mellitus is associated with **higher maternal and perinatal morbidity and mortality rates.**
- **Folate supplementation reduces the incidence of fetal neural tube defects, which occur with greater frequency in fetuses of diabetic mothers.**
- In addition, optimizing glucose control during key periods of organogenesis reduces other congenital anomalies including **sacral agenesis, caudal dysplasia, renal agenesis, and ventricular septal defect.**
- Once pregnancy is established, **glucose control should be managed more aggressively** than in the nonpregnant state.
- **Fetal macrosomia** is associated with an increased risk of maternal and fetal birth trauma. Pregnant women with diabetes have an increased risk of developing **preeclampsia**, and those with vascular disease are at greater risk for developing **intrauterine growth restriction**, which is associated with an increased risk of **fetal and neonatal death.**
- Because of **delayed pulmonary maturation** of the fetuses of diabetic mothers, **early delivery should be avoided** unless there is biochemical evidence of fetal lung maturity.
- All pregnant women should be screened for gestational diabetes unless they are in a low-risk group.
- Pregnant women with gestational diabetes are at **increased risk of preeclampsia**, delivering infants who are large for their gestational age, and birth lacerations.

Their fetuses are at risk of hypoglycemia and birth trauma (Brachial Plexus) injury.

Maternal Complications	Fetal Complications
❒ Abortion	❒ Fetal macrosomia
❒ Infections	❒ Neonatal malformations (CVS and Neural Tube defects)
❒ Preeclampsia	❒ Renal Agenesis
❒ Hydraminos	❒ Hypoglycemia ❒ Hypomagnesemia ❒ Hypocalcemia

❒ Maternal Distress	❒ RDS
❒ Increased complications of labor	❒ Hyper viscosity Syndrome
❒ Shoulder Dystocia	❒ Hyperbilirubinemia
❒ PPH	❒ Hyper trophic Cardiomyopathy
❒ Perineal Injuries	❒ Polycythemia
	❒ Erbs, Klumpkes palsy

➲ Heart Disease and Pregnancy

CLARKE'S classification for risk of maternal mortality caused by various heart diseases

Group-1: Minimal Risk 0-1

- ✓ ASD, VSD, PDA,
- ✓ Pulmonic or tricuspid disease
- ✓ Fallot tetralogy (corrected)
- ✓ Bioprosthetic valve
- ✓ Mitral stenosis, NYHA classes I and II

Group-2: Moderate Risk 5-15

- ✓ Mitral stenosis, NYHA classes III and IV
- ✓ Aortic stenosis
- ✓ Aortic Coarctation without valvular involvement
- ✓ Fallot tetralogy, uncorrected
- ✓ Previous myocardial infarction
- ✓ Marfan's syndrome, normal aorta
- ✓ Mitral stenosis with atrial fibrillation
- ✓ Artificial valve

Group-3: Major Risk 25-50 (Contraindications to Pregnancy)

- ✓ Pulmonary hypertension (primary and secondary)
- ✓ Aortic coarctation with valvular involvement
- ✓ Marfan's syndrome with aortic involvement

Mitral Stenosis: MS:

- Most common heart disease associated with pregnancy. **AI 1997**
- This is the **valvular disease most likely to cause death during pregnancy.**
- The pregnancy-induced increase in blood volume and cardiac output can cause pulmonary edema in women with mitral stenosis.
- Pregnancy associated with long-standing mitral stenosis may result in **pulmonary hypertension. Sudden death** has been reported when hypovolemia has been allowed to occur in this condition.
- Pregnant women with mitral stenosis are at **increased risk for the development of atrial fibrillation and other tachyarrythmias.**
- Medical management of severe mitral stenosis and atrial fibrillation with **digoxin and beta blockers is recommended.**

Balloon valvulotomy can be carried out during pregnancy.

Mitral Regurgitation and Aortic Regurgitation These are **both generally well tolerated** during pregnancy.

The pregnancy-induced decrease in systemic vascular resistance reduces the risk of cardiac failure with these conditions.

As a rule, mitral valve prolapse does not present problems for the pregnant patient and aortic stenosis, unless very severe, is also well tolerated. In the most severe cases of aortic stenosis, limitation of activity or balloon valvuloplasty may be indicated.

For women with artificial valves contemplating pregnancy, it is important that **warfarin be stopped and heparin initiated prior to conception.**

Warfarin therapy during the first trimester of pregnancy has been associated with **fetal chondrodysplasia punctata.** In the second and third trimester of pregnancy, warfarin may cause **fetal optic atrophy and mental retardation.**

- **Aortic stenosis** carries **worst prognosis** in pregnancy. AIIMS 2007, 2006
- **Highest mortality** in pregnancy is seen in Eisenmegers complex. AI 1997
- Maximum strain on heart during parturition occurs in **immediate postpartum period.** AI 2007
- **Diastolic murmur** is a feature of heart disease in pregnancy PGI 2003
- **Absolute indications for termination:** AIIMS 2009
  - ✓ **Primary pulmonary hypertension**
  - ✓ **Eisenmegers syndrome**
  - ✓ **Pulmonary venoocclusive disease**

⇨ HIV and Pregnancy: AIIMS 2008

Perinatal Transmission of HIV

- Vertical transmission
- Transplacental transmission
- Vertical transmission is more in cases with preterm birth and with prolonged membrane rupture.
- Risks of vertical transmission directly related to the maternal viral load and inversely related to the maternal immune status.
- Maternal anti retroviral therapy reduces the risk of vertical transmission.
- Pregnancy has got no effect on HIV progression. Increased incidence of abortion, prematurity, IUGR and perinatal mortality in HIV seropositive mothers still remains inconclusive. Maternal mortality and morbidity are not increased.

Management:

Perinatal care:

- Voluntary serologic testing for HIV
- In seropositive cases, tests for other STDs
- Counselling about the risk of HIV transmission
- Progression of disease assessed by the CD4+ count and viral (HIV RNA) load
- Antiretroviral therapy: Triple chemotherapy is preffered as a first line defences and to be started any time between 14 and 34 weeks and then continued throughout pregnancy, labors and postpartum period.

Intrapartum Care:

- Zidovudine given IV infusion starting at the onset of labor (vaginal delivery) or 4 hrs before Cesariean Section (CS). Loading dose 2mg/kg/hr and maintenance dose 1 mg/kg/hr until cord is clamped.
- **Elective CS reduces the risk of vertical transmission by about 50%** Cord should be clamped.
- **Elective CS reduces the risk or vertical transmission by about 50%.** Cord shoud be clamped as early as possible and the baby should be bathed immediately.
- Avoid procedures that result in break in the skin or mucous membrane of the infants. Amniotomy, attachment of scalp eletrode and determination of scalp blood pH should be avoided.
- Caps, masks, gowns and double gloves should be worn. Protective eye wear (gogglels) should be used).
- Blunt tipped needle should be used and appropriate sterilization of instreuments and linens should be done.
- Post exposure prophylaxis with triple therapy for 4 week reduces the risk of seroconversion by more than 80%.

Guidelines for management of HIV in pregnancy is as follows:

- If maternal HIV RNA level is more than 1000copies/mL, the combination antiretroviral therapy is indicated.
- For women with no treatment prior to labor, intrapartum prophylaxis is appropriate with Zidovudine, zidovudine with lamivudine, zidovudine with nevirapine, or nevirapine alone.
- LSCS is recommended for HIV infected women whose HIV-1 RNA load exceeds 1000 copies/mL.
- There is no need to omit ergometrine and it can be given safely to HIV positive mother.
- Breastfeeding should be avoided.

HIV can be transmitted in pregnancy:

- ✓ During delivery (Most Common)
- ✓ In utero
- ✓ During breastfeeding

Highest risk is associated with:

- ✓ High maternal viral load
- ✓ Low CD 4 T cell count
- ✓ Chorioamnionitis
- ✓ Vitamin A deficiency

Lower risk is associated with

- ✓ LSCS. AI 2010
- ✓ Antiretroviral prophylaxis (Zidoviduine) AIIMS 2008
- ✓ Avoiding breastfeeding AIIMS 2008
- ✓ Vitamin A prophylaxis AIIMS 2008
- ✓ Intrapartum nevirapine AI 2010

⇨ Hypertension in Pregnancy:

Pregnancy induced HTN:

Predicted by: AI 1997

- ✓ Rolling over test done at 20 weeks. PGMEE 2006
- ✓ Serum uric acid ↑
- ✓ Weight gain > 2 kg/ month
- ✓ Earliest sign is ↑ BP. AIIMS 1994

➲ Preeclampsia: (High Yield for 2011/2012)

- ▶ Preeclampsia: Hypertension+proteinuria+edema. JK BOPEE 2011
- ▶ Hypertension with proteinuria in a previously normotensive and non proteinuric patient.
- ▶ Mild preeclampsia: Systolic BP>140 or Diastolic BP>90 mm Hg on two or more occasions and proteinuria>300 mg/24 hours.
- ▶ Severe preeclampsia: Systolic BP>160 or Diastolic BP>110 mm Hg on two or more occasions and proteinuria>5gms/24 hours
- ▶ Eclampsia is preeclampsia + convulsions.
- ▶ Imminent eclampsia is heralded by:
  - ✓ Headache
  - ✓ Blurring of vision
  - ✓ Epigastric pain
  - ✓ Brisk deep tendon reflexes.
  - ✓ Diminished urinary output
- ▶ Delivery of fetus is the definitive treatment

- ❒ **Control of hypertension** is the most important factor in management of preeclampsia
- ❒ **LOW GFR is a feature.** AIPGME 2012
- ❒ Eclampsia is **preeclampsia + convulsions.**
- ❒ Eclampsia is mostly seen **antepartum** Calcutta 2000
- ❒ Causes of convulsions in eclampsia is **cerebral anoxia.** Kerala 1996
- ❒ PIH is **hypertension developing after 20 weeks of pregnancy**
- ❒ **Giants roll over test** is done in PIH at **28-32 weeks** Orissa 2000
- ❒ **Rapid gain in weight** is the **earliest sign** of PIH.
- ❒ In pregnancy induced hypertension, sudden loss of vision is due to **Retinal detachment** JIPMER 1999
- ❒ **Magnesium sulfate is effective in eclampsia.** AMU 1985
- ❒ **Mg sulfate toxicity is monitored by: Urinary output, knee jerk, respiratory rate** UPSC 1996

Complications of preeclampsia are: AI 2009

- ✓ Cerebral Hemorrhage
- ✓ Pulmonary edema
- ✓ ARF

- ❒ Drugs considered safe in pregnancy are:
- ❒ **Hydralazine and Methyl dopa.**
- ❒ The drug of choice for "**Hypertension**" in pregnancy is Methyl dopa.
- ❒ The drug of choice for "**Hypertensive crisis**" in Pregnancy is Hydralazine.
- ❒ The drug of choice for "**SEVERE preeclampsia**" in Pregnancy is Labetelol. **AI 2008**
- ❒ The drug of choice to control "**seizures**" in pregnancy is Magnesium sulfate.
- ❒ ACE inhibitors are absolutely contraindicated in pregnancy. **AI 2004, UP 2004**

⇨ Indications for Immediate Termination in Severe Pre-eclampsia: AIIMS 2010

a. Uncontrolled hypertension
b. Imminent eclampsia or eclampsia
c. Abnormal Renal function
d. Abnormal liver function
e. Coagulopathy
f. HELLP syndrome
g. Fetal distress
h. Severe IUGR
i. Abruption
j. Attainment of 34 weeks.

➲ HELLP Syndrome:

- ✓ The HELLP (Hemolysis, Elevated liver enzymes, Low platelets) Syndrome. **KCET 2012**
- ✓ Microangiopathic hemolysis occurs.
- ✓ AST↑
- ✓ LDH↑
- ✓ Acute fatty liver of pregnancy, cholestasis of pregnancy, eclampsia, and the **HELLP** syndrome (can be confused with viral hepatitis during pregnancy).

➲ Antepartum Hemorrhage

⇨ Placenta Previa:

Abnormal implantation of placenta usually near cervical os.

Risk factors:

- ✓ **Prior cesarean**
- ✓ **Grand multipara**
- ✓ **Multiple gestations**
- ✓ **Prior placenta previa**

- ❒ Painless. ☛☛
- ❒ No tenderness☛☛
- ❒ Soft uterus☛☛
- ❒ No uterine irritability
- ❒ Malpresentation ☛☛
- ❒ FHR normal usually☛☛
- ❒ Coagulopathy uncommon☛☛

Placenta praevia is diagnosed by:

- **Transabdominal usg** — **PGI 2011**
- **Transvaginal usg** — **PGI 2011**
- **Transperineal usg** — **PGI 2011**
- **MRI**
- **Color doppler study**

Expectant line of management in placenta previa: (Mcafee and Johnson) **AIIMS 2010**

⇨ Prerequisites

a. For expectant management maternal and fetal condition good.
b. Gestational age < 37 weeks.
c. Fully equipped maternity hospital facilities for emergency section.

When to terminate expectant management:

a) Thirty seven completed weeks
b) Onset of active labor
c) Fetus is dead
d) Profuse bleeding at anytime
e) Maternal or fetal jeopardy **AIIMS 2010**

⇨ Abruption Placenta

Premature separation of a normally placed placenta. ☛☛

Risk factors:

- ✓ **Hypertension**
- ✓ **Trauma to abdomen**
- ✓ **Smoking**
- ✓ **Cocaine use**

- ❒ Painful☛☛
- ❒ Tenderness☛☛
- ❒ Increased uterine tone☛☛
- ❒ Uterine irritability☛☛

❒ Malpresentation none usually☛☛
❒ FHR abnormal usually☛☛
❒ Coagulopathy common☛☛

Abruptio Placentae has Two Classifications:
- **Page classification**
- **Sher's classification**

Page Classification:
- Stage 0 - A diagnosis purely on pathology without symptoms
- Stage I - Quiescent forms with live baby
- Stage II - Mild forms with onset of clotting problem
- Stage III - Severe forms with coagulation deficits and fetal deathin utero

Sher's Classification

It has three stages:
- Stage I - Mild with unexplained vaginal bleeding and retrospective diagnosis of small hematoma postpartum.
- Stage II - Is the intermediate forms with a hypertonic uterus and a live baby.
- Stage III - Is the severe forum with an intrauterine death, subdivided with-**III A-without coagulopapthy-IIIB-with coagulopathy.**

⇨ Vasa Previa

❒ Fetal vessels crossing cervical os. ☛☛
❒ Associated with **velemantous cord insertion.**
❒ Higher incidence in twins.
❒ **Painless vaginal bleeding +fetal distress.** ☛☛
❒ **APT test + look for nucleated cells in cord blood by wrights stain.**
❒ **Emergency cesaren is TOC.**

➲ PPH (High Yield for 2011/2012)

"Any amount of bleeding from or into the genital tract following birth of baby until the end of puerperium which adversely effects the general condition of the patient evidenced by rise in pulse rate and falling BP is called PPH." ☛☛

Commonest cause of PPH is: **Atonic Uterus**

Due to Atonic Uterus: MC **AIIMS 97**
- Grand multipara ☛☛ **PGI 1997**
- Over distension of Uterus☛☛
- Malnutrition and Anemia☛☛
- APH☛☛
- Prolonged labor ☛☛

- Uterine Malformation☛☛
- Mismanaged third stage☛☛
- Constriction ring☛☛

Due to Trauma:

- Instrumental Delivery, (cervical lacerations)
- Face to Pubis Delivery,
- Precipitate labor,
- Macrosomia

Due to Blood coagulopathies:

- Abruption
- Sepsis
- IUD
- HELLP Syndrome

✓ **PPH** occurs when blood loss is **>500 cc.** **DNB 99, KAR 1996**

✓ **Atonic uterus** is more common in **multipara.** ☛☛

✓ Drugs used for PPH are: **Misoprostol, carboprost, methergine, ergometrine**
AI 2008, Manipal 2006, I 2006, DNB 2005, DNB 2003

✓ **B lynch suture is applied on uterus.** **AI 2003**

- **Placenta accerta: Chorionic villi attached to superficial myometrium.**
- **Placenta incerta: Villi invade myometrium.**
- **Placenta percerta: Villi penetrate full thickness of myometrium up to serosa.**

Heterotopic or Heterotropic Pregnancy

- Heterotopic or heterotropic pregnancy **is rare**, but the incidents of it are **on the rise.**
- Heterotopic pregnancy is a multiple pregnancy with **one embryo viably implanted in the uterus and the other implanted elsewhere as an ectopic pregnancy.** ☛☛
- This type of pregnancy does occur very rarely in natural conception, at the rate of 1 in 30,000.
- However, **in pregnancies conceived through assisted reproduction (ART, GIFT, IVF)**, the rate of heterotopic pregnancies jumps to as many as 1 in 100 pregnancies. ☛☛
- Today's rate of heterotopic pregnancies has increased dramatically partly due to a rise in **pelvic inflammatory disease (PID)**, and partly due to a number of other issues. **Previous pelvic surgery, congenital or acquired abnormalities of the uterine cavity and fallopian tubes may contribute to the condition, as does tubal microsurgery, drug ovulation stimulation, and ART.** ☛☛
- When it comes to women who have undergone IVF (in vitro fertilization), the rise in occurrence is largely due to the transfer of multiple embryos to the uterus.
- When **more than five embryos are implanted**, the risk of heterotopic pregnancy increases from 1 in 100 to 1 in 45.

⇨ Uterine Inversion

- ✓ Inside out turning of uterus. ☛☛
- ✓ Results from mismanaged third stage of labor. **Delhi 1998**
- ✓ Patient presents with intense shock. ☛☛
- ✓ On examination of abdomen, fundus of uterus cant be felt. ☛☛
- ✓ Hemorrage (mc), neurogenic shock, pulmonary embolism, uterine sepsis and sub involution are complications. **JIPMER 2003**

Acute Inversion of Uterus

a. 1st degree - fundus inverts but does not herniated through the internal os.

b. Second degree-fundus passes through cervix lies within vagina.

c. Third degree-entire uterus turned inside out and hangs outside the vagina.

Management:

- Replacement
- Manual reposition
- Spinelli procedure
- Kestner procedure
- Huntingtons procedure
- Hantham procedure

➲ Idiopathic Cholestasis of Pregnancy: ☛☛ (High Yield for 2011/2012)

- ► Usually in last (3rd) trimester **PGI 2005, PGI 2002**
- ► Slight jaundice
- ► Generalized pruritis is the commonest symptom, often severe. **PGI 2002**
- ► Disease recurs in next pregnancies.
- ► Marked
  - ✓ ↑ In alkaline phosphatase.
  - ✓ ↑ ALT, **PGI 2002**
  - ✓ ↑ AST,
  - ✓ ↑ Bile acids,
  - ✓ ↑ Bilirubin,
  - ✓ ↑ GTT.
  - ✓ Liver biopsy is the test of choice.
  - ✓ Uresodoxycholic acid is used in treatment. **PGI 2005**
  - ✓ UROSIDOL is used for treatment **AI 2010**

⇨ Antiphospholipid Antibody Syndrome

- Autoimmune disorder.
- Due to **lupus anti coagulant/anticardiolipin antibody.**
- Predominantly **venous thrombosis**
- Associated with **recurrent fetal loss**
- ✓ ↑ **PT**
- ✓ ↑ **PTT**
- ✓ ↑ **Kaolin clotting time.**
- ✓ ↑ **Dilute Russel viper venom time**

⇨ Monitoring of Growth Restricted Fetus

The tests useful for monitoring of Growth restricted fetus are:

- ❐ **Biophysical profile**
- ❐ **Cardiotocography**
- ❐ **Umblical artery Doppler.**

⇨ NST: Non Stress Test

- Is determination of fetal heart rate (FHR) tracing using Doppler to assess FHR and its relationship to fetal movements.
- It is indicated in uteroplacental insufficency/fetal distress.
- Normal result is called **reassuring NST:** At least 2 accelerations of FHR>15 beats per minute lasting >15seconds in 20 minutes.
- Abnormal result is called **non reassuring NST:** <2 accelerations of FHR>15 beats per minute lasting >15seconds in 40 minutes
- In case of non reassuring NST **do BPP.**

➲ FHR

⇨ Normal Pattern

- ❐ Base line heart rate: 120-160 bpm
- ❐ Base line variability: 5-25 bpm
- ❐ Two accelerations in 20 minutes
- ❐ No deceleration

⇨ Abnormal Pattern

- ❐ Unexplained tachycardia
- ❐ Unexplained bradycardia
- ❐ Base line variability <5 bpm
- ❐ Repetitive early or variable decelerations
- ❐ Repetetive late decelerations
- ❐ Sinusoidal pattern

⇨ Deceleration

► Early deceleration: ☚☚ head compression	GI 1997
► Late deceleration: ☚☚ placental insufficiency	I 1998
► Variable deceleration: ☚☚ cord compression.	

The biophysical profile (BPP) is a **noninvasive test that predicts the presence or absence of fetal asphyxia and, ultimately, the risk of fetal death in the antenatal period.** When the BPP identifies a compromised fetus, measures can be taken to intervene before progressive metabolic acidosis leads to fetal death. ☚☚

The BPP combines data from 2 sources (i.e., ultrasound imaging and fetal heart rate [FHR] monitoring). Dynamic realtime B-mode ultrasound is used to measure the amniotic fluid volume (AFV) and to observe several types of fetal movement. The FHR is obtained using a pulsed Doppler transducer integrated with a high-speed microprocessor, which provides a continuously updated reading.

Originally described by **Manning and colleagues**, the BPP has become a standard tool for providing antepartum fetal surveillance. The BPP integrates 5 parameters to yield a biophysical profile score (BPS) and includes

(1) The non stress test (NST), ☚☚

(2) Ultrasound measurement of the AFV, (Amniotic fluid volume) ☚☚

(3) Fetal breathing movements PGI 2002

(4) Fetal body movements, and PGI 2002

(5) Tone. ☚☚

The BPP allows 2 points for each parameter that is present, yielding a maximum score of 10

- ❐ **Reassuring score is 8-10**
- ❐ **<6 is fetal distress.**

➲ BPP

Bpp is a Screening Test for Utero-Placental Insufficiency. The Following Biophysical Tests Are Used:

- **Fetal movement count**
- **Cardiotocography**
- **Non stress test (NST)**
- **Fetal biophysical profile (BPP)**
- **Doppler ultrasound**
- **Vibroacoustic stinulation test**
- **Contraction stress test (CST)**

Cardiotocography:

- Monitoring the baby's heartbeat is one way of checking babies' well-being in labor. By listening to, or recording the baby's heartbeat, it is hoped to identify babies who are hypoxic and who may benefit from caesarean section or instrumental vaginal birth.
- The heartbeat can also be checked continuously by using **a CTG machine.**
- This method is sometimes known as **electronic fetal monitoring (EFM)** and produces a paper recording of the baby's heart rate and their mother's labor contractions.

⇨ Risk facors for Neural Tube Defects

- Family history of NTD
- Insufficient folate
- Maternal diabetes
- Maternal use of antiepeleptics

⇨ Causative Organisms of

Donovaniosis	Calymmatobacter granulomatosis
LGV	Chlamydia trachomatis
Chancroid	H. ducreyi, Herpes hominis
Condyloma acuminate	HPV 6, 11, 16, 18
Yaws	T, pertune
Pinta	T. caratenum

Chorioamnionitis:

- ✓ Fever+maternal tachycardia
- ✓ Uterine tenderness
- ✓ Foul odor of amniotic fluid.
- ✓ Leukocytosis

Complications are: premature rupture of membranes.

- Premature labor
- Endometritis
- Parametritis
- Abruption placenta.

Vaginal delivery is the mainstay of treatment.

Remember:

✓ **ACE inhibitors** are **contraindicated in pregnancy**	**UP 1999**
✓ **Yellow fever vaccine is contraindicated in pregnancy.**	**UP 2000**
✓ **Propyl thiouracil is drug of choice** among antithyroid drugs in pregnancy.	**DNB 2008**
✓ **INH** is **safe** in pregnancy.	**AI 95**

✓	**Streptomycin** is **not given** in pregnancy.	AI 1996
✓	**Primaquine** is **contraindicated** in pregnancy.	DNB 2001
✓	**Valproic acid** in pregnancy causes **Neural tube defects.**	UP 2001

- ✓ **Alcohol: Fetal alcohol syndrome**
- ✓ **Warfarin: Fetal warfarin syndrome**
- ✓ **Phenytoin: Fetal hydantoin syndrome**
- ✓ **Tetracycline: Discoloration of teeth**

►	Methotrexate is **unsafe in pregnancy:**	AI 2009
►	**Propothiouracil is safe** in pregnancy.	AI 2009
►	Varicella can cause **focal skin lesions and hypoplastic limbs.**	AI 2009

►	**Couvelaire uterus** seen in: Abruption placenta	UP 2007
►	**Rule of Hasse:** Determines age of fetus	AIIMS 2003
►	**Banana and lemon sign:** Seen in neural tube defects	PGI 2005
►	**Hartmans sign** is implantation bleeding	AI 98
►	**Chemical pregnancy** means positive beta hCG, negative gestational sac.	UPSC 1997

Causes of Symmetrical Enlargement of Uterus

- ❒ Pregnancy
- ❒ Submucous or Intramural (Solitary) fibroid
- ❒ Adenomyosis
- ❒ Myohyperplasia
- ❒ Pyometra
- ❒ Hematometra
- ❒ Lochiometra
- ❒ Malignancy
- ❒ CA of uterine body
- ❒ Choriocarcinoma

Remember:

- ► **Mons Pubis: Pad of subcutaneous adipose connective tissue.**
- ► **Labia Majora: Are homologous to scrotum and have hair follicles, sweat glands and sebaceous glands.**

► **Labia minora:**	✓ **Don't contain hair follicles.**
► **Clitoris:**	✓ **Is analogous to penis in males**
► **Anterior perineal triangle is:**	✓ **Urogenital triangle.**
► **Posterior perineal triangle is:**	✓ **Anal triangle**
► **Central point of perineum is:**	✓ **Perineal body**
► **Rectoutreine pouch is:**	✓ **Pouch of douglas.**

Embryonic structure	Female
▶ Genital ridge❋	Ovary
▶ Genital swelling❋	L. majora
▶ Genital fold❋	L. minora
▶ Genital tubercle❋	Clitoris

⇨ Fallopian Tube

- ✓ Has 4 parts
- ✓ Lined by ciliated columnar epithelium
- ✓ Has peg cells
- ✓ Measures 10 cms

⇨ Female Urethra

- ✓ 4 cms in length
- ✓ 6 mm in diameter
- ✓ Posterior urethrovesical angle is 100°
- ✓ Has transistional epithelium

- ▶ Uterine artery arises from internal iliac artery.
- ▶ Vaginal artery arises from uterine artery
- ▶ Ovarian artery arises from aorta

Thelarche, pubarche and menarche is the order of sexual development in girls. **PGI 2002**

⇨ Estrogen

- ❒ Produced by the **Syncytiotrophoblast**☛☛
- ❒ Its synthesis depends much on the precursor derived mainly from the fetus.
- ❒ In late pregnancy, **estriol** is the most important estrogen. ☛☛
- ❒ Estrogen increases the **secretion and ciliary beating in fallopian tubes.**
- ❒ Estrogen changes the **cuboidal lining of vagina to stratified.**
- ❒ Estrogen changes the **break down of glycogen into lactate in vagina.**
- ❒ Estrogen **initiates breast development.** ☛☛
- ❒ Estrogen causes **early epiphyseal closure.** ☛☛
- ❒ Estrogen causes **water retention**☛☛

⇨ Progesterone

- Produced by **Syncytiotrophoblast**☛☛
- Chief hormone of **Corpus luteum**☛☛
- Precursors from fetal origin are not necessary
- After delivery, its level decreases rapidly and is **not** detectable **after 24 hours**☛☛.

⇨ Corpus Luteum Secretes DNB 2004

- ✓ Progesterone
- ✓ Estrogen
- ✓ Inhibin
- ✓ Relaxin

➲ Ovulation (High Yield for 2011/2012)

► Best predictor of ovulation is: preovulatory rise in progesterone.	COMED 2008
► Source of progesterone in normal menstrual cycle is: corpus luteum	MAHE 2007
► Inhibin is secreted by Graffian follicle	KAR 2006
► Ovulation coincides with LH surge	UPSC, PGI
► LH surge preceeds ovulation by 24 hours	MAHE 08
► Ovulatory period corresponds to 14 days before menstruation.	TN, 90, 98

► Proliferative phase:	► Estrogen stimulation☛☛
► Secretory phase:	► Progesterone stimulation☛☛
► Estrogen:	► Produced by granulosa cells☛☛
► Progesterone:	► Produced by corpus luteum☛☛
► FSH: ☛☛ AIIMS 08	► Stimulates growth of granulosa cells. Measure of ovarian reserve.
► LH:	► Stimulates follicle rupture and ovulation

⇨ Supports of Uterus All 1999

- ✓ Perineal body
- ✓ Pelvic diaphragm
- ✓ Transcervical ligament
- ✓ Pubocervical ligament
- ✓ Uterosacral ligament
- ✓ Uterine axis
- ✓ Round ligament of uterus
- ✓ Broad ligament is not a support of uterus☛☛

⇨ Anomalies of Uterus

- ► Uterus bicornis bicollis: Two uterine cavities, double cervix
- ► Uterus bicornis unicollis: Two uterine cavities, single cervix
- ► Septate uterus: Septum between two fused mullerian ducts
- ► Retroverted uterus: Long axis of body of uterus and cervix are in line instead of normal anteverted and anteflexed uterus.

⇨ Supports of Vagina

AIIMS 2004

- ✓ Perineal body☛☛
- ✓ Pelvic diaphragm☛☛
- ✓ Levator ani muscle ☛☛

⇨ Important Points about Vagina

- ▶ Vagina lacks mucus secreting glands. UPSC 2007
- ▶ pH of normal adult vagina: 4.5 - 5.5
- ▶ pH of pregnant vagina: 3.5-4.5
- ▶ Epithelium of vagina: stratified squamous

Lymphatic Drainage of Uterus☛☛

- From **fundus** and **upper part of body** → **Pre aortic** and **Lateral aortic** group of nodes
- Cornu of uterus→ **Superficial inguinal lymph** nodes
- Lower part of body → **Internal iliac group** of lymph nodes

Lymphatic drainage of cervix ☛☛

- **External iliac** nodes and **obturator** lymph nodes either directly or through para-cervical lymph nodes.
- **Internal iliac** group of lymph nodes
- **Sacral group**

Lymphatic drainage of fallopian tube☛☛

- **Para -aortic** group along the ovarian vessels.

Lymphatic drainage of vagina

- **Upper 1/3**→ **Lliac** group
- **Middle 1/3 upto hymen**→ **Internal iliac** group
- **Below hymen**→ **Superficial inguinal** lymph nodes.

Lymphatics of clitoris: Superficial inguinal, deep inguinal, Cloquets node ☛☛ PGI 2000

BARTHOLIN'S GLAND

- Correspondes to **bulbourethral glands of male☛☛**
- Situated in the **superficial perineal pouch☛☛**
- Lies **close** to the **posterior end** of vestibular bulb.
- Are **pea** sized.
- Lie near the junction of the **anterior 2/3 and posterior 1/3of labium majus. ☛☛**
- It is a Compound **Racemose** Gland and its duct measures about **2 cm**,lined with **columnar**
- **Epithelium.**
- Its duct passes forward and inward to open **external to the hymen** on **inner side of Labium minus**
- Infection of these glands or their ducts result in **Bartholinitis.**

Acute Bartholinitis (High Yield for 2011/2012)

- ❐ Although Gonococcus is always in mind but more commonly **E.coli, Staphlococcus,**
- ❐ **Streptococcus or Chlamydia trachomatis** are involved
- ❐ The end results of acute bartholinitis are
- ✓ Complete resolution
- ✓ Recurrence
- ✓ Abscess formation
- ✓ Cyst formation.

Recurrent Bartholinitis

- ✓ Periodic painful attacks cause annoyance to the patient. ☚☚
- ✓ Treatment:**Active Phase**: Hot compress, Analgesics and Antibiotics after proper culture
- ✓ **Quiescent Phase**: Excision of the gland along with its duct.

Bartholins Abscess

- ✓ It is the **end result** of acute bartholinitis
- ✓ Duct is blocked by fibrosis, exudates pent up inside to produce abscess.
- ✓ Treatment: Same as for bartholinitis .Abscess should be drained at the earliest before it bursts.
- ✓ **Marsupialization:** Not only helps in drainage of pus but prevents recurrence of abscess☚☚
- ✓ And future cyst formation.
- ✓ It should be done under **General Anesthesia.**
- ✓ Reccurrent Bartholins abscess Rx _____**Excision in Quiescent Stage**

Bartholins Cyst

- ❐ It commonly involves the **duct** and **not** the gland☚☚.
- ❐ Cyst of the duct or the gland can be **differentiated** by the **lining epithelium**
- ❐ Sometimes the cyst becomes large up to the size of **Hens egg**
- ❐ The shape of vulval cleft changes to **S-shaped**
- ❐ Rx: **Marsupialization**☚☚

Advatages of Marsupialization over traditional excision☚☚

- ✓ **Simple**
- ✓ **Can be done even under local anesthesia**
- ✓ **Shorter hospital stay.**
- ✓ **Postoperative complications almost nil.**
- ✓ **Gland function remain intact.**

GARTNER'S DUCT

- ❐ Remnant of **wolfian duct.** ☚☚
- ❐ Runs below but **parallel** to the fallopian tube in the **mesosalpinx.**
- ❐ The tubules of the gartners duct may be **cystic,**

- The outer ones are **Kobelts tubules**, ☛☛
- The **Middle** set, the **Epoophoron**☛☛
- The **proximal** set, the **Paroopohoron.** ☛☛

- Small cyst may arise from any of the tubules.
- A cystic swelling from the Gartners duct may appear in the anter -lateral wall of the
- Vagina **confusing** with cystocele. Cystic swelling is present at the **junction of lower 1/3 and upper 2/3 of vaginal wall.**

GARTNER'S CYST	CYSTOCELE
▶ Situated **anteriorly** or **anterolateral**	➠ Situated **anteriorly**
▶ Size is **variable**	➠ Size **increases** on straining☛☛
▶ Rugosities of the overlying vaginal. Mucosa is **lost.** Vaginal mucosa over it becomes **Tense and shiny.**	➠ Mucosa over the bulge has **Transverse rugosity**
▶ Margins are **well defined.**	➠ **No such** thing is seen.
▶ **Not** reducible	➠ Margins are **diffuse.**
▶ **No** impulse on coughing	➠ Reducible.
	➠ Impulse on coughing is present.

▶ **Length of female urethra:** 40mm	**DNB 1995**
▶ **Uterine cervix ratio up to 10 years: 1:2**	**PGI 1989**
▶ Uterine cervix ratio **in adult** : 3:1	
▶ **Normal Urethrovesical angle** : 100°	
▶ **Size of Graffian follicle:** 2mm	

⇨ Important Facts about Vulva

▶ Leukoplakia of vulva is treated by **simple vulvectomy.**	
▶ Lymphatics of vulva go to **inguinal lymph nodes.**	
▶ Vulval carcinoma metastasizes to **superficial inguinal lymph nodes.**	
▶ **Sentinel biopsy is used in vulval cancer.**	**AI 2010**

⇨ Important Facts about Vagina

❒ **Straw berry vagina: trichomoniasis vaginalis**	
❒ **Clue cells in vagina, fishy odoue, positive whiff test: hemophilus vaginalis**	**UPSC 2007**
❒ **pH of vagina is lowest in pregnancy.**	
❒ **Senile vaginitis is due to estrogen deficiency**	**COMED 2007**
❒ **Vagina has no mucus secreting glands.**	**UPSC 2007**
❒ **Lactobacillus is the protective bacterium in normal vagina**	**JK 2001**

➲ Kartagener's Syndrome (High Yield for 2011/2012)

Infertility is common, due to defective ciliary action in the fallopian tube in affected females or diminished sperm motility in affected males.

In Kartagener's syndrome (KS), primary **defects of the ciliary axoneme cause dyskinetic ciliary motion.** Because ciliary motion is an **important factor in normal ovum transport, ciliary dyskinesia may cause infertility.** In active regions, beat frequency ranged from 5 to 10 Hz, approximately 30% of normal.

- Electron microscopy shows morphological **defects in** tubal mucosa.
- The number of cilia per cell is ↓
- The major ultrastructural abnormality was an absence of the central microtubules.

Electron microscopy demonstrated that the majority of cilia **lack dynein arms** and radial spokes and that various defects of microorgans existed in the sperm.

➲ Pelvic Inflammatory Diseases PID

⇨ Vaginal Discharge:❋

Yellow, pH>5, clue cells, amine odor:	**Bacterial vaginosis**
Cottage cheese discharge, pruritis, Vulvovaginitis:	**Candida**
Frothy, Foamy discharge and motile trophozites seen:	**Trichomonas vaginalis**

Gram **negative diplococcic** in PMNs in urethral Exudate:	**Nisseria gonorrhea**
Culture negative specimen with **inclusion bodies:**	**Chlamydiae trachomatis**
Organisms **without cell wall** and **urease positive:**	**Ureaplasma Urealyticum**
Flagellate protozoa with motility :	**Trichomonas vaginalis**

⇨ Predisposing Factors of Candidiasis — AIIMS 2010

- Use of broad spectrum antibiotics
- Other genital infections causing local inflammation
- Late pregnancy
- Immunosuppressed states
- Steroid therapy
- Diabetes mellitus
- Endocrine problems (thyroid and adrenal)
- Continue oral contraceptive pill

➲ Chancroid: (High Yield for 2011/2012)

- **Hemophilus ducreyi.**
- **Painful ulcer, genital ulceration and inguinal adenitis.** PGI 2002
- **Painful lymphadenopathy seen**

▶ Associated with **infection with HIV**	
▶ **School of fish appearance**	AI 1989
▶ H. ducreyi is a highly fastidious coccobacillary gram-negative bacterium **whose growth requires X factor (hemin).**	
▶ **Chancroid** can be treated effectively with several regimens, including (1) **Ceftriaxone**, 250 mg intramuscularly as a single dose; (2) Azithromycin, 1 g orally as a single dose; (3) Erythromycin, 500 mg orally four times daily for7days; and (4) Ciprofloxacin, 500 mg orally twice daily for 3 days	

⇨ Candida

▶ Caused by **candida albicans.**	
▶ **Recurrent vulvovaginalis: 4 or more episodes per year.**	
▶ It is a **gram-positive fungus.**	
▶ **Common in pregnancy, diabetes mellitus**	
▶ Commonly seen in **pregnancy, diabetes, antibiotics, OCP use, Corticosteroids.**	
✓ **Profuse curdy white curdy** discharge or **cottage cheese appearance.**	AI 2000
✓ Dyspareunia	
✓ Burning sensation.	
✓ Intense pruritis	PGI 2000

⇨ Trichomoniasis

▶ **Most common vaginal infection.**	
▶ **Caused by flagellate parasite "trichomonas vaginalis"**	PGI 2005
▶ **Profuse, thin, greeny discharge which is malodorous.**	PGI 2008
▶ **Straw berry vagina/colpitis macularis appearance.**	AIIMS 1998
▶ **Best test: Culture**	
▶ **Metronadizole is DOC.**	PGI 2000
▶ **Treat sexual partener concurrently**	

➲ Bacterial Vaginosis: (High Yield for 2011/2012)

Poly Microbial Caused by:	
✓ **Gardenella vaginalis**	
✓ **Hemophilus vaginalis**	K 2008
✓ **Mobilincus**	
✓ **Ureaplasma urealyticum**	
✓ **Mycoplasma hominis**	
▶ ↓ **lactobacilli**	
▶ ↓ **leucocytes**	
▶ **Alkaline pH**	PGI 2002

- "**Clue cells**" are epithelial cells with bacteria adhering to their surface and sometimes obscuring their borders. Clue cells indicate bacterial vaginosis. **AIIMS 2008**
- Clue cells were first described by **Gardner and Dukes** in 1955 and were so named **as these cells give an important "clue" to the diagnosis of bacterial vaginosis (BV).**
- Clue cells are vaginal squamous epithelial cells coated with anaerobic Gram-variable coccobacilli Gardnerella vaginalis.

Pathogenesis:

The detection of clue cells is the most useful single procedure for the diagnosis of BV. Presence of more than 20% clue cells in vaginal discharge is included in **Amsel's criteria** for the diagnosis of BV. Other criteria for the diagnosis of BV include:

Milky, homogeneous, adherent discharge; **PGI 2005**

Vaginal pH greater than 4.5;

Positive Whiff test, i.e., typical fishy odor on addition of one or two drops of 10% KOH to vaginal discharge **DNB 2011**

Few or no lactobacilli.

Metronadizole (DOC) or clindamycin is used in treatment. **PGI 2002**

Metronadizole is used in pregnancy.

- "**Clue cells**" are epithelial cells with bacteria adhering to their surface and sometimes obscuring their borders. Clue cells indicate bacterial vaginosis. **AIIMS 2008**

LGV

- **Chlamydia trachomatis L type**
- **Painless ulcer.**
- **Esthiomine seen in LGV** **P 1988**
- **Groove sign. (double genitocrural fold)** **KCET 2012**
- **Genital elephantiasis is seen.** **AI 2002**
- Incubation period = 3 days to 3 weeks
- **Painless,** vesicle, often transient, followed by **suppurative LAP**
- **Sign of Groove +** (LAP present both above and below inguinal ligament) **AI 1989**
- **Elephaintiasis** of vulva + Vaginal and rectal strictures seen
- **Frei's** intadermal test +
- **Doxycycline is DOC** **KAR1994**

⇨ Donovaniosis (Granuloma Inguinale)

- Calymatobacterium granulomaosis
- Painless ulcer
- Painless beffy red ulcer with fresh granulation tissue.

⇨ Herpes Genitalis

- HSV II virus usual
- Painful vesicular lesions

⇨ Condyloma Acuminata

- **Most common** viral STD.
- Caused by HPV: **6, 16, 18**
- Immunosuppression, diabetes, pregnancy are predisposing factors
- **Cauliflower like masses**, pedunculated

Treated by:

- **Podophyllin, podophox** ☛☛ **OMED 2007**
- **Trichloroacetic acid,** ☛☛
- **Imiquimoid**☛☛
- **Cryo,**
- **LASER,**
- **Surgical excision.**

Condyloma lata are seen in secondary syphilis☛☛

➲ Chlamydia (High Yield for 2011/2012)

- Purulent discharge, urethritis, arthritis, conjuctivitis
- **Infertility** associated with fallopian-tube scarring. It appears that subclinical tubal infection ("Silent salpingitis") may produce scarring.
- **Ectopic pregnancy,**
- **Perihepatitis, or the Fitz-Hugh-Curtis syndrome,** this syndrome should be suspected whenever a young, sexually active woman presents with an illness resembling cholecystitis (fever and right-upper-quadrant pain of subacute or acute onset). Symptoms and signs of salpingitis may be minimal. High titers of antibodies to C. trachomatis are generally present.
- **PCR is gold standard for diagnosis**
- **Azithromycin is DOC for uncomplicated chlamydiae.**
- **Azithromycin is DOC for chlamydiae in pregnancy.**
- **Erythromycin is safe in pregnancy** AI 2010
- **Azithromycin and contact tracing is the most effective for chlamydiae infections** AI 2002

Genital TB (High Yield for 2011/2012)

- Genital TB is almost always **secondary** to focus elsewhere.
- Primary focus is in **lungs (50%),** lymph nodes (40%) cases. UP 2003
- **Hematogeneous spread** is the commonest mode followed by direct spread and ascending route.
- **Major forms:**
  - ✓ Tuberculous endosalpingitis
  - ✓ Tuberculous exosalpingitis
  - ✓ Interstitial salpingitis
- Only about 10% of genital TB cases have children.
- First site of affection are the **fallopian tubes.** AIIMS 1993
- Commonest site of affection are the **fallopian tubes** AI 1998
- **"Tobacco pouch appearance"** of fallopian tubes is a feature.
- **"Salpingitis isthimica nodosa"** is nodular thickening of tubes in genital TB.
- **Endometrium** of uterus **is involved in 60% cases.**
- **Cervix** is involved in **10-15% of cases.**
- Infertility is due to blockage of fallopian tubes. In the form of TB endosalpingitis.
- The first line of treatment is **ATT** (Anti tubercular therapy).

Endometriosis

- **Commonest site: Ovary** DNB 2011, KCET 2012
- **Followed by: pouch of douglas, uterosacral ligaments, rectovaginal septum.**
- Peak age: 30-40 years
- Common in nullipara Kerala 94
- Chocolate cysts PGI 2002
- Tenderness and nodularity of uterosacral ligaments.
- **Sampsons theory of retrograde menstruation. (most accepted) SGPGI 2005**
- **Meyer and ivanoffs coelomic metaplasia theory**
- **Direct implantation theory**
- **Halbans lymphatic theory**
- Rare in negroes
  - ✓ Pelvic pain (Commonest manifestation) UPSC
  - ✓ **Painful periods** Dysmenorrhea
  - ✓ **Painful intercourse** Dyspareunia
  - ✓ **Painful bowel movements** Dyschezia

- ✓ Menorrhagia,
- ✓ Polymenorrhea,
- ✓ Infertility
- ✓ Treatment

▶ **Progesterone**	**UPSC 2004**
▶ **OCP**	
▶ **CLOMIPHENE (In Infertile Women)**	**MAHE 2003**
▶ **Danazol**	
▶ **GnRH analogues (leupolide)**	**UPSC 2007**
▶ **Ovarian cystectomy/oopherectomy/ Wedge resection**	**UPSC 2006**
▶ **Paratubal lysis by laproscopy.**	
▶ **Total hysterectomy: For diffuse endometriosis interna**	

⇨ Endometriosis: Atypical Sites

- ▶ Abdominal scar
- ▶ Bladder/ ureter
- ▶ Cervix/vagina
- ▶ Umbilicus
- ▶ Gut
- ▶ Lungs

⇨ Naked Eye Appearances

- ❒ Powder burns
- ❒ Red flame shaped areas
- ❒ Yellow brown patches
- ❒ White areas and circular peritoneal defects

Pseudoxanthoma cells: adjacent to lining of endometriosis, presence of polyhedral, phagocytic, pigmented cells with hemosiderin:

➲ Adenomyosis: (High Yield for 2011/2012)

- ▶ Endometrial glands within Myometrium of uterine wall.
- ▶ Secondary dysmenorrhea and menorrhagia are common.
- ▶ Uterus is enlarged and tender.
- ▶ Treatment: Hysterectomy.

Contraception

Gossypol:

Male contraceptive.
Direct suppression of semineferous tubules causing azoospermia.
Suppresses LH.

Intrauterine Contraceptive Device (IUCD)

Act by ovulation inhibition, causing aseptic endometritis	JIPMER, AIIMS
Act by prevention of fertilization	AI 2006
Act by interfering with implantation	AI 2006
Contraindications:	
✓ PID	
✓ Diabetes mellitus	
✓ Congenital uterine anomalies	
✓ Heart disease	
✓ Pelvic TB	
✓ HIV Positive	
✓ Suspected pregnancy	
✓ Previous ectopic	
✓ Menorrhagia	
Commonest side effect is bleeding.	

Nova T has a silver core but contains both copper and silver — PGI 2005

▶ In CuT_{200}, 200 means 200 mm^2 of copper.	
▶ CuT_{200} is inserted postnatally after 8 weeks	KAR 2005
▶ If CuT_{200} is implanted in Myometrium treatment is hysteroscopic removal	CUPGEE 2K
▶ CuT_{200} should be replaced after every 10 years.	COMED 2008

Contraceptive TODAY	APPG 2006
▶ Contains 9 NON OXYNOL	
▶ Is a barrier contraceptive	
▶ Effective for 24 hours after insertion	
▶ Spermicidal in nature.	

▶ NORPLANT contains levonorgesterol.	
▶ **Centrochroman** is anti estrogenic, anti progestogenic non teratogenic, long acting pill.	
▶ **Mifeprestone** is an anti progestogen.	
▶ **MINERA** is progesterone IUCD.	AIIMS 2007

➲ Uses of OCP (High Yield for 2011/2012)

- **Contraception, emergency postcoital (prophylaxis)** A combination of levonorgestrel 50 or norgestrel with ethinyl estradiol is used as emergency contraception (also called intraception, morning-after treatment, or postcoital contraception) for postcoital birth control, after pregnancy has been ruled out. The dosing method using high doses of estrogen-progestin hormones is commonly called the **Yuzpe method.**
- **Acne vulgaris**
- **Amenorrhea**
- **Dysfunctional uterine bleeding (DUB)**
- **Dysmenorrhea**
- **Hypermenorrhea**
- **Endometriosis (prophylaxis and treatment)**
- **Hirsutism, female**
- **Hyperandrogenism, ovarian**
- **Polycystic ovary syndrome**

⇨ WHO Categories Contraindications for Estrogens/OCPS

- ✓ Age >40 years
- ✓ Smoker <35 years
- ✓ History of Jaundice
- ✓ Mild Hypertension
- ✓ Gallbladder disease
- ✓ Diabetes.
- ✓ Sickle Cell anemia
- ✓ Headache
- ✓ CIN or Ca Cervix

- ✓ Unexplained Vaginal bleeding
- ✓ Hyperlipidemia
- ✓ Past Breast Cancer
- ✓ Benign Liver tumors
- ✓ Heavy smoker
- ✓ Breast feeding

- OCPS protect against **endometrial cancer, Ovarian cancer.**
- **OCP of choice in Lactating females is Mini Pill.** COMED 2008
- **Fertility returns 6 months after OCP use.** UPSC 2007

2

OBSTETRICS AND GYNECOLOGY

⇨ Drugs Decreasing Effectiveness of OCP

- Barbiturates
- Carbamezapine
- Phenytoin
- Rifampicin

⇨ Levonorgestrel

- Levonorgestrel is a **synthetic progestogen** used as an active ingredient in hormonal contraception.
- **Makes endometrium unreceptive.** **UPSC 2007**
- **Makes cervical mucus thick.**
- It is used effectively in emergency contraception both **in combined form with estrogens as well as levonorgestrel only method.**
- Levonorgestrel only method uses **"1500 μgm single dose"** or **"750 μgm" doses twelve hours** apart within 3 days of unprotected sexual activity.

⇨ Progastasert

- ✓ Third generation IUCD containing progestrone
- ✓ Decreases blood loss
- ✓ Decreases dysmenorrhea
- ✓ BUT ↑ risk of ectopics

⇨ Choices of Contraception

▶ **Newly married**	Pill
▶ **Postabortal**	Pill
▶ **Postpartum Non lactating**	Pill
▶ **Diabetic**	IUCD
▶ **Pulm. TB**	Barrier
▶ **Emergency**	LNG

⇨ Lifespan

- Nova T: 5 YEARS
- Cu T 380A: **10 YEARS** **MAH 2012**
- Progastasert: 1 YEAR
- Cu T 200B: 4 YEARS
- LNG IUCD: 5 YEARS

⇨ LNG-IUS (Levonorgestrel Intrauterine System)

- Is a hormone releasing IUCD.
- It is replaced every 5 yrs.
- Its efficacy is comparable to sterilisation. The non-contraceptive benefits are:

✓ **Risk of ectopic pregnancy significantly reduced**

✓ **Risk of PID reduced**

✓ **Significan reduction in menstrual blood loss, menorrhagia, dysmenorrhea and prementstrual tension syndrome (PSM) and anemia improves**

✓ **Treatment of edommetrial hyperplasia, adenomyosis, uterine fibroids and endometrial cancer**

✓ **Can be used as an alternative to hysterectomy for menorrhagia**

✓ **It provides excellent benefits of hormone replacement therapy (HRT) when used over the transition years of reproduction to perimenopause.**

⇨ Depo Medroxy Progesterone Acetate (DMPA)

Is an injectable steroid contraceptive used in a dose of 150 mg every three months or 300 mg every six monts.

Advantages:

✓ It eliminates the regular medication as imposed by oral pil

✓ Can be used safely during lactation. It increases milk secretion without altering its composition

✓ No estrogen related side effects

✓ Menstrual symptoms e.g menorrhagia, dysmenorrhea are reduced, anemia imporoves

✓ Protective against endometrial cancer

✓ Can be used as an interim contraceptive before vasectomy becomes effective

✓ Reduction in PID, endometriosis, ectopic pregnancy and ovarian cancer.

Drawbacks:

- Failure rate 0-0.3 HWY
- Irregular bleeding and occasional phase of amenorrhea
- Return of fertility after discontinuation is usually delayed for 4-8 months.

⇨ Third Generation OCP

Contain 3rd generation progesterone

✓ **Desogestrel**

✓ **Norgestimate**

✓ **Gestodene**

Lower risk of arterial thrombosis

Higher risk of venous thrombosis

Lipid friendly UPSC 2002

➲ OCP

Helps in protection against:

- **Uterine ca** AIIMS 2002

➡ Ovarian ca	AIIMS 2002
➡ Ovarian cysts	
➡ Endomteriosis	
➡ PID	
➡ Ectopics (indirectly)	
➡ Menorrhagia	
➡ Polymenorrhea	
➡ Rheumatoid arthritis	AI 2007
➡ Endometriosis	AI 2007
OCP can cause	
➡ Hepatic adenomas	PGI 2006
➡ Cancer cervix	
Drugs which can reduce effectiveness of OCP:	
✓ Rifampicin	AIIMS 2007
✓ Carbamezapines	
✓ Phenobarbitone	
✓ Phenytoin	
✓ Griseofulvin	
✓ Tetracyclines	

⇨ Criterion for Sterilization — UPSC 2006

- Age of female >22 years
- Age of male<60 years.
- Couple should have at least 2 children.

⇨ Minilap Methods

- Pomeroys method
- Madlener method
- Fimbriectomy

⇨ Laproscopic Sterilization

- ► Here fallopian tube is identified and clipped by Fallope ring, Hulka clip, Filsche clip.
- ► Most common site for female sterilization is Isthmus. AIIMS 2007, AI 2007
- ► In Pomeroys method of female sterilization, isthimo ampullary porition is ligated. UPSC 2007

⇨ Emergency Contraception is by — UPSC 2006

- ✓ OCP
- ✓ CuT
- ✓ Levonorgestel

⇨ Indications for Emergency Contraception

- In protected sex
- Condom rupture
- Missed pill
- Sexual assault
- Rape

➲ Infertility: (High Yield for 2011/2012)

- **Failure to conceive within one or more years of regular unprotected sex.**
- **Male responsible for 30% cases.**
- **Female responsible for 30% cases.**

⇨ Intrauterine insemination

Indications:

- ✓ **Hostile cervical mucus**
- ✓ **Cervical stenosis**
- ✓ **Oligospermia**
- ✓ **Immune factors**
- ✓ **Unexplained fertility**

⇨ Intracervical Insemination

Indications

- ✓ **Hypospadias**
- ✓ **Retrograde ejaculation**
- ✓ **Impotence**
- ✓ **Third degree retroversion of uterus.**

⇨ In Vitro Fertilization

Indications

- ✓ **Tubal disease** — **PGI 1988, PGI 1990, PGI 1989**
- ✓ **Unexplained infertility**
- ✓ **Cervical hostility**
- ✓ **Failed ovulation induction**
- ✓ **Endometriosis**
- ✓ **Male factor infertility**

⇨ Other Assisted Reproduction Techniques

GIFT : Gamete intrafallopian transfer	AI 1995
ZIFT: Zygote intrafallopian transfer	AI 1995
MIST: Microinsemination sperm transfer	

⇨ Indications for Artificial Insemination

- Oligospermia
- Impotency
- Premature ejaculation
- Retrograde ejaculation
- Hypospadias
- Antisperm antibodies in cervical mucus
- Unexplained infertility

➲ Artifical Insemination Techniques: (High Yield for 2011/2012)

- IVF: In vitro fertilization and Embryo transfer
- GIFT: Gamete intrafallopian transfer
- ZIFT: Zygote intrafallopian transfer
- POST: Peritoneal oocyte and sperm transfer
- SUZI: Subzonal insemination
- ICSI: Intra cytoplasmic sperm injection

⇨ Indications for Donor Insemination

- Azoospermia
- Vasectomy (Failure of reversal)
- Untreatable oligospermia
- Ineradicable STD in case of males
- Genetic disorder of male partner
- Incorrectable ejaculatory dysfunction

⇨ Sperm recovery can be done using:

❒ MESA: Microsurgical epidydmal sperm aspiration	
❒ PESA: Percutaneous epidydmal sperm aspiration	
❒ TESE: Testicular Sperm Extraction	
❒ TESA: Percutaneous Testicular Sperm fine needle aspiration	AI 2007

Aspiration of sperms is done in TESA.	AI 2007
In Post testicular azospermia technique used is PESA/MESA	Orissa 2005
Ferning pattern of cervical mucus is because of: estrogen	UPSC 1985
Palm leaf patter cervix is due to estrogen.	JIPMER 1980
Spinbarkiet phenomenon is maximum in ovulatory phase	AIIMS 1984
Post coital test determines cervical factor	TN 1987

⇨ Prolapse

❒ **Cystocele:** Prolapse of upper 2/3 of anterior vaginal wall. Formed by **base** of bladder	UPSC, PGI
❒ **Uerethrocele:** Prolapse of lower 1/3 of anterior vaginal wall	
❒ **Enterocele:** Prolapse of upper 1/3 of posterior vaginal wall	
❒ **Rectocele** Prolapse of lower 2/3 of posterior vaginal wall	
❒ **Uterine prolapse:** Abnormal descent of uterus through vagina	
❒ **Procedentia:** Complete uterine prolapse outside vulva	

➨ Prolapse in pregnant women in **Ist Trimester: Pessary**	UPSC 2006
➨ Prolapse in pregnant women in **2nd Trimester: Resolves itself**	
➨ Prolapse in young women: **Sling operation, Perineal exercise**	UPSC 2007, KAR 2001
➨ Prolapse in Women **<40 years with family complete** **wanting to retain** menstrual function: **Fother gills operation**	MAH 2012
➨ Prolapse in **Women >40 years with family complete** **Not wanting to retain** menstrual function: **Vaginal Hysterectomy**	
➨ Prolapse in **old Women who cant sustain surgery: Le Fortes surgery**	

⇨ Complications

Elongation of cervix	
Cystocele	
Decubitus ulcer	
Decubitus ulcer is because of venous congestion	PGI

▶ **MC urinary fistula: Vesico vaginal**	
▶ **MC cause of VVF in india: obstructed labor (DOC cystoscopy)**	AI 2010
▶ **MC cause of Uretro vaginal fistula: injury to ureter in Hysterectomy**	
▶ **MC cause of vesico uterinefistula: cesarean section**	
▶ **MC cause of Recto Vaginal fistula: complete perineal tear**	

➲ VVF

Commonest Causes (High Yield for 2011/2012)

Obstetrical causes are commoner in developing countries.

- Obstructed and prolonged Delivery
- Traumatic Instrumental like with forceps
- During LSCS
- Operative
- Traumatic
- Malignancy
- Radiation
- Infective chronic granulomatous lesions like
  - ✓ TB, LGV
  - ✓ Schistosomiasis
  - ✓ actinomycosis

Presentation: A continuous dribbling of urine with sodden and excoriated vulval skin

Confirmation of diagnosis

- **Speculum examination**
- **EUA**
- **Dye test using Methylene blue**
- **Three swab test** Three swab test is done to differentiate between VVF, ureterovaginal and urethrovaginal fistula.
- **Indigo carnine test (given IV) to pick up an ureterine fistula**
- **Cysto-urethroscopy**

Treatment

Preventive Antenatal care

Intrapartum care Prophylactic catheterization in case of doubt

Most obstetric fistulas can be operated upon immediately however postsurgical cases are repaired **after 3-6 months.**

Prolonged and obstructed labor is the MC cause of VVF in India.

- ✓ History and clinical examination are very important.
- ✓ Urine routine and culture should be done to rule out concomitant infection.
- ✓ If ureter involvement is suspected then IVP can be performed.
- ✓ Dye test can be done. Methylene blue dye is inserted in bladder and vaginal examination is done. Appearance of blue dye in vagina indicates a VVF.

The most useful investigation is cystoscopy. All patients should undergo cystourethroscopy prior to surgery

➲ Menstrual Disorders

- **Menarche"** (First Menstruation) occurs between **11-15 years.**
- Normal duration of menstrual period is **4-5 days.**
- Peak Secretory activity is seen on **Day 22** of menstrual cycle

- Amount of blood loss is **20-80 ml.** **DNB 2003, DNB 1998**
- **AVERAGE** blood loss in normal periods is **50 ml.** **PGI 2005**
- **Precocious menstruation** occurs in females aged less than 10 years.
- **"Menopause"** means permanent cessation of menstruation at an average age of 50 years.
- **"Premature menopause"** is when menstruation stops at or below 40 years of age. **MAHE 2007**
- **"Delayed Menopause"** is when menopause fails to occur even beyond 55 years.

Polymenorrhea is cyclic bleeding where cycle length is reduced to less than 21 days and remains constant at that frequency.

Metorrhagia is irregular, acyclic bleeding.

Menomettorhagia is irregular and excessive bleeding to the extent that menstrual period is not recognized at all.

Hypomenorrhea is scant bleeding lasting for less than 2 days

- **Most common cause of postmenopausal bleeding in India is ca cervix.** **AIIMS 2007, AI 2007**
- **Most common cause of secondary amonorrhea in India I: endometrial tuberculosis.** **AI 2005**

Amenorrhea means absence of periods for 6 months or more

Causes of **Cryptomenorrhea:**

- Imperforate hymen
- Transverse septum in vagina
- Non canalization of cervix
- Cervical canal stenosis

Primary Amenorrhea: (High Yield for 2011/2012)

Failure of onset of menses in a girl by 16 years of age.

Causes:

- **Aplasia/hypoplasia of uterus**
- **Turners syndrome**
- **Pseudohermaphroditism**
- **Cretinism**

Syndromes Causing Amonorrhea

- **Kallamans syndrome**
- **Prader willi syndrome**
- **Laurence moon biddel syndrome**
- **Frohlichs syndrome**
- **Turners syndrome**

- Sheehans syndrome
- Sweyers syndrome
- Ashermans syndrome

Dysfunctional Uterine Bleeding: (High Yield for 2011/2012)

Menorrhagia without extra genital cause and normal pelvic examination.

Associated with metropathia hemorrhagica — UP 2003, DELHI 1997, DNB 1996

Endometrium can be:

- Normal
- Hyperplastic (Commonest) — JIPMER 1992
- Irregular shedding, irregular ripening — MAHE 1998
- Tubercular endometritis
- Chronic endometritis
- Progesterone is usually deficient.↑Estrogen — DELHI 1999

Treatment of DUB:

- NSAIDS
- Progesterone — PGI 2011
- Traxenemic acid — PGI 2011
- Low dose OCP
- Conjugated estrogens — PGI 2011
- Gn RH analogues
- Desmopressin

Premenstrual Syndrome: PMS

Depression, irritability, anxiety, breast tendernesslethargy, insomnia/Hypersomnia, swelling, weight gain on monthly basis and disappearing with menses.

More severe form is premenstrual dysmorphic disorder.

Symptoms should occur for 3 consecutive cycles.

Must interfere with normal functioning.

Must resolve with onset of menses.

Mittelschmerz — AI 2003

- Lower abdominal pain cyclically 2 weeks before menstruation.
- In mid menstrual period
- Nausea and constipation invariably absent
- May be associated with mucoid discharge

PCOD

Hirusitism, Obesity, Acne, Acanthosis Nigricans, Infertility
Associated with endometrial hyperplasia and endometrial cancer.
↑Testosterone
↑LH/FSH
Bilaterally Enlarged Ovaries
✓ OCPS
✓ Metformin
✓ Clomiphene citrate
✓ Spironolactone are used in treatment.

Treatment Options in PCOD: AIIMS 2010

Unmarried with irregular period, acne, hirsuitism
a. Exercise
b. Diet
c. Metformin
d. Cyproterone acetate + ethinyl estrodial
Married with infertility (Anovulation)
a. Exercise
b. Diet
c. Clomiphine
Not responding to treatment:
a. Laparoscopic ovarian drilling
b. Wedge resection

Maturation Index

An index indicating the degree of maturation attained by the vaginal epithelium as adjudged by the cell types being exfoliated;

- Serves as an objective means of evaluating hormonal secretion or response; represents the percentage of parabasal cells/intermediate cells/superficials, in that order;
- **"Shift to the left"** indicates more immature cells on the surface (atrophy),
- **"Shift to the right"** indicates more mature epithelium.

An MI is a ratio obtained through performing a random count of three major cell types (**parabasal cells, intermediate cells and superficial cells)** that are shed from the squamous epithelium.

The cell count is expressed as a percentage that reads as follows: **MI= % parabasal cells, % intermediate cells, % superficial cells.**

- **Parabasal cells are the least mature cells** having not been affected by estrogen or progesterone.
- **Intermediate cells display mild maturation,** having been affected by progesterone, and
- **Superficial cells display the most maturity,** having been affected by estrogen.

A patient's **MI can vary on a daily basis**, and of course MIs vary from patient to patient. The Maturation Index provides practitioners with a simply obtained (samples are taken during the course of obtaining a pap smear) sample that is easily analyzed to detect hormonal changes in the vagina that are age-appropriate or an early sign of possible hormonal related disease processes.

Meyer Rokintansky Hauser Syndrome	Testicular Feminization Syndrome
❒ 46 XX	❒ 46 XY
❒ Phenotype: female	❒ Phenotype: female
❒ Aplasia/hypoplasia of vagina	❒ Blind vaginal pouch with absent uterus
❒ Ovary present	
❒ Female Secondary sexual characters normally developed	

➲ Mullerian Agenesis (High Yield for 2011/2012) AIIMS 2009

- Mullerian agenesis **(the Mayer-Rokitansky-Kuster-Hauser syndrome** second in frequency only to gonadal Dysgenesis as a cause of primary amenorrhea.
- Caused by mutations in the genes encoding **anti-mullerian hormone (AMH) or its receptor (AMHR).**
- **Women** with this syndrome have a
  - ✓ **46, XX karyotype**,
  - ✓ **Female secondary sex characteristics**, and
  - ✓ **Normal ovarian function**, including cyclic ovulation. AI 2010
  - ✓ **Absence or hypoplasia of the vagina.** AI 2010
- **The uterus** usually consists of only rudimentary bicornuate cords, but if the uterus contains endometrium, cyclic abdominal pain and accumulation of blood may occur, as in other forms of outlet obstruction.
- One-third of women with this syndrome have **abnormalities of the urogenital tract**, and one-tenth have **skeletal anomalies**, usually involving the spine.
- **Demonstration of a 46, XX karyotype, the biphasic basal body temperature curve characteristic of ovulation, and elevated levels of progesterone during the luteal phase establish the diagnosis of mullerian agenesis.**

⇨ Testicular Feminization Syndrome

- The major diagnostic problem is distinguishing mullerian agenesis from complete testicular feminization.
- **46, XY genetic males with testes** differentiate as phenotypic women but with a **blind vaginal pouch and no uterus.**
- Women with testicular feminization have **feminized breasts but a paucity of pubic and axillary hair.** The disorder is X-linked and is caused by mutations in the androgen receptor that result in profound **resistance to the action of testosterone**
- Testicular feminization can be diagnosed by demonstrating a
  - ✓ **Male level of serum testosterone**
  - ✓ **46, XY karyotype**

❐ A Girl with

Primary amenorrhea with normal ovaries,

Absent internal genitalia, normal external genitalia

Has most likely: Mullerian agenesis — AI 2010

❐ A 16 year old female has

Primary amenoorhea with bilateral inguinal hernia normal sexual development but no pubic hair.

USG shows no uterus and ovaries and blind vagina.

Most likely diagnosis is: Androgen insensitivity syndrome — AIIMS 2007

❐ A 10 year old girl has

Primary amenorrhea,

Absent breast,

Malformed uterus.

Most likely diagnosis is: Turners syndrome — AIIMS 2008

❐ A 16 year old female has

Primary amenoorhea.

Her breasts are Tanner 4 but no pubic hair.

USG shows no uterus and ovaries and blind vagina.

Most likely diagnosis is: Testicular feminization syndrome — AI 2006

❐ A girl presents with

Cystic swelling at the junction of lower 1/3 and upper 2/3 of anterior vaginal wall at 10 O clock position.

Most likely diagnosis is: Gartners cyst — AI 2000

- ► **Doderleins bacillus** is protective bacterium in normal vagina. — JK 2001
- ► **Nabothian follicles** are seen in cervical erosion. — TN 1991
- ► **Lipshutz ulcer effects**: vagina — PGI 1984

⇨ Various Surgeries

► Chassar moir operation:	VVF	UP 2007
► Ward Mayo operation:	Vaginal hysterectomy	HPU 2001
► Balls operation:	Pruritis vulva	ORISSA
► Strass man operation:	For septate uterus	AIIMS 1988
► Jones operation:	For septate uterus	
► Thompkins meteroplasty:	For septate uterus	
► Marshall Marchetti Krantz surgery:	Stress incontinence	
► Manchester repair:	Prolapse uterus	
► Fother gills surgery	Prolapse uterus MAH 2012	

⇨ Cancer Cervix

Predisposing Factors:

- Early age of coitus
- Multiple sex partners
- Multiparity
- Poor hygiene
- Poor socioeconomic status
- Smoking, alcohol, drug abuse
- Associated STDS
- Immunosupression

✓ **Most common virus associated with squamous cell carcinoma: HPV 16**

✓ **Most common virus associated with Adeno carcinoma: HPV 18**

✓ **Most common virus associated with Verrucous carcinoma: HPV 6**

▶ Commonest Presenting symptom: **bleeding pv**	
▶ Arises from **squamo columnar junction.**	PGI 1999
▶ Earliest symptom is **post coital bleeding.**	PGI 1999
▶ **MC site is ectocervix**	UP 2004
▶ Caused By **HPV Virus.**	
▶ Mc agent HPV 16	AI 2010
▶ Types associated with **cervical** carcinoma are **16, 18**, 31, 45, and 51 to 53.	KAR 2005, AMU 2005
▶ Predisposing factors are: **HSV, HIV, HPV infections**	PGI 2001
▶ **Obturator, hypogastric and external iliac lymph nodes** are affected	PGI 2002
▶ Time taken for conversion of **CIN TO INVASIVE CANCER: 10 YEARS**	JK 2001

Uncomplicated HPV lower genital tract infection and condylomatous atypia of the cervix can progress to CIN. This lesion precedes invasive **cervical** carcinoma and is classified as low-grade squamous intraepithelial lesion (SIL), high-grade SIL, and carcinoma in situ

Approximately 80% of invasive cervix carcinomas are **squamous cell tumors,** COMED 2008

10 to 15% are adenocarcinomas, 2 to 5% are adenosquamous with epithelial and glandular structures, and 1 to 2% are clear cell mesonephric tumors.

Patients with cervix **cancer** generally present with **abnormal bleeding or postcoital spotting** that may increase to intermenstrual or prominent menstrual bleeding. Yellowish vaginal discharge, lumbosacral back pain, and urinary symptoms can also be seen.

The staging of **cervical** carcinoma is clinical and generally completed with a pelvic examination under anesthesia with cystoscopy and proctoscopy. **Chest X-rays, intravenous pyelograms, and computed tomography are generally required, and magnetic resonance imaging (MRI) may be used to assess extracervical extension.** **AIIMS 1996**

- **Stage 0** is **carcinoma in situ,**
- **Stage I** is disease **confined to the cervix,**
- **Stage II** disease invades **beyond the cervix but not to the pelvic wall** or lower third of the vagina,
- **Stage III** disease **extends to the pelvic wall or lower third of the vagina** or causes hydronephrosis,
- **Stage IV** is present when the **tumor invades the mucosa of bladder or rectum or extends beyond the true pelvis.**

▶ Cervical biopsy is the **best method of diagnosing** cervical cancer.	**AI 2008**
▶ Pap smear is the **best method of screening**	**AI 02, 1992**
▶ Renal failure is the **commonest cause of death.**	**AI 1991**
▶ **100% cure rates** are seen in carcinoma situ.	**TN 1997**

▶ Treatment of stage II is: Extended hysterectomy, chemotherapy and intracavitary brachy therapy.	**Delhi 1997**
▶ Treatment of stage III B is: Radiotherapy and chemotherapy.	**DELHI 2003, AI 1998**

➲ Cone Biopsy: (High Yield for 2011/2012)

Indications:

✓ **Cervical lesion cannot be visualized by coloposcope.**

✓ **Squamo columnar junction is not seen by coloposcope.**

✓ **Endocervical curettage demonstrates findings positive for CIN II, CINIII.**

✓ **Lack of coorelation between bipsy and coloposcopy.**

✓ **Microinvasive carcinoma or adenocarcinoma in situ on coloposcopy.**

✓ **Theraupatic in case of CIN III (Best approach in elderly is hysterectomy)** **AI 2010**

Done under general anesthesia ideally

Complications:

- Hemorrhage
- Infection
- Cervical stenosis

PAP smear is useful in diagnosis of:

➦ CIN	
➦ Trichomonas vaginalis infection	**AIIMS 2002**
➦ Bacterial vaginosis	**AIIMS 2002**

- HSV infections
- Radiation induced cellular changes
- Actinomycosis
- Candidiasis
- IUD induced cellular change
- Atrophy

Coloposcopy: (High Yield for 2011/2012)

- Is a method devised to evaluate changes in the terminal vascular network of the vaginal part of cervix, transformation zone, vagina and fornix.
- Lower one-third of cervix is visualized.
- Acetic acid is used as 3-5%.
- The process is adided by coloposcope which has a maginification of 5-15 times.

✓ **Used for evaluating:**

✓ **Dysplasias**

✓ **Metaplasia**

✓ **CIN**

Hysteroscopy

Visualizing the interior of uterine cavity directly by aid of hysterescope.

Used to diagnose:

- **Congenital uterine malformations**
- **Uterine synechiae**
- **Misplaced IUD**
- **Submucous fibroid**
- **Evaluate cause of recurrent pregnancy loss**
- **Evaluate intrauterine abnormalities leading to infertility**

Treatment Options for CIN III are:

LEEP/LLETZ in young patients who are desirous of future childbearing.

If the patient is old or family is complete then this is treated by simple hysterectomy.

A 40-year-old woman presenting with CIN III on pap smear treatment of choice is...... HYSTERECTOMY

In case of visible mass: Punch biopsy.

In case of no mass: Coloposcopic directed biopsy.

⇨ Fibroid (Uterine Leiomyoma)

FIBROID (UTERINE LEIOMYOMA)

- They are **proliferative**, well- **circumscribed, pseudoencapsulated, benign tumors** composed of smooth muscle and fibrous connective tissue.
- They are the **most common** uterine mass found in the **female pelvis.**
- Most common **neoplasm** found in the female pelvis.
- Most common **benign solid tumor** in females.
- They are present in **15-20%** of women especially after **30-35 years** of age.
- They vary in diameter from **1mm** to more than **20 cm**.
- They are **more** common in **nulliparous.**
- The prevalence is highest between **35-45** years.

ETIOLOGY

- Fibroids are **monoclonal tumors** resulting from **somatic mutation.** They arise from
- Single neoplastic smooth muscle cell.
- Abnormalities in **chromosomes 6,7,12 and 14** have been identified.
- Disruption or Dysregulation of the high mobility group genes on **chromosome 12** contribute to fibroid development.

ROLE OF HORMONES:

- Estrogen is a promoter of fibroid growth **and not** its causal factor
- Fibroids rarely found **before puberty.**
- They stop growing **after menopause.**
- New fibroids rarely appear **after menopause.**
- They often grow rapidly during **pregnancy and amongst Pill Users.**
- **GnRH agonists** create a hypoestrogenic environment that results in a reduction of the size of fibroid.
- Some **Peptide growth factors** play a role in etiology
- Epidermal Growth Factor (**EGF**) induces DNA synthesis in fibroids and myometrial cells.
- Estrogen exerts its effect through **EGF**.
- **PIRFENIDONE**, an antifibrotic agent suppresses fibroid growth as it inhibits fibrogenic cytokines including basic **FGF, PDGF, TGF-beta** and **EGF.**

INTRAMURAL OR INTERSTITIAL FIBROID:

- **Most common** variety
- Occur within the walls of uterus as isolated, encapsulated nodules of varying size.
- When they grow, they distort uterine cavity or external surface and are pushed inwards or outwards.
- They cause **symmetrical enlargement** of the uterus when they occur singly (**Solitary**)

SUBMUCOUS FIBROID

- Located beneath the endometrium and can grow into the uterine cavity.
- Least common (**about 5%**) BUT **maximum** symptoms.

Fate of Submucous Fibroid

- ✓ Surface necrosis (abnormal bleeding and anemia)
- ✓ Polypoid change following pedicle formation
- ✓ Infection
- ✓ Degenerations including Sarcomatous change

SUBSEROUS FIBROID (SUBPERITONEAL)

- Located just **beneath the serosal surface** and grow out towards the peritoneal cavity, causing bulging of the peritoneal surface of the uterus.
- They may develop a pedicle, become pedunculated and reach a large size within the peritoneal cavity without producing symptoms.

OTHER TYPES OF FIBROID

Wandering fibroid: In Subserous variety, on rare occasion, the pedicle may be torn through; the fibroid gets its nourishment from the **omentum**, **mesentery** or **bowel** and develop a secondary blood supply. The resulting structure is known as **Wandering fibroid** or **Parasitic fibroid.**

Intraligamentary fibroid (false or pseudo fibroid): The **Intramural** fibroid may be pushed out in between the layers of Broad Ligament and is called **Intraligamentary fibroid** or **Broad ligament fibroid.**

CERVICAL FIBROID:

- Rare (1-2%)
- **SITE**: Supravaginal part of cervix
- **INTERSTITIAL** variety may displace the cervix or expand it so much that **external os** is difficult to recognize.
- All these disturb the pelvic anatomy, specially the **ureter**. In the vaginal cervix, the fibroid is usually **pedunculated** and rarely sessile.

Pseudocervical fibroid: A Fibroid polyp arising from the uterine body when occupies and distends the cervical canal, it is called **Pseudo cervical Fibroid**

⇨ Pathological changes

1) Fibroids are **pseudoencapsulated** solid tumors.
2) **Well demarcated** from surrounding myometrium.
3) The **false capsule** have more parallel arrangement while the tumor have Whorled appearance.
4) The capsule is pinkish in color in contrast to Whitish appearance of the tumor.
5) The capsule is separated from the tumor by **A THIN LOOSE AREOLAR TISSUE.**
6) The blood vessels run through this plane to supply the tumor.
7) The tumor is shelled out during Myomectomy through this plane.

8) The periphery of tumor is more vascular and have more growth potentiality.
9) The center of the tumor is least vascular and likely to degenerate.
CELLULAR LEIOMYOMAS: Are tumors with mitotic counts of **five to ten per 10** consecutive **high power fields** that **lack** cytological atypia.
LEIOMYOSARCOMAS: Previously diagnosed on the basis of mitotic count of 10 mitotic figures per 10 high-power fields.The new factors recently recognized are **CELLULAR ATYPIA** and **COAGULATIVE NECROSIS** of tumor cells.

SECONDARY CHANGES IN FIBROIDS

(1) Degeneration
(2) Atrophy
(3) Necrosis
(4) Infection
(5) Vascular changes
(6) Sarcomatous changes

➲ Red Degeneration of Fibroid (High Yield for 2011/2012)

❒ Occurs mainly in **large** fibroids.	
❒ **Tumor is red/purple in color.**	
❒ **It is due to thrombosis of large veins in the tumor.**	**UPSC 1986**
❒ **It has a peculiar fishy odor**	
❒ Occurs during **Second half** of pregnancy or **puerperium.**	**SGPGI 2005**
❒ Most **frequent complication** of myoma during pregnancy.	
❒ The tumor assumes a peculiar **purple-red color.**	
❒ Cause is **vascular** in nature (Thrombosis of large veins in the tumor).	
❒ Infection has **no** role and the process is an **aseptic** one.	**MP 1998**
❒ Presentation as a case of an **acute abdomen**	
❒ It produces **pain and tenderness** (hyaline degeneration **does not**)	
❒ Clinical features include **fever**, moderate **leucocytosis** and **increased ESR.**	
❒ It has a peculiar **fishy odor.**	
❒ Management is **conservative** and include:	
✓ Bedrest	
✓ Analgesics and Sedatives	**MAHE 2005**
✓ The symptoms usually clear off within **10** days.	
✓ **Laparotomy** if done with **mistaken diagnosis**, the abdomen is to be **closed** immediately.	

⇨ Sarcomatous Change in Fibroid

- **Rarest** among all other secondary changes in the fibroid. (**0.5%** of all myomas)
- Seen in **women > 40 years** age.
- **Postmenopausal.**
- **Intramural and submucous fibroid > Sub-serous (Least Common)**
- Treatment is total hysterectomy and bilateral salpingoopherectomy followed by radiotherapy. **AIIMS 1982**

GUIDELINES FOR THE MANAGEMENT OF MYOMAS

1) **ASYMPTOMATIC: No** treatment required

2) **SYMPTOMATIC**

A. YOUNG

B. OLD and FAMILY COMPLETE

1) Medical Treatment

2) Hysterectomy

✓ Ru 486 (Mifepristone)

✓ GnRH analogues.

3) Surgical (Myomectomy)

➲ Myomectomy

A. **INDICATIONS**

1) **Infertile Women** in her reproductive period desirous of having a baby.

2) **Recurrent pregnancy wastage** due to fibroid

B. **PRE REQUISITES PRIOR TO MYOMECTOMY**

1) Examination of **Husband** (From fertility point of view)

2) **Hysterosalpingography** (to detect a fibroid encroaching the uterine cavity OR polyp OR tube)

3) **Diagnostic D+C** (in cases of irregular cycles to exclude endometrial carcinoma)

C. **FACTS TO BE IN MIND PRIOR TO CONSIDERATION OF MYOMECTOMY**

- ❒ It should be done mainly to **preserve** the reproductive function
- ❒ The wish to preserve the menstrual function in parous women should be judiciously complied
- ❒ More **risky** operation when the fibroid **is too big** and **too many**.
- ❒ Chance **of recurrence (5-10%)**
- ❒ Chance of **persistence** of menorrhagia **(1-5%)**
- ❒ Increased rate of **relaparotomy** to the extent of **20-25%.**
- ❒ Pregnancy rate is about **40-50%**
- ❒ Pregnancy following myomectomy should have a **mandatory hospital delivery,** although the chance of scar rupture is rare.

Contraindications

- ✓ Husband proved **infertile.** In the face of advent of ART, counseling is imperative.
- ✓ Associated **bilateral infective tubo-ovarian** mass
- ✓ **Infected** fibroid

TECHNICALLY DIFFICULT CASES WITH POOR REPRODUCTIVE OUTCOME

1) **Big** broad ligament fibroid
2) Too many fibroids

ADVANTAGES OF HYSTERECTOMY OVER MYOMECTOMY

1) There is no chance of recurrence
2) Adnexal pathology and the unhealthy cervix can also be removed.

ROLE OF VAGINAL HYSTERECTOMY IN FIBROID SURGERY

– Fibroids with size of **10-12 weeks** of pregnancy and **associated with uterine prolapse** are better dealt by **Vaginal Hysterectomy** with repair of pelvic floor ☛☛

INDICATIONS OF SURGERY IN ASYMPTOMATIC FIBROID☛☛

- ❒ Size > **12 weeks** of pregnancy. ☛☛
- ❒ Diagnosis is **not** certain☛☛
- ❒ Fibroid **grows during follow up.**
- ❒ **Subserous pedunculated fibroid**☛☛
- ❒ **Unexplained infertility** with distortion of the uterine cavity. ☛☛
- ❒ **Unexplained recurrent abortion**☛☛
- ❒ Situated in the **lower part of uterus** and likely to complicate delivery.

INDICATIONS OF EMERGENCY SURGERY IN FIBROID

- ❒ **Torsion of subserous pedunculated fibroid**
- ❒ **Massive intraperitoneal hemorrhage following rupture of veins over subserous fibroid.**
- ❒ **Uncontrolled infected fibroid**
- ❒ **Uncontrolled bleeding fibroid.**

➲ Important Questions Repeated

- ► Fibroids are the **commonest benign solid tumors in females.**
- ► Most common variety of fibroid is **intramural/interstitial.** — AIIMS 1991
- ► They are estrogen dependent.
- ► **Most common type of degeneration** is the **"Hyaline Type"** which starts from the center. — UPSC 1988
- ► **Red degeneration** of fibroid is seen with pregnancy.
- ► **Sarcomatous change** or malignant change is rare (0.5%).
- ► **Malignant potential** is most in **intramural fibroids** — AIIMS 1998

► **Calcerous degeneration** is most with **sub serous fibroid**	**PGI 1997**
► Most fibroids start as **Interstitial fibroids**	**PGI 1998**
► **Uterine fibroids are associated with endometriosis**	PGI 2002
► **Wandering or parasitic fibroid is sub serous fibroid**	
► **MC symptom is menorrhagia**	

⇨ Fibroids are Associated with **PGI 2002**

✓ **Follicular ovarian cysts**
✓ **Endometriosis**
✓ **Endometrial Hyperplasia**
✓ **Endometrial Ca**

⇨ Endometrial Hyperplasia

➡ **Women near menopause or, less frequently, in early adolescence are most frequently affected.**
➡ **The basic problem is anovulation and failure of corpus luteum formation without production of progesterone.**
➡ **Continued stimulation of the endometrium by estrogen brings about proliferation, overgrowth, and hyperplasia of the endometrium.**
➡ **Areas of thickened endometrium may form polyps. Cycles become irregular, with intervals of amenorrhea associated with other intervals of intermenstrual spotting or bleeding. Pelvic examination is usually nonrevealing, and curettage produces copious amounts of endometrial scrapings.**
➡ **Microscopic examination shows hyperplasia of the epithelium and stroma. The cells lining the glands are nonsecretory, and the stroma often contains cells with frequent mitotic figures. Cystic changes of the glands may be present.**
➡ **Curettage is useful in diagnosis and for treatment, because it removes the hypertrophied endometrium and leaves a fresh surface for endometrial regeneration.**
➡ **Because of the frequency of recurrence of hyperplasia, the administration of cyclic progesterone often aids in prevention of recurrence and promotes cyclic menses.**
➡ **If endometrial hyperplasia recurs, it may proceed to atypical or adenomatous hyperplasia and then to carcinoma in situ, which may lead to endometrial cancer.**
➡ **Recurrent abnormal bleeding requires repeated curettage for diagnosis and proper therapy.**
➡ **Adenomatous hyperplasia is diagnosed when there is marked proliferation, with the glands being closely packed and the stroma quite dense and hyperplastic.**
➡ **This adenomatous pattern closely resembles adenocarcinoma and is thought to be a precancerous lesion.**
➡ **Diagnosis of lesion is by curettage.**

➲ Endometrial Carcinoma (High Yield for 2011/2012)

Occurs most often in the **sixth and seventh decades of life.**

Symptoms often include ☛☛

- **Abnormal vaginal discharge** ☛☛
- **Abnormal bleeding which is usually postmenopausal;** ☛☛
- **And leukorrhea** ☛☛

Between **75 and 80%** of all endometrial carcinomas are **adenocarcinomas.** KERALA 1994, AIIMS 1984

Adenocarcinoma with squamous differentiation is seen in 10% of patients; the most differentiated form is known as **adenoacanthoma,** and the poorly differentiated form is called **adenosquamous carcinoma.**

Most Malignant: Clear Cell carcinoma JIPMER 2003

Other less common pathologies include

- ✓ **Carcinoma (5%)** and **papillary serous carcinoma**
- ✓ **Secretory (2%),**
- ✓ **Ciliated, clear cell,**
- ✓ **And undifferentiated carcinomas.**

Lymph nodes involved are: AIIMS 1997

- ✓ **Paraaortic**
- ✓ **Presacral**
- ✓ **Inguinal**

⇨ Predisposing Factors for Endometrial Cancer: PGI 1988, JK 2007, JK 2008

❒ **Family History** ☛☛	AI 2003
❒ **Hypertension** ☛☛	
❒ **Obesity**	PGI 2004
❒ **Late Menopause**	
❒ **Diabetes**	PGI 2001
❒ **Atypical Endometrial Hyperplasia**	
❒ **Unopposed Estrogen**	
❒ **Nulliparity**	
❒ **Tamoxifen therapy**	AI 99, 98, PGI 2000
❒ **PCOD**	PGI 2004

The prognosis of endometrial Ca depends on:

- **Age at diagnosis (Old Age: Worse prognosis)**
- **Stage of disease**
- **Histological subtype**

2

OBSTETRICS AND GYNECOLOGY

⇨ Histological Grade

- ❐ Myometrial invasion
- ❐ Lymph node metastasis
- ❐ **Cervical extension** (Cervical involvement is associated with increased risk of extrauterine disease and Lymph node metastasis)
- ❐ Tumor size
- ❐ **Hormone receptor status** (Receptor positive-better prognosis)
- ❐ **Ploidy status** (Aneuploid tumors have better prognosis than diploid tumors)
- ❐ **Oncogene expression/mutation** (HER 2/neu, k ras: poor prognosis)

⇨ Progression of Hyperplasia to Endometrial Ca

Simple Hyperplasia without atypia	1%
Complex Hyperplasia without atypia	3%
Simple Hyperplasia with Atypia	8%
Complex Hyperplasia with atypia	30%

Risk factors for endometrial Hyperplasia are:

- ❐ Obesity
- ❐ Anovulation
- ❐ Low fertility index

"The Lynch syndrome" occurs in families with an autosomal dominant mutation of mismatch repair genes MLH1, MSH2, MSH6, and PMS2, which predispose to non polyposis colon cancer as well as endometrial and ovarian cancer

➲ Abdominal Hysterectomy (Indications)

- **Total abdominal hysterectomy**
  - DUB
  - Uterine fibroid
  - Tubo-ovarian mass (TO MASS)
  - Endometriosis
- **Sub-total hysterectomy**
  - Difficult TO mass
  - Endometriosis (Rectovaginal septum)
  - Obstetric causes
- **Panhysterectomy**
  - Indications for total hysterectomy in perimenopausal age.
- **Extended hysterectomy**
  - Carcinoma Endometrium
- **Radical hysterectomy**
  - Carcinoma **cervix I and II**

⇨ Adjuvant Radiotherapy in Cancer Endometrium is Given in Case of PGI 2005

- Cervical enlargement
- Lymph node involvement
- Carcinoma in situ
- Poor differentiation
- Deep myometrial involvement AIIMS 2007

- **Commonest cause of ca endometrium: Unopposed estrogen** UP 2005
- **Ca endometrium is associated with PCOD** UP 2004
- **Most malignant endometrial cancer is: Clear cell cancer** JIPMER 2003
- **Atypical endometrial hyperplasiais treated by hysterectomy** DELHI 2000
- **Treatment of choice in elderly female with endometrial hyperplasia is Pan hysterectomy** UPSC, PGI 1988

⇨ Important Points about Endometrial Ca

- Combination of Hypertension, Diabetes, Obesity in association with endometrial Ca is called as" **Corpus Cancer Syndrome."**
- Most common type of endometrial Ca is "**Adenocarcinoma/Endometroid** "Ca.
- "**Postmenopausal bleeding**" is the most common clinical feature.
- "**Simpsons sign**" in endometrial Ca is Referred pain in Hypogastrium or iliac fossae.
- Endometrial aspiration biopsy is the investigation of choice for "**screening** "endometrial Ca

➲ Vulvar Cancer (High Yield for 2011/2012)

- **A malignant invasive growth in the vulva,**
- Accounts for about 4% **of all gynecological cancers** and typically affects women in later life.
- **Vulvar carcinoma is separated from vulvar intraepithelial noeplasia (VIN), a non-invasive lesion of the epithelium that can progress via carcinoma-in-situ to squamous cell cancer, and from Paget disease of the vulva.**

Pathology:

- **Vulvar intraepithelial neoplasia (VIN)** predisposes to vulvar cancer.
- **Lichen sclerosis** is not generally considered to be a premalignant condition.
- **Squamous cell hyperplasia** is often found in regions adjacent to vulvar cancer, but the relationship of this lesion to invasive cancer is unclear.
- **Pagets's disease** is a special type of VIN and associated adenocarcinoma of apocrine gland is present in about 10% cases.
- There is high incidence (30%) of associated **carcinomas of other organs (breast, cervix, ovary and bladder).**

Aetiology:
✓ Increased association with **obesity, hypertension, diabetes and nulliparity**
✓ Associated local lesions like **chronic vulval dystrophy**
✓ Human papilloma virus (HPV) DNA **(type 16, 18)** has been detected in patients with invasive vulval cancer.
✓ Causal relation with **Condyloma accuminata (HPV 6, 11), Herpes Simplex virus type 2 (HSV-2), Syphilis and Lymphogranuloma venereum.**
✓ **Chronic pruritus** usually precedes invasive cancer
✓ **Chronic irritation** by chemical or physical trauma with poor hygiene
✓ Other primary malignancies have been observed in about 20% of cases with vulval cancer.
✓ **Cervix is most commonly affected**; other sites are breast, skin or colon.

➲ Ovarian Tumors

⇨ Benign Ovarian Tumors

SEROUS CYSTADENOMA
➨ **Most common benign** tumor of ovary. ☛☛
➨ **Most common benign** ovarian tumor which **turns** into malignancy. ☛☛
➨ **Psammoma body** is present in fast growing tumor☛☛
➨ **Intracystic hemorrhage** and **Malignancy (ADENOCARCINOMA)** are highest in **papillary variety of serous** cystadenoma
➨ Epithelium **resembles** Epithelium of Endosalpinx (Fallopian tube)
REMEMBER 30%
✓ **Accounts for 30% of ovarian tumor.**
✓ **Bilateral in 30% of cases.**
✓ **Chance of malignancy is 30%.**

➲ Mucinous Cystadenoma

➨ **Largest benign** ovarian tumor. ☛☛
➨ **Most common ovarian tumor** which can lead to **Pseudomyxoma peritoni**☛☛
➨ Usually **unilateral**☛☛
➨ Epithelium **resembles** Epithelium of Endocervix.
➨ Occasionally, **associated** with **Dermoid cysts** or **Brenners tumor.**
➨ **Torsion is most frequently** seen with this tumor

➲ Dermoid Cysts (Benign Cystic Teratoma)

➨ **Most common Germ** cell tumor of Ovary. ☛☛
➨ **Most common** ovarian tumor found **during pregnancy.** ☛☛
➨ Chance of malignancy is **lowest** in this type of Benign ovarian tumor (Usually Squamous cell carcinoma)
➨ **Rokitanskys Protruberence** is seen. ☛☛

➠ **Most common type** of cyst lying anterior to uterus.	
➠ **Most common complication** is Torsion.	UPSC 2007
➠ Frequently in **association** with **Mucinous Cystadenoma** to form a Combined tumor.	
➠ The inner surface of the cyst is always irregular and contains **Embryonic Node** from which the hairs project and in which the teeth and bone are usually found.	
➠ **Malignancy** which may develop in Dermoid cyst are:	
✓ **Squamous cell carcinoma**	
✓ **Mammary cancer**	
✓ **Malignant thyroid tumors**	

➲ FIBROMA

- ✓ Most common **benign** ovarian tumor of **connective tissue origin.**
- ✓ Most common ovarian tumor **associated** with **Meigs Syndrome.**
- ✓ They resemble **histologically** with **Brenner Tumor.**

⇨ Meig's Syndrome — AIIMS 1997, AI 1995, PGI 1995, PGI 1999

- ▶ Ascites
- ▶ Hydrothorax (Right Sided)
- ▶ **Benign** tumor of ovary (FIBROMA)

➲ Pseudo-Meigs Syndrome (High Yield for 2011/2012)

- ▶ Ascites
- ▶ Hydrothorax (Right Sided)
- ▶ **Malignant** ovarian tumor of ovary.

➲ Remember Other Points about Benign Ovarian Tumors

- ▶ **Struma Ovarii** is a highly specialized, containing Thyroid tissue, which often leads to Thyrotoxicosis.
- ▶ **Thecomas** (Pure Theca Cell Tumors) are benign but those with Granulosa cell element may be malignant.

➲ Malignant Ovarian Tumors

Remember:

- ✓ Among Gynecological cancers it **Ranks 3 rd**
- ✓ **Among all** Gynecological cancers in India it accounts **for 5%.**
- ✓ **Among all** deaths due to Gynecologic cancers, **most common** cause is due to **ovarian cancer.**
- ✓ **Most common** Ovarian cancer is **Papillary Serous Cystadenocarcinoma.**
- ✓ **Second most common** ovarian cancer is **Endometroid Carcinoma**
- ✓ **Most common** in women **< 20 years** of age is **Dysgerminoma**
- ✓ **Most Common hormonally active** ovarian tumor is **Granulosa-Theca cell Tumors**

2

OBSTETRICS AND GYNECOLOGY

⇨ Epithelial Cancers

Remember:

- ❒ Constitute about **80%** of all Primary ovarian carcinomas ☛☛
- ❒ Bilateral **50%** cases.
- ❒ **Cystic type** is more common than solid type.
- ❒ **Most common histological type** is **Papillary Serous Cystadenocarcinoma.** ☛☛
- ❒ Median age **60 years**
- ❒ The **single most important risk factor** for Epithelial ovarian cancer is **Age > 40 years**☛☛

⇨ Ovarian Functional and Neoplastic Tumors

TUMOR	Features
Follicle Cysts☛☛	❒ Rare in childhood ❒ Frequent in menstrual years ❒ Never in postmenopausal years ❒ Size < **6cm**,often bilateral ❒ Occasional anovulation with persistently proliferative endometrium
Corpus Luteum Cysts	❒ Occur in menstrual years ❒ Size: **4-6 cm**, unilateral.
Thecalutein Cysts	❒ Occurs with **H.mole, Chorio Carcinoma, Gonadotrophin** or **clomiphene therapy**☛☛ ❒ **4-5 cm**, multiple, bilaterally. ❒ Ovaries may be **>20 cm** in dia ❒ Tense consistency, amenorrhea ❒ HCG elevated as a result of Trophoblastic proliferation☛☛

⇨ Krukenberg's Tumor

- ❒ Are Secondary tumor of the ovary.
- ❒ They are invariably bilateral solid tumors.
- ❒ The primary of these tumors are: Carcinoma of stomach (70%) (**Most Common Site**), Carcinoma of large bowel (15%), Carcinoma breast (6%)☛☛

Gross Features

- ❒ **SURFACE**: Smooth with no tendency to form adhesions; No infilteration of capsule
- ❒ **SHAPE**: Retains the shape of normal ovary
- ❒ **CONSISTANCY**: Solid waxy; Cystic spaces may be seen due to degeneration
- ❒ **MOBILITY**: Freely movable in the pelvis.

Microscopy

- ❒ Cellular or myxomatous stroma with Scattered **SIGNET RING CELLS.** (Mucin Secreting cells) ☛☛
- ❒ Involvement of Ovary is by Retrograde Lymphatics.
- ❒ The first halt of tumor cells between **Stomach and Ovary is Superior Gastric Lymph Nodes.** ☛☛

⇨ Primary Ovarian Cancers

- **Epithelial ovarian cancer (80%)**
- **Non-epithelial ovarian (10%)**

A. Epithelial Ovarian Cancer: arise from the epithelial surface of the ovary.

B. Non-epithelial Ovarian Cancer: arise from -

- ✓ **Ovarian germ cells**
- ✓ **Sex cord cells**
- ✓ **Stromal cells**

⇨ Malignant Ovarian Tumors

- In Menopausal, Postmenopausal woman (**> 50 yrs**) the chance of malignancy **> 50%** (In premenopausal it is **15%).**
- Tumors in childhood are usually malignant.
- In **Nulliparous**, more commonly seen. Multiparity, to some extent, protects a woman against ovarian malignancy.
- Pain pressure pain can occur with any tumor; but referred pain suggests malignant involvement of N. root
- **Abnormal** uterine bleeding
- **Rapidly growing** tumor
- **Unilateral** oedema
- **Cachexia, loss of appetite and loss of weight** (late stage)

⇨ Clinical Findings of Malignant Ovarian Tumor

- Bilateral (**About 50%) Solid tumor** except Fibroma, Brenner tumor and few Feminizing tumors like Thecoma and Granulosa cell tumor.
- **Fixed** tumor
- **Presence of Ascites** (Meigs Syndrome)
- **Hepatomegaly** due to metastasis
- **Unilateral non-pitting edema of leg or vulva (characteristic of malignancy)**
- The **nodules in Pouch of Douglas** associated to a pelvic mass is highly suggestive of ovarian malignancy.

PRIMARY EPITHELIAL TUMORS 80% MAHE 2007, UPSC 2007	NON-EPITHELIAL TUMORS	HORMONE-PRODUCING TUMORS
❒ **Mucinous Cystadenoma** or Cystadenocarcinoma☛☛ ❒ **Serous Cystadenoma** or Cystadenocarcinoma☛☛ ❒ **Endometrioma** or Endometriod Carcinoma☛☛ ❒ **Clear cell carcinoma**☛☛ ❒ **Brenner Tumor**☛☛	❒ Fibroma Dysgerminoma ❒ Teratoma ❒ Gonadoblastoma ❒ Yolk-sac tumor	❒ **Estrogen- producing**☛☛ ✓ Granulosa cell tumor ✓ Thecoma ❒ **Androgen -producing**☛☛ ✓ Sertoli-Leydig cell tumor ✓ (Arrhenoblastoma) ✓ Hilar cell tumor ✓ Lipoid cell tumor (Ovoblastoma,Musculinovoblastoma, ✓ Adrenal-like tumor) ❒ **OTHERS** ✓ Carcinoid (Seratonin- producing) ✓ Thyroid tumor (Struma Ovarii) ✓ Choriocarcinoma of the ovary

⇨ **Complications of Ovarian Tumor** ☛☛

- ► **Torsion of Pedicle**
- ► **Intra-Cysic hemorrhage**
- ► **Infection**
- ► **Rupture**
- ► **Psedomyxoma peritonei**
- ► **Malignancy**

TORSION: Torsion of the Pedicle (**Axial Rotation**) is very common during pregnancy (**12%**) cases.

Structers forming the Ovarian Pedicle

Laterally: Infundibulopelvic ligament containing structures there in i.e, Ovarian vessels, nerves and lymphatics.

Medially:-

- ✓ Ovarian ligament
- ✓ Medial end of fallopian tube
- ✓ Mesosalpinx containing utero-ovarian anastomotic vessels

Middle:- Broad ligament

Torsion is common in tumors having: ☛☛

- ✓ Moderate Size, preferably with round contor.
- ✓ Free mobility
- ✓ Long pedicle

Predisposing factors for torsion

- ✓ Trauma☛☛
- ✓ Violent physical movement☛☛
- ✓ Contractions of pregnant uterus☛☛

Summary of torsion of ovarian pedicle

- ❐ Common in **Dermoid** or **Simple Serous Cystadenoma** — UPSC 2003
- ❐ Partial axial rotation followed by complete torsion is explained by **Hemodynamic theory.**
- ❐ Symptoms of **acute pain** lower abdomen **with a lump.**
- ❐ General condition remain **unaffected.**
- ❐ Abdominal examination reveals a **tense cystic tender mass** in the **hypogastrium** arising from the pelvis.
- ❐ Pelvic examination reveals the **mass separated** from the uterus
- ❐ Treatment is **Laparotomy** and **Ovariotomy.**

⇨ Staging of Ovarian Tumor — AIIMS, 2001, AIPGME 2003

STAGE I Lesion confined to Ovaries

- ► **Ia** One Ovary; No Ascites)
- ► **Ib** Both Ovary; No Ascites)
- ► **Ic** (One or two Ovaries with Ascites)

STAGE II One or two ovaries with extension to Pelvis

STAGE III Widespread intraperitoneal metastases (Omentum commonly involved)

STAGE IV Distant Metastases

➲ Treatment

Surgically Debulk **all Stages** of tumor that involves:

Total AbdominalHysterectomy **(TAH)** + **BSO + Omentectomy + any other tumor > 2 cm diameter size.**

In Stage III and Stage IV Debulking Surgery is done or **at least** biopsy of the tumor is obtained.

ADJUVANT THERAPY

1) Radiotherapy **STAGE Ib and Ic**

2) Chemotherapy **STAGE II, III, IV**

➲ Other Facts about Ovarian Cancer (High Yield for 2011/2012)

- ► Accounts for **5%** of all Gynecological cancers in India. ☛☛
- ► **Most common cause of death** due to Gynecological cancers is **Ovarian Carcinoma**☛☛

- ▶ Most common Cancer is Papillary Serous Cystadenocarcinoma
- ▶ Second most common ovarian cancer is Endometroid Carcinoma

2

OBSTETRICS AND GYNECOLOGY

⇨ Clinical Associations of Malignant Ovarian Tumors

- ✓ Nulliparity
- ✓ Infertility
- ✓ Most common ovarian cancer in women **under the age of 20** is dysgerminoma
- ✓ Most common **hormonally active ovarian tumor is Granulosa-Theca cell tumors.**
- ✓ Incidence **is higher** amongst women from the affluent classes (due to high fat content in their diet)
- ✓ An enlargement of the ovary in women of **menopausal or postmenopausal** age should be regarded as **malignant until Proved Otherwise.**

⇨ Masculinizing Ovarian Tumors are:

❒ Arrhenoblastoma/Androblastoma	
❒ Sertoli Leyding cell tumor	
❒ Sertoli cell tumor	AIIMS 1985
❒ Leyding cell tumor	AIIMS 1985
❒ Hilus cell tumor	AIIMS 1985
❒ Adrenocortical tumor	
❒ Gynandroblastoma	

⇨ Feminizing Tumors are:

❒ Granulosa cell tumor	PGI 1986
❒ Theca cell tumor	PGI 1986
❒ Fibromas	

Call Exner Bodies:	PGI 2003	▶ Granulosa cell tumor	AIIMS 2001
Renkies Crystals:		▶ Hilus cell tumor	AIIMS 1995
Signet ring cells:		▶ Krukenbergs tumor	
Schiller Duval bodies:		▶ Endodermal sinus tumor	AMU 2005
Psommoma bodies:		▶ Serous tumors	
Meigs syndrome:		▶ Fibroma ovary	
Pseudomeigs syndrome:		▶ Brenner cell tumor	
Walthard cell nest:		▶ Brenner tumor	
Rokintansky bodies:		▶ Teratoma	AMU 2005

Tumors may arise from any of the major components of the ovary:

Surface epithelium, ovarian stromal and follicle lining granulosa cells, or germ cells.

- **Epithelial tumors** are the most common malignant ovarian tumorsand are more common in women older than 40 years of age.
- The major types of **epithelial tumors** are serous, endometrioid, and mucinous.
- **Germ-cell tumors** (dysgerminoma), (embryonal), (endodermal sinus tumor), (choriocarcinoma), (teratoma).
- **Sex cord stromal tumors** may display differentiation toward **granulosa**, Sertoli, Leydig. **AIPGME 2012**

INCREASED RISK ASSOCIATED	DECREASED RISK ASSOCIATED
▶ Early menarche	▶ Pregnancy☛☛
▶ Nulliparity	▶ Lactation☛☛
▶ Late menopause	▶ OCPs☛☛

Guideline for the management of ovarian tumor in pregnancy

(A) During Pregnancy

UNCOMPLICATED	COMPLICATED
Principle: To remove the tumor as soon as the diagnosis is made. ☛☛ **Best Time:**For Elective Operation is **14-18th week**☛☛ ➢ If the diagnosis is made **before** this time, the patient should be kept **under observation.** ➢ If the diagnosis is made in **3rd trimester** **Immediate removal** is done ➢ If the diagnosis is made **beyond 36**weeks, The operation is **withheld till delivery** and the tumor is **removed as early in puerperium** as possible.	The tumor is **removed** irrespective of the period of Gestation☛☛

(B) During Labor

▶ **If the tumor is well above the presenting part**☛☛	▶ **If the tumor is impacted in the pelvis causing obstruction**☛☛
A Watchful Expectancy hoping for Vaginal delivery☛☛	Caesarean Section followed by removal of tumor in the same sitting. ☛☛

(C) During Puerperium

On Occasion, the diagnosis is made following delivery. The tumor should be removed as early in puerperium as possible. ☛☛

⇨ **Remember Risk of Malignancy Index (RMI)**

RMI=U x M x CA125

➢ U=USG Score determined by:

✓ Multilocular cyst,
✓ Solid area,
✓ Metastasis,
✓ Ascites,
✓ b/l lesions

1 point for each

M = 3 for post menopauasal women

CA125 level in units/ml

- ► Low-risk: RMI<25
- ► Moderate risk: RMI25-250
- ► High-risk: RMI>250

⇨ **Regarding Ovarian Tumors**

Most common (overall) ovarian tumor:	Epithelial cell tumor	
Most common in less than 20 years of age	Dysgerminoma	AI 2005
Most common Benign tumor of ovary:	Dermoid Cyst	
Most common tumor in young women:	Germ cell tumor	
Most common Malignant tumor:	Serous Cystadenoma	
Most common tumor diagnosed in pregnancy:	Dermoid Cyst	
Most common tumor to undergo torsion:	Dermoid Cyst	
Most radiosensitive ovarian tumor:	Dysgerminoma	AIIMS 1997

► Marker for ovarian cancer: **CA 125**	AIIMS 1997, 1998
► Marker for granulosa cell tumor: **inhibin**	AIIMS 2008
► Marker for dysgerminoma: **serum LDH**	AI 2008
► Marker for dysgerminoma: **Placental alkaline phosphatase**	PGI 1996

⇨ **CA 125**

Is a monoclonal antibody that recognizes an antigen secreted by Ovarian and other cancers. Analogous to CEA in colon cancer, the serum CA 125 is **neither sensitive nor specific for the diagnosis of ovarian cancer.** Thus, the CA 125 may increase in patients **with breast, lung, pancreas, and colorectal cancers.** In addition, CA 125 elevations are not limited to patients with malignant disease; increased levels have been found in patients with **endometriosis, pelvic inflammatory disease, benign ovarian cysts, the first trimester of pregnancy, menstruation, and liver disease.**

⇨ Pseudomyxoma Peritonei

This is a rare condition resulting from

- **Rupture of a mucocele of the appendix,**
- **A mucinous ovarian cyst, or**
- **Mucin-secreting intestinal or ovarian adenocarcinoma.**

✓ The abdomen becomes filled with masses of **jelly-like mucus.**

✓ Colloid carcinoma arising from the stomach or colon with peritoneal implants may resemble pseudomyxoma at laparotomy.

✓ The course of this type of highly malignant tumor is one of rapid cachexia and early death.

✓ The diagnosis usually can be made by the appearance of many **highly malignant cells in the peritoneal implants.**

⇨ Ovarian Hyperstimulation Syndrome (OHSS)

Is enlargement of ovary with multiple follicles after stimulation "<u>Necklace sign</u>" of ovaries is seen on USG.

- Common with FSH/LH therapy.
- Clomiphene therapy
- Pulsatile GnRH therapy. **Features are:**

❑ **Ascites, hydrothorax**

❑ **Cerebrovascular events, DVT, thromboembolism.**

❑ **Abdominal pain**

❑ **Renal failure**

❑ **Torsion of ovarian cysts**

❑ **Liver dysfunction**

❑ **Coagulopathy**

⇨ Ovarian Remanent Syndrome

Persistence of ovarian function even after B/L Oopherectomy presenting with Chronic pelvic pain and dyspareunia due to remaining ovarian tissue.

⇨ Trapped Residual Ovarian Syndrome

Presenting with Chronic pelvic pain and dyspareunia due to tension within developing follicles with periovarian adhesions or because of perioophritis.

⇨ Genital Malignancies

❑ MC Type of vulval carcinoma:	Squamous cell carcinoma
❑ MC Type of vaginal carcinoma:	Squamous cell carcinoma
❑ MC Type of cervical carcinoma:	Squamous cell carcinoma
❑ MC Type of endometrial carcinoma:	Adeno carcinoma

➲ Differentiate: (High Yield for 2011/2012)

Vaginismus	Dyspareunia	Desire disorder	Arousal disorder	Anorgasmia
Painful reflex spasm of paravaginal thigh adductors. Diagnosed by physical examination. Almost always pshycogenic. Vaginal dilators useful as therapy.	Pain related to sexual intercourse	Apathy for and lack of enjoyment of sex.	Failure of vaginal lubrication and lack of pelvic engorgement	Women never has had orgasm by any means

Remember:

- ▶ **Hirusitism:** Male pattern hair growth in females☛☛
- ▶ **Virilization:** Male pattern hair growth in females **+Clitoromegaly/Baldness/Loss of female body contours/Lowering of voice/↑Muscle mass.**
- ▶ **↑DHEA:** Adrenal tumor ☛☛
- ▶ **↑Testosterone: PCOD**☛☛
- ▶ **↑↑↑Testosterone:** Ovarian Tumor (Sertoli leyding , Hilus cell tumor) ☛☛
- ▶ **↑Serum 17 OH Progesterone levels:** Congenital Adrenal Hyperplasia
- ▶ **Maternal virilizing tumor of pregnancy** is called **luteoma of pregnancy** can result in masculinization of female fetus.

⇨ Hirsutism

Hirsutism is the presence of excess hair in women. This is usually an androgen-dependent process. ETIOLOGY. Hirsutism may be divided into androgen-dependent and androgen-independent causes.

Androgen-dependent hirsutism is restricted to areas where men typically become hirsute and often begins with adolescence. In women, androgens arise from the ovaries, the adrenal glands, or exogenous sources such as anabolic steroids

- ✓ Androgen-independent hirsutism is caused by drugs
- ✓ Cyclosporine,
- ✓ Glucocorticoids,
- ✓ Minoxidil, PGI 2011
- ✓ Diazoxide, PGI 2011
- ✓ Phenytoin or PGI 2011
- ✓ Starvation (anorexia nervosa);

⇨ Clomiphene

- Antiestrogen with weak agonistic activity as well
- Enclomiphene has antiestrogenic effect — AP 1997
- Is indicated in the **treatment of anovulation or oligo-ovulation** in patients desiring pregnancy, whose sexual partners have adequate sperm, and who have potentially functional hypothalamic-hypophyseal-ovarian systems and adequate endogenous estrogen.
- **Chances of pregnancy are 3 fold** as compared to placebo — AIIMS 2009
- Risk of **multiple pregnancy is 6-10 fold** — AIIMS 2009
- May be used to treat **corpus luteum dysfunction**
- Is used to detect **abnormalities of the hypothalamic-pituitary-gonadal axis in males**
- Used in **Stein Levinthal syndrome** — AIIMS 1984
- Is used to **treat infertility in males with oligospermia.** — AIIMS 2009
- Is sometimes given as a **test dose to aid in predicting whether an ovulatory response might occur**

⇨ Tamoxifen

- Non steroidal antiestrogenic — UP 2007
- Is indicated for adjuvant treatment of **axillary node-negative breast cancer** in women following total mastectomy or segmental mastectomy, axillary dissection, and breast irradiation
- Indicated for adjuvant treatment of **axillary node-positive breast cancer in postmenopausal women following total mastectomy or segmental mastectomy, axillary dissection, and breast irradiation**
- That women whose tumors **are estrogen receptor-positive are more likely to benefit** from **tamoxifen** therapy
- Is indicated to **reduce the risk of developing breast cancer in women who have been determined to be at high risk for developing this cancer.**

⇨ Danazol

Androgen derivative, Gonadotropin inhibitor — CUPGEE 2001

Indications

- **Endometriosis treatment** — PGI 1988
- Fibrocystic Breast disease,
- **Cyclic mastalgia, non cyclic mastalgia** — AIIMS 2002
- Angioedema, hereditary (prophylaxis)
- **Menorrhagia, primary** — JIPMER 1991
- Gynecomastia
- **Puberty precocious** — DNB 1999

⇨ GnRH Analogues

AP 1997

- Goserelien
- Buserelin
- Naferelein
- Historelein
- Triptorelin

⇨ Used for

- ✓ Precocious puberty
- ✓ Infertility
- ✓ Ca breast
- ✓ DUB
- ✓ Endometriosis
- ✓ Fibromyoma uterus
- ✓ Hirsutism

⇨ Important Syndromes

▶ Sheehans syndrome:	➨ Postpartum pituitary necrosis
▶ Ashermans syndrome:	➨ Overzealous curettage resulting in endometrial synechiae
▶ Stein levinthal syndrome:	➨ PCOD
▶ Kallamans syndrome:	➨ Primary amonorrhea, hyposmia, failure of secondary sexual features

➲ Important Points Repeated

Antitubercular drugs contraindicated in pregnancy: PGI 2005

- Streptomycin
- Pyrazinamide

Reversible methods of contraception are: PGI 2005

- ❒ OCP
- ❒ IUCD
- ❒ Barrier
- ❒ Depot injection

Contraceptive advice in lactating mother: PGI 2005

- Mini pill
- Barrier method
- Depot injection

Evaluation in Adolescent Abnormal Uterine Bleeding: PGI 2006

- Hemogram
- Platelet count
- USG
- D and C

True about Bacterial Vaginosis: PGI 2006

- Grey discharge
- Clue cells found
- Fishy odor discharge
- Caused by Gardnerella vaginalis

A woman in second trimester was found to have over distended uterus. Common causes include: PGI 2006

- Wrong date
- Hydramnios
- Distended bladder
- Twins
- Fibromyoma

Glucose tolerance test is indicated in a pregnant lady in case of: PGI 2006

- Big baby
- Repeated abortion
- Previous GDM
- H/O diabetes in maternal uncle

In placenta previa conservative treatment not done in case of: PGI 2006

- Active labor
- Anencephaly
- Dead baby
- Severe placenta previa

Spermicidal agent are: PGI 2006

- Nonoxynol
- Menfegol

True about Tubal Pregnancy: PGI 2008

- Prior History of tubal surgery
- Prior tubal pregnancy
- Prior history of PID
- IUCD predisposes
- OCP predisposes

In PCOD Symptoms and Signs Seen are: PGI 2007

- Amenorrhea
- Theca cell hyperplasia
- Hyperandrogenism
- Anovulation

Emergency Contraception is by: PGI 2008

- Combination of estrogen and progesterone
- Mifepristone MAH 2012
- Levonorgestrol
- IUCD

Causes of Hydrops Fetalis: PGI 2008

- Parvo virus infection
- HZV infection
- Down's syndrome
- Toxoplasma

A woman of 50 yrs who attained menopause, coming with one episode of bleeding P/V. Which of the following to be done: PGI 2009

- Assess History of HRT
- Hysterectomy
- PA P Smear
- Endometrial biopsy
- DUB

Contraindications for IUCD: PGI 2009

- PID
- HIV
- Uterine malformation
- Previous ectopic

Bishop's Score Includes: PGI 2009

- Cervical dilatation
- Cervical effacement
- Cervical softening
- Condition of os
- Position of head

Dysgerminomas are: PGI 2009

- Radiosensitive
- MC malignant germ cell tumor
- Bilateral

The effects of diabetic mother on infants are: PGI 2009

- First trimester abortion
- Unexplained fetal death
- Caudal regression

True labor pain includes: PGI 2011

- ❐ Painful uterine contractions at regular intervals
- ❐ Increased contractions with increased intensity
- ❐ Increased contractions with increased duration
- ❐ Show
- ❐ Progressive effacement of cervix
- ❐ Progressive dilatation of cervix
- ❐ Formation of bag of waters.

True about PCOD: PGI 2009

- ↑ LH
- Hyperinsulinemia

Mother to baby transmission of HIV can be minimised by AIPGEE 2011, From Platinum 2010

- Zidovudine
- Vitamin A
- Avoidance of breastfeeding

Regarding PCOD Lab values true are: AIPGEE 2011, From Platinum 2010

A. High LH/FSH

B. High DHEAS

C. High prolactin

D. Raised LH

Erythema nodosum is seen in AIPGEE 2011, From Platinum 2010

- Tuberculosis
- SLE
- Pregnancy

➲ Clinical Wrap Up

❐ A 20 year old **obese** female with **irregular menstrual periods, acne, insulin resistance and elevated LH: FSH ratio**	✓ **PCOD**
❐ A 30 year old female with **foul smelling, frothy, light green colored vaginal dischare with vaginal erythema and straw berry cervix**	✓ **Trichomonas vaginalis**
❐ A female of 25 years with **parasthesias, burning pain in perineal area and vesicles showing Cowdry inclusions. Painful inguinal Lymphadenopathy** is also noticed	✓ **Herpes Simplex II (Herpes Genitalis)**
❐ A 30 year old female with **profuse watery, dirty grey discharge giving positive whiff test**	✓ **Bacterial vaginosis**
❐ A 55 year old female with **constipation, abdominal and pelvic swelling increased CA 125 levels**	✓ **Ovarian Ca**
❐ A **22 year** old female with **irritability, breast tenderness, fatigue, headache and bloating week before menstrual cycles**	✓ **Premenstrual dysmorphic disorder**
❐ A female of **35** years complaing of **dysmenorrheal, dyspareunia and dyschezia with fixed retroverted uterus and nodularity of uterosacral ligaments.**	✓ **Endometriosis**
❐ A female 36 years old with **dysmenorrhea, menorrhagia, chronic pelvic pain and symmetrically, enlarged smooth uteru**s tender to palpation	✓ **Adenomyosis**
❐ A **16 year old girl** with **missing periods, failure to gain weight, emaciated with low LH, FSH and Estrogens.**	✓ **Anorexia Nervosa**
❐ A female with **fever, diarrhea, skin rash, headache with hypotension** and altered mental status who **used vaginal tampon.**	✓ **Toxic shock syndrome**
❐ A 30 year old female with **soft, pinkish, cauliflower like lesions** with **multiple sex partners responding to Imiquimod**	✓ **HPV (Condyloma acuminata)**
❐ A 25 year female **2 weeks after normal delivery inability to breast feed her child, nausea, weakness and fatigue with low ACTH, LH, FSH**	✓ **Sheehans syndrome**
❐ A 33 year old who is **38 weeks pregnant with rupture membranes** comes in emergency **with respiratory distress, hypotension with ↓platelets and ↑FDD with fetal cells in maternal blood sample**	✓ Amniotic fluid embolism
❐ A 57 year old **obese, hypertensive and diabetic female with vaginal bleeding**	✓ Endometrial cancer
❐ A 16 year old **female with ammonorrhea, webbed neck, low hair line and widely spaced nipples.** USG shows **streak ovaries**	✓ Turners Syndrome
❐ A 24 year old **female with abdominal pain and adenexal mass.** Pelvic USG showing **heterogenous, well circumscribed mass with solid and cystic components with dense calcification.**	✓ Teratoma

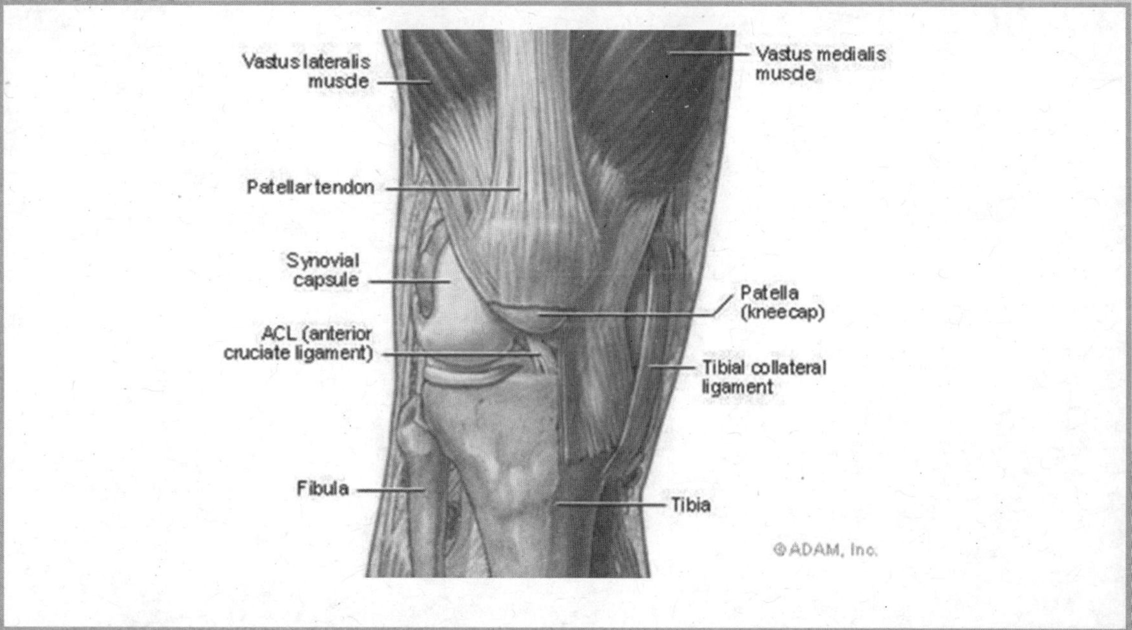

ORTHOPEDICS

Term "orthopedics" was coined by Nicholas Andrey (JIPMER 92)

➲ Basic points in orthopedics

- Bone is the **hardest tissue** of the human body, and is second only to cartilage in its ability to withstand stress
- **Periosteum:** It is a CT Covering seen on the outer aspect of the bone and is bilayered formed of:
- Outer Fibrous Layer of CT Fibers and CT Cells.
- Inner Osteogenic Layer formed of Osteoblasts
- **Endosteum:** It lines the bone marrow cavities. It is formed of CT (Connective tissue) and Osteocytes
- The structural unit of a bone is the **Osteon or the Haversian system.**
- It is composed of **Haversian Canal** which runs parallel to the long axis of the bone around which lie 5-25 concentric lamellae of bone composed of osteocytes. The lamellae are the
- **External circumferential lamellae** (in relation to periosteum)
- **Internal circumferential lamellae** (in relation to endosteum)
- **Interstitial lamellae** (in between haversian systems)
- **Volkmann's canals** are special canals present transversely connecting the haversian systems with periosteum with the bone marrow cavity.
- **Perforating fibers of Sharpey**: They are collagenous fibers connecting tendons of muscles with periosteum.

➲ Hormones and Bones

☐ SEX STEROIDS

Sex steroids, particularly estrogens, have slow but extremely important anabolic effects on bone. The effects are exerted directly on the bone organ, perhaps through receptors in the osteoblast. Estrogen deficiency results in accelerated bone remodeling with disproportionate bone resorption, particularly in trabecular bone.

☐ GLUCOCORTICOIDS

Glucocorticoids affect many of the cells that contribute to mineral metabolism.The most striking effect is bone thinning that results from high glucocorticoid concentrations. This thinning is probably a consequence mainly of inhibited osteoblasts. In addition, glucocorticoids antagonize the actions of vitamin D metabolites by unknown mechanisms.

☐ THYROID HORMONE

Thyroid hormones also have direct effects on bone cells. Excess of thyroid hormones causes increased release of calcium from bone. The skeletal consequences of deficient thyroid hormone are most evident in the disordered growth of cartilaginous epiphyses associated with congenital hypothyroidism.

☐ GROWTH HORMONE

Growth hormone stimulates the growth of bone and cartilage, in part by stimulating local production of IGF-1 by osteoblasts and chondrocytes.

➲ Biochemical Markers in Bone Metabolism High Yield for Exams

Role in "Bone mineralization"***

- Bone Specific Alkaline Phosphatase.☚
- Osteocalcin (bone-GLA protein) ☚
- Propeptide of Type I Collagen ☚
- Osteonectin☚
- Osteopontin ☚

⇨ Urinary markers for "Bone resorption" are

Urinary and serum cross linked N Telopeptide☚

- Urinary and serum cross linked C Telopeptide☚ MAH 2012
- Urine hydroxyproline,☚
- Serum bone sialoprotein☚
- Serum Tartarate acid Phosphatase (TRAP)☚

➲ Classification of Fractures

- A single fracture line is referred to as a **"Simple" fracture**☚
- When multiple fracture lines and bone fragments exist, the fracture is said to be **"Comminuted" fracture.**
- Penetrating injury producing a fracture, or fracture fragments protruding through the skin, constitute an **"Open" fracture.**☚
- When no such wound is present, the fracture is classified as **"Closed" fracture.**☚
- More subtle trauma such as the activities of daily living may also produce fractures in elderly patients with osteoporosis, in patients with metabolic bone-wasting disease, or in patients with tumor of the bone. Such injuries are referred to as **Pathologic fractures**. The most common causes of pathologic fracture are osteoporosis and metastatic carcinoma.☚
- Healthy bone may fracture with the repetitive application of minor trauma, as in **"Fatigue" or "Stress" fractures**. These fractures are seen in the metatarsals after a long hike or in the tibia, fibula, femur, or other skeletal locations in individuals involved in regular athletic activities.☚☚
- **In India Nutritional causes tend to be the most common cause for Fracture development.** AIPGME 2012

➲ Fractures in children

- The **periosteum is extremely strong** in children
- Children's **bones are much more resilient** and less brittle than those of adults
- Bending moments applied to the bone of a child may cause a **Greenstick fracture**, in which there is distraction of the cortex on the convex side and compression of bone on the concave side. **(Cortex intact)**

  PSC 07

Buckle Fractures:

- "**Torus**" **fracture** is also called as "**Buckle fracture**" (JK BOPEE 09)
- It occurs most often in **children**
- Bones in children are soft and do not break but **buckle under pressure**
- It occurs when there is a fall **on outstretched hand**
- It refers usually to fracture of distal radius and distal ulna
- It heals quickly
- Distal humeral # is commonest in childhood. BHU 1988

Commonly asked Terminology

- **Dislocation** means that the articular surfaces are not opposed or congruous and that the restraining ligaments and probably the capsule have been partially or completely torn.
- **Subluxation** means a partial displacement of one side of the joint on the other, but with less severe distortion than a dislocation. Soft tissue interposition may prevent complete reduction in either instance.
- **Reduction** refers to the action required to obtain anatomic alignment.
- **Arthoplasty:** Joint is Excised and bones are so kept to avoid fusion (PGI 83)

Commonly asked Fractures

Aviators #:	Neck of Talus
BOXERS #:	Neck of fifth metacarpal
Bennets #	(Intra Articular) Base of Ist Metacarpal (UP 88)
Rolandos#	(Extra articular) Base of Ist Metacarpal
Chauffers #:	Radius above styloid process (AMU 05)
Chance #:	Horizontal # through vertebrae due to sudden deceleration
Clay shovellers #:	Spinous process of T1
Cottons #:	Trimalleolar #
Galezzi #:	Distal radius with dislocation of distal radio Ulnar joint
Jeffersons#:	Burst fracture of Atlas (C1) (AI 99)
Jones #:	Base of 5th metatarsal
Hangmans #:	Axis
Monteggias #:	Proximal ulna with dislocation head of radius JK BOPEE 2011

■ March #:	Stress # shaft of second or third Metatarsal	(Kar 06) KCET 2012
■ Masonneres #:	Neck of fibula	
■ Potts #	Bimalleolar ankle	(APPGE 1995)
■ Smiths#:	Reverse of colles	
■ Pond #	Depressed Skull # in infants	
■ Toddlers #	Spiral # of Tibia	
■ Crescent #	Iliac bone with sacroiliac disruption	(AIIMS 09)

⇨ Factors effecting fracture healing are

- **Degree of immobilization** is the **"most important factor"**. Repeated disruptions of repaired tissue significantly impairs healing☛☛☛ JK BOPEE 08
- **Age:** Young patients heal rapidly
- **Nutrition:** Good nutrition plays a vital role
- **Diseases** like Diabetes Mellitus, Osteoporosis, Immunocompromised states, Marfans syndrome, Ehler Danhlos Syndrome cause delayed healing.
- **Hormones:** Growth Hormone, Calcitonin promote growth healing. Corticosteroids delay healing of fractures.
- **Type of bone:** Cancellous bones heal quickly due to increased vascularity.
- **Severe Degree of trauma** and secondary infection cause delayed fracture healing.
- **Inadequate blood supply** near talus, NOF cause delayed fracture healing.
- **Intraarticular fractures** communicate with synovial fluid which contains collagenases retards fracture healing.
- **Separation of bone ends:** Normal apposition is also important, inadequate reduction, excessive traction or interposition of soft tissue prevents healing.
- **Infection:** infections cause necrosis and edema, impair healing and increase mobility of fracture site.

Most common bone fractured in body: clavicle.	KERALA 1996
Most common bone fractured during birth : humerus	MP 1998

➲ Important Bursitis

➨ Prepatellar Bursitis☛☛	House Maids Knee	
➨ Infrapatellar Bursitis☛☛	Clergy mans Knee/ Vicars Knee	(PGI 97)
➨ Olecranon Bursitis☛	Students elbow	

➠ Ischial Bursitis☚	Weavers Bottom
➠ Lateral Malleolus Bursitis	Tailors Ankle
➠ Great Toe Bursitis☚	Bunion

➲ Important Casts in orthopedics

▶ Minerva cast	Cervical spine disease☚☚	
▶ Turn Buckle cast Scoliosis☚		
▶ Rissers cast Scoliosis☚		
▶ Milwaukees brace Scoliosis ☚		PGMEE 2005
▶ Boston brace Scoliosis☚		DNB 04
▶ Frog leg cast	CDH☚	
▶ Cylinder cast	# Patella☚	
▶ Hip spica	# Femur☚	
▶ Hanging cast	# Humerus☚	
▶ Tube cast Knee ☚☚☚		(AI 07)

⇨ Important Splints

I.	Thomas splint	# Femur☚☚	
II.	Dennis Brown splint	CTEV☚	
III.	Cock-up splint	Radial nerve palsy ☚☚☚	(AIIMS 95)
IV.	Knuckle bender splint	Ulnar Nerve Palsy☚	
V.	Aeroplane splint	Brachial Plexus injury ☚	(CUPGEE 02)
VI.	Von Rosen Splint	CDH ☚	(PGI 97)

⇨ Important Osteotomies

• Mc Murrays Osteotomy: ❋ # NOF	
• Mc Ewans Genu valgum	DNB 1990
• Pauwels ❋ # NOF	
• French ❋ Correction of Gun stock deformity	
• Salters • Chiaris • Pembertons❋	CDH

⇨ Common Tractions

A. Gallows/Bryants Traction: # shaft of femur — AIIMS 2010, 2011
B. Russels Traction: Trochanteric #
C. Perkins traction: # shaft femur in adults
D. Dunlop/Smith Traction: Supracondylar # femur
E. Bucks Traction: Skin traction
F. Head Halter Traction/ Crutch field Traction: cervical spine injuries

⇨ Extra Tractions Used

- Well-leg traction Correction of adduction or abduction deformity of hip
- Dunlop traction Supracondylar fracture of humerus
- Smith's traction Supracondylar fracture of humerus
- Calcaneal traction Open fractures of ankle or leg
- Metacarpal traction Open forearm fractures
- Head-halter traction Cervical spine injuries
- Crutchfield traction Cervical spine injuries
- Halo-pelvic traction Scoliosis

➲ Order of Repair in Orthopedics

After all structures have been thoroughly cleansed, debrided and identified, repair is begun.

Shorten and internally fix bone

— Repair extensor tendons
— Repair flexion tendons
— Arteries
— Nerves
— Veins
— Close or cover wound.

➲ Nerve Injuries of Upper Limb

⇨ Ulnar nerve "Musicians Nerve"❋❋❋

- Ulnar nerve supplies medial 1/3 of palm **(Hypothenar area)**
- Ulnar nerve in hand supplies:
  - ✓ **3, 4 Lumbricals**
  - ✓ **Palmar and dorsal interosei**
  - ✓ **Adductor pollicis**
  - ✓ **Hypothenar muscles**
- Ulnar nerve in hand supplies
  - ✓ **Flexor carpi ulnaris and**
  - ✓ **Medial half of flexor digitorum profundus**
- Lesion of ulnar nerve causes
- **Weakness of ulnar deviation**
- **Weakness of wrist flexion**
- **Adductor pollicis paralysis with loss of thumb adduction.**

⇨ **In ulnar nerve palsy there is**

- ▶ **Positive card test** ☛☛ **(UPSC 95)**
- ▶ **Positive book test/Froment sign**
- ▶ **Positive Egawa's test**
- ▶ **Ulnar claw hand** ☛☛ **(AIIMS 07)**

⇨ Median nerve: "Laborers nerve" ❋❋ (PGI 99)

- Does not supply arm.
- Supplies all flexors except Flexor carpi ulnaris and medial half of flexor digitorum profundus in forearm
- Supplies:
  - ✓ Lumbrical 1 and 2
  - ✓ Opponens pollicis
  - ✓ Abductor pollicis brevis
  - ✓ Flexor pollicis brevis in hand **(LOAF).**
- **Implicated in:**
  - ▶ **Ape thumb deformity** ☛
  - ▶ **Carpal tunnel syndrome** ☛☛ **(PGI 99)**
  - ▶ **Pointing index** **(Kerala 88)**
  - ▶ **Loss of opposition and abduction of thumb** ☛☛
  - ▶ **Pen test is positive in median nerve injury**

Radial Nerve❋❋

- Supplies **Extensor** Compartment of Arm And Forearm
- Commonly involved in **"Spiral groove/Radial groove"**
- **Accompanied by Profunda Brachii vessels**
- **Supplies:**
- **BEAST** Muscles (Brachioradialis, Extensors of wrist and fingers, Anconeus, Supinator, Triceps)

- ▶ Implicated in **"Crutch Palsy"** ☛ **(PGI 99)**
- ▶ Implicated in **"Saturday night Palsy"** ☛
- ▶ **Implicated in "Wrist Drop"** ☛

⇨ Important "sites" of Injury

— Injury to Upper end of Humerus ☛	Axillary nerve damage	(UPSC 07)
— Injury (Anterior Dislocation of Shoulder) ☛	Axillary nerve damage	(COMED 07)
— Injury to Mid Humerus☛☛	Radial Nerve	
— Injury to Lower end (Medial)of Humerus☛☛	Ulnar Nerve	
— Injury to Supra Condylar area of Humerus	Median Nerve	
— Injury to upper trunk of Brachial Plexus☛	Erb Palsy	
— Injury to Lower trunk of Brachial Plexus☛	Klumpkes Palsy	

⇨ Important conditions affecting Upper Limb

- ✓ Infections from thumb and index finger spread to thenar spaces.❋
- ✓ Infections from middle and ring fingers spread to mid palmar spaces.❋
- ✓ Infections from little finger spread to ulnar bursa and forearm space of Parona❋❋

⇨ "Absent radii" is a feature of

- Fanconis Anemia
- VATER Syndrome
- TAR Syndrome
- Holt Oram syndrome

⇨ Carpal Tunnel Syndrome

- ▶ Entrapment of **Median Nerve** in Carpal Tunnel leading to tingling, parasthesias, weakness in hand.
- ▶ Painful.
- ▶ Associated with
- — Trauma,
- — Pregnancy,
- — Acromegaly,
- — Rheumatoid arthritis,
- — Amyloidosis,
- — Multiple Myeloma,
- — Hypothyroidism.
- ▶ Tinnels sign +
- ▶ Phalens sign + PGI 1998
- ▶ Electrodiagnostic tests, USG imaging and MRI are useful adjuncts

⇨ Dupuyterns contracture: ❋❋

- Progressive
- Painless
- Puckering of skin of Palmar Fascia
- Flexion of MCP joints of ring and little fingers

⇨ Colles Fracture: ❋❋❋❋

- ✓ Fall on outstretched hands☛
- ✓ Common in elderly women☛
- ✓ Distal fragment displaced dorsally, Angulated dorsally, supinated — JK BOPEE 2011
- ✓ "Dinner Fork "Deformity ☛☛
- ✓ Commonest complication is "Stiffness of fingers"☛

- ✓ Commonest # after 40 years of age: **Colles #**
- ✓ Commonest cause of sudecks atrophy in upper limb: **Colles #**
- ✓ **Position of immobilization in Colles #:** pronation, palmar deviation, ulnar deviation

➲ Scaphoid Fracture: ❋❋❋❋

- Scaphoid is one of the Carpal bones which undergo fracture commonly as well as avascular necrosis. — PGI 2011
- Avascular necrosis of "proximal" fragment is seen. — AIPGME 2012
- Injury occurs by fall on outstretched hands
- MC site of injury is "Waist". — MAH 2012
- Tenderness in "Anatomical snuff box" may be seen.
- Best Radiological view is Oblique view.
- In absence of Radiological findings, suspect scaphoid fracture.
- Most common site is between proximal 1/3 and distal 2/3.

➲ Nerve Injuries

Nerve Injuries:

- ► **Neurapraxia:** Complete recovery Possible — (UP 07)
- ► **Axonotmesis:** Rupture of nerve fiber with intact sheath
- ► **Neurontmesis:** Rupture of nerve fiber and sheath.

- ✓ Best recovery is seen in **pure motor nerve (Radial Nerve).**
- ✓ In mixed nerve recovery is poor because sensory and motor fibers may unite with each other.

⇨ Important Nerves Involved in:

► Wrist drop:❋	✓ Radial nerve palsy
► Foot drop:❋	✓ Common peroneal nerve palsy
► Meralgia parasthetica:❋	✓ Lateral cutaneous nerve of thigh (AI 07)
► Winging of scapula: ❋	✓ Long thoracic nerve of Bell (UPSC 07)
► Erbs Palsy: ❋	✓ Upper trunk of brachial plexus
► Klumpkes palsy:❋	✓ Lower trunk of brachial plexus

Nerves injured in supracondylar fracture humerus

- Interosseus Nerve (most common) **AIPGMEE 2011**
  - Median
  - Radial
  - Ulnar

⇨ Common Peroneal Nerve **AIPGMEE 2011**

It is relatively unprotected as it **traverses the lateral aspect of the neck of fibula** - **hence is prone to injury** at this area. The clinical features of common peroneal nerve injury are:

- Foot drop
- Weakness of **dorsiflexion of foot**
- Weakness of extensor hallucis longus
- Weakness of **eversion of foot**
- Sensory loss on **lateral aspect of leg** which extends to dorsum of foot

➲ Dislocation of Shoulder Joint❋❋❋

- **Shoulder is the "most common" joint to dislocate in human body.**
- **"Subcoracoid" dislocation/Inferior dislocation is the commonest type.** **MAH 2012**
- **Posterior dislocation of shoulder is rare and associated with epileptic convulsions.** **(AIIMS 04)**
- **Bankharts (Glenoid Labrum) and Hill Sacks lesion (Humeral Head) are seen.** **(AIIMS 02)**
  - ► **Hamilton ruler Test,**
  - ► **Dugas Test**
  - ► **Callaways Test are used** **PGMEE 2006**
- **Reduction is by Kochers Manouver.** **(Kar 96)**
- **Recurrent dislocation is treated by Putti Plaut and Bankhart Operation.**

➲ Adhesive capsulitis High Yield for 2011-2012

Often referred to as "**frozen shoulder,**"

Adhesive capsulitis is characterized by pain and restricted movement of the shoulder, usually in the Absence of intrinsic shoulder disease.

Adhesive capsulitis, may follow :

- **Bursitis or tendinitis of the shoulder or**
- **Chronic pulmonary disease,**
- **Myocardial infarction, and**
- **Diabetes mellitus.**

Prolonged immobility of the arm contributes to the development of adhesive capsulitis, and reflex sympathetic dystrophy is thought to be a pathogenic factor. The capsule of the shoulder is thickened, and a mild chronic inflammatory infiltrate and fibrosis may be present.

- Adhesive capsulitis occurs more commonly in women after age 50. Pain and stiffness usually develop gradually over several months to a year but progress rapidly in some patients.
- Pain may interfere with sleep.
- The shoulder is tender to palpation, and both active and passive movement are restricted. Radiographs of the shoulder show osteopenia.
- The diagnosis is confirmed by arthrography, in that only a limited amount of contrast material, usually 15 mL, can be injected under pressure into the shoulder joint.

➲ Rotator Cuff Tendinitis and Impingement Syndrome High yield for 2011-2012

Tendinitis of the rotator cuff is the major cause of a painful shoulder and is currently thought to be caused by inflammation of the tendon(s).

The rotator cuff consists of the tendons of the

- **Supraspinatus,**
- **Infraspinatus,**
- **Subscapularis and**
- **Teres minor muscles**, and inserts on the humeral tuberosities.
  - ✓ Of the tendons forming the rotator cuff, the supraspinatus **tendon is the most often affected**, probably because of its repeated impingement (impingement syndrome) between the humeral head and the undersurface of the anterior third of the acromion and coracoacromial ligament above as well as the reduction in its blood supply that occurs with abduction of the arm.
  - ✓ **Symptoms usually appear after injury or overuse, especially with activities involving elevation of the arm with some degree of forward flexion.**
  - ✓ Impingement syndrome occurs **in persons participating in baseball, tennis, swimming, or occupations that require repeated elevation of the arm.**
  - ✓ Tenderness is present over the lateral aspect of the humeral head just below the acromion.
  - ✓ NSAIDs, local glucocorticoid injection, and physical therapy may relieve symptoms.

⇨ Calcific Tendinitis:

- ✓ This condition is characterized by deposition **of calcium salts, primarily hydroxyapatite**, within a tendon. The exact mechanism of calcification is not known but may be initiated by ischemia or degeneration of the tendon.
- ✓ The **supraspinatus tendon is most often affected** because it is frequently impinged on and has a reduced blood supply when the arm is abducted.
- ✓ The condition usually develops after age 40.
- ✓ Calcification within the tendon may evoke acute inflammation, producing sudden and severe pain in the shoulder. However, it may be asymptomatic or not related to the patient's symptoms.

➲ Bicipital Tendinitis and Rupture High yield for 2011-2012

- ➢ Bicipital tendinitis, or tenosynovitis, is produced by friction on the tendon of the **long head of the biceps as it passes through the bicipital groove.**
- ➢ When the inflammation is acute, patients experience **anterior shoulder pain that radiates down the biceps into the forearm.**
- ➢ **Abduction and external rotation** of the arm are painful and limited. The bicipital groove is very tender to palpation.
- ➢ Pain may be elicited along the course of the tendon by resisting supination of the forearm with the elbow at 90° **(Yergason's supination sign).**
- ➢ Acute rupture of the tendon may occur with vigorous exercise of the arm and is often painful. In a young patient, it should be repaired surgically.
- ➢ Rupture of the tendon in an older person may be associated with little or no pain and is recognized by the presence of persistent swelling of the biceps **("Popeye" muscle)** produced by the retraction of the long head of the biceps. Surgery is usually not necessary in this setting.

➲ Congenital Dislocation of Hip:✱✱✱✱

- It is a developmental Anomaly.
- Associated with "oligohydraminos". AI 2006
- Females are more prone.
- Most common in western race. AIGEE 2003
- Shallow acetabulum is predisposing factor PGI 1997
- Common in first born baby☛☛
- Incidence is common in Frank breech☛
- Tests used:☛☛☛
- ► *Ortolanis Test (Click of entrance)* UP 2007
- ► *Von Rosens sign,*
- ► *Barlows sign are useful in Diagnosis*
- Lurching gait (Unilateral CDH)
- Waddling Gait (Bilateral CDH)
- Ultrasonography is used for Diagnosis☛☛
- Shentons line is broken☛ PGI 1989
- Von Rosen Splint is used in Treatment☛ UP 2007

▶ Commonest type of hip dislocation: posterior.	UPSC 1988
▶ Flexion, adduction and internal rotation are a feature.	JIPMER 1985
▶ Posterior dislocation Can be seen on per rectal examination.	AP 1998

⇨ Tarsal Tunnel Syndrome:

- Is entrapment of "Posterior Tibial nerve" in the Tarsal tunnel. (AIIMS 09)❋❋
- Occurs in association with
  - ✓ "Rheumatoid arthritis",❋❋❋
  - ✓ Ankylosing spondylitis, ❋❋
  - ✓ Neural tumors or Perineural fibrosis❋
- Pain and sensory disturbances over plantar aspect of foot is seen.

➲ Congenital Talipes Equino Varus❋❋ (CTEV)

- Also called as Club Foot.
- IE Deformity:
- ▶ *Inversion deformity*
- ▶ *Equinus deformity*
- Associated with :
  - ✓ Idiopathic causes
  - ✓ Neurological disorders
  - ✓ Spina bifida
  - ✓ Arthrogyrophosis multiplex (PGI 01)
- Foot in Equines, Varus and Adduction
- Usually bilateral
- Manipulation should begin "immediately after birth by mother (UP 93, KAR 94)
- At 2 years treatment is "Posteromedial soft tissue release" (PGI 99)
- Treatment of chronic cases is "Triple Arthodesis" (JIPMER 95)

⇨ Conservative Management of CTEV

- **Kite's method:** Serial manipulation and cast correction in order beginning with forefoot adduction and proceeding to correction of heel varus and finally equinus. Today kite's method is rarely used because of inability of others to match his results and excessive amount of time required for infants to remain in casts.
- **Ponseti method:** Order of deformity correction—cavus, adduction, varus and equnimus **(CAVE)** Is the most followed conservative method.
- French physiotherapy method.

3

ORTHOPEDICS

⇨ Options for Treatment of CTEV

✓ <3 years:	Soft tissue release✱
✓ 4-8 years:	Evans surgery✱
✓ 8-11 years:	Wedge Tarsectomy✱
✓ >12 years:	Triple arthrodesis✱
✓ Already operated:	Ilizarov technique✱

⇨ Important Terms:

▶ Tennis Elbow is Medial Epicondylitis	(Affects Common Flexor Origin)
▶ Golfers Elbow is Lateral Epincondylitis	(Affects Common Extensor Origin)
▶ Students elbow	Olecranon bursitis
▶ Painful arc Syndrome	Supraspinatus Tendinitis in which patient cant abduct his arm beyond 30° without pain
▶ Frozen Shoulder	Active movement at shoulder is not possible at all.

➲ Different Types of Pelvis

▶ Triradiate pelvis ☛☛ is seen in	✓ Osteomalacia COMED 2008
▶ Beaked pelvis☛☛ is seen in	✓ Osteomalacia
▶ Funnel shaped pelvis☛☛ is seen in	✓ **Android** type of pelvis
▶ **True pelvis** ☛☛ refers to	✓ **Lower pelvis**
▶ Rachitic pelvis ☛☛ is seen in	✓ Rickets **(R-R)**
▶ Nageles pelvis ☛☛ is	✓ **One ala absent**
▶ Roberts pelvis ☛☛ is	✓ **Both ala absent**
▶ **Kyphotic/Funnel** Shaped pelvis is also seen in	✓ **Tuberculosis/Rickets**

➲ Important Classifications in Orthopedics:

Garden's classification of Fracture Neck of Femur	
▶ Stage I	**Incomplete** #NOF
▶ Stage II	Complete #NOF **without** displacement
▶ Stage III	Complete #NOF with **partial** displacement ORISSA 03
▶ Stage IV	Complete #NOF with **complete** displacement

Enneking's Classification of Malignant Tumors:	AIIMS 2007
▶ **Stage IA:**	Low Grade **Intracompartment**
▶ **Stage IB:**	Low Grade **Extracompartment**
▶ **Stage IIA:**	**High Grade** Intracompartment
▶ **Stage IIB:**	**High Grade** Extracompartment
▶ **Stage III:**	**Either Grade** With metastasis

⇨ Salter Harris Classification of Epiphyseal Injuries: Classification of Epiphyseal injuries was given by: Salter Harris — MAH 2012

- ▶ Type I: **Epiphyseal separation** through epiphyseal plate with or without displacement
- ▶ Type II: Fractures have metaphyseal spike attached to separated epiphysis with separation through epiphyseal plate
- ▶ Type III: Separation of epiphyseal plate with fracture through epiphysis into the joint
- ▶ Type IV: Fractures through **Metaphysis, Epiphyseal plate, epiphysis** into the joint
- ▶ Type V: **Compression fracture of Epiphyseal plate** where permanent damage is done to plate
- ▶ Type VI: Bruise or Contusion to periphery of Epiphyseal plate

⇨ Classification of Sutures:

- ▶ **Monofilament Absorbable:** ❋ Surgical gut (**Cat gut**) and Collagen
- ▶ **Monofilament Non Absorbable:** ❋ Polyamide, Poly propolene, Steel, Polyster
- ▶ **Multi filament Absorbable:** ❋ **Poly glycolic and Poly glactin**
- ▶ **Multi Non filament Absorbable:** ❋ Silk, Polyester Braided, Polyamide Braided

Remember "new" Important points in Orthopedics

- ▶ **Guyons canal**: Fibroosseous canal bound by hamate and pisiform bone through which **ulnar artery and nerve pass.❋**
- ▶ **Bowlers thumb**: Traumatic neuropathy of **ulnar digital nerve to thumb❋**

3

ORTHOPEDICS

- **Pronator syndrome: High Carpal tunnel syndrome:** Entrapment of **Median nerve nerve at elbow.**
- **Anterior interosseous syndrome:** Compression of AIN (**Anterior interosseous Nerve)** 4-6 cms below elbow causing weakness of FPL, FDP and pronator quadrates
- **Cubital Tunnel Syndrome:** Compression of **ulnar nerve** during its passage around medial aspect of elbow☛
- **Radial tunnel Syndrome:** Resistant Tennis Elbow due to entrapment **of Posterior Interosseous nerve** in the lateral aspect of Proximal forearm☛
- **Wartenburgs Syndrome:** Entrapment of **Sensory branch of Radial nerve** as it emerges beneath Brachioradialis proximal to Radial Styloid process.
- **Meralgia Parasthetica : Lateral cutaneous nerve of Thigh**☛
- **Anterior Tarsal Tunnel Syndrome: Deep peroneal nerve** ☛
- **Tarsal Tunnel syndrome: Posterior Tibial nerve** ☛ **(AIIMS 09)**
- **Joggers Foot: Medial plantar nerve**☛
- **Hip Pointer: Iliac Crest**☛
- **Tennis Leg: Gastrocnemius Soleus strain**❋

Prolapse of Intervertebral Disk:

- ✓ Most common site **L4-L5.**
- ✓ Burst # occurs due to **compression.** **AI 2007**
- ✓ Most common cause is **Trauma.**
- ✓ Extrusion of Nucleus pulposus into body of vertebrae is **Schmorls node**

Spondylosis

- ✓ is **Degeneration** of Intervertebral disk☛
- ✓ Spondylolysis is a **bony defect in the <u>pars interarticularis</u>** (a segment near the junction of the pedicle with the lamina) of the vertebra; ☛

Spondylolisthesis

- ✓ It is the **anterior slippage of the vertebral body, pedicles, and superior articular facets,** leaving the posterior elements behind. ☛
- ✓ Spondylolisthesis is **associated with spondylolysis** and degenerative spine disease and occurs more frequently in women.☛
- ✓ The slippage may be asymptomatic but may also cause low back pain, nerve root injury (the L5 root most frequently), or symptomatic spinal stenosis.
- ✓ A **"step"** may be present on deep palpation of the posterior elements of the segment above the spondylolisthetic joint. ☛

- ✓ The trunk may be shortened and the abdomen protuberant as a result of extreme forward displacement of L4 on L5 in severe degrees of spondylolisthesis.
- ✓ **Spondylolesithesis** is **slipping** of one vertebrae over other. ☚
- ✓ Beheaded Scottish Terrier sign is seen.☚ **JIPMER 1988**
- ✓ Beheaded Scottish Terrier sign is seen in oblique view. **JIPMER 1990**
- ✓ Myelography, CT, or MRI is indicated preoperatively to establish definitively the nature and extent of disease as well as the level of vertebral involvement. **AIIMS 2011**

⇨ Tests Suggesting Disk Prolapse:

- ▶ **Naffeziers test**☚
- ▶ **Miligrams test**☚
- ▶ **Sitting root test**☚

➲ Vertebrae and Corresponding Spinal Level

— Cervical region	**C1-C7 Add1**
— Upper Thoracic Lesion	**T1 -T6 Add 2**
— Lower Thoracic Lesion	**T7-T9 Add 3**
— T 10	**Corresponds to L1-L2**
— T12-L1	**Corresponds to L5-S1**

➲ Eponym Bone Diseases

▶ **Marble bone disease**	• **Osteopetrosis**
▶ **Spotted bone disease**	• **Osteopoikilosis**
▶ **Stripped bone disease**	• **Osteopathia striata**
▶ **Candle bone disease**	• **Melorrheostosis** **(JK BOPEE 09)**

⇨ Gait

Phases of Normal Gait:

- ▶ **Stance phase:** 60% of cycle: When foot is on the **ground heel strike**
- ▶ **Swing phase:** 40% of cycle: When foot is **moving forward**

⌗ **Tredlenburg gait:**

Due to weakness of gluteus medius muscle. Seen in **coxa vara, # Greater Trochanter, polio**✱

⌗ **Antalgic gait:**

Patient avoids pain in foot and takes off his weight as early as possible during stance phase❋

⌗ **Steppage gait**

It is produced by weakness of ankle dorsiflexion. Because of the partial or complete foot drop, the leg must be lifted higher than usual to avoid catching the toe on the floor during the forward swing of the leg. ❋

- **Normal carrying angle Males: 10-15 Degrees, Females:15-18 Degrees**☚
- **Cubitus Varus** Reduction in normal carrying angle☚
- **Cubitus Valgus** Increase in carrying angle☚
- **Cubitus rectus** No valgus or varus angulation☚

➲ Slipped femoral Epiphysis (SCFE)❋❋

- It is displacement of "Proximal Femoral Epiphysis".☚
- Common in children (Obese) in 2nd decade.☚ AI 1988
- Pain is the initial and most common complaint.☚
- "Epiphysis" slips "downwards and posteriorly".
- Limping is associated feature ☚
- Flexion, Abduction and Medial Rotation are limited☚
- Diagnosis is by:
  - ✓ Trethowans sign,
  - ✓ Capeners sign ☚
  - ✓ Tredlenburgs sign may be positive.☚

⇨ Perthe's Disease ❋❋

- Is chronic disease with ischemia of upper end of femur causing "avascular necrosis." PGI 2011
- Osteochondritis of Femoral head AI 1991
- Boys are affected more
- Adduction of limb is unaffected SGPGI 2005
- Not obese
- Pain is the initial and most common complaint.
- Limping is associated feature
- MRI is the investigation of choice AI 2005

⇨ Coxa Vara

Term used to describe a hip in which angle between neck and shaft of femur is less than 125°

- ✸ Localized bony dysplasia of the femoral neck
- ✸ Characterized by a decreased neck shaft angle and the presence of a triangular ossification defect (Fairbanks Triangle) of the inferior femoral neck MAH 2012
- ✸ Results in decreased length of the involved limb

➲ Osteochondritis: ✸✸ ✸

▶ Perthes disease:	▶ Osteochondritis of Femoral head AI 1991
▶ Panners disease:	▶ Osteochondritis of Capitulum
▶ Keinbocks disease:	▶ Osteochondritis of Lunate COMED 2008
▶ OsGood Scalters disease:	▶ Osteochondritis of Tibial tubercle PGI 2007
▶ Severs disease:	▶ Osteochondritis of Calcaneum NIMHANS 1996
▶ Kohlers disease	▶ Osteochondritis of Navicular
▶ Friebergs disease:	▶ Osteochondritis of Metatarsal head
▶ Scheurmanns disease:	▶ Osteochondritis of Vertebrae MAH 2012

➲ Different vertebral Types in Different Diseases

▶ Picture frame vertebrae:	✓ Pagets disease (P-P)
▶ Square-shaped vertebrae:	✓ Ankylosing Spondylitis
▶ Hamburger vertebrae:	✓ Osteopetrosis
▶ Beak-shaped vertebrae:	✓ Mucopolysacchroidoses
▶ Wedge-shaped vertebrae: ▶ Fish head vertebrae:	✓ Osteoporosis ✓ Osteoporosis AIIMS 1987
▶ Fish mouth vertebrae:	✓ Osteogenesis imperfect AI 1989 ✓ Ehlaer Danhlos syndrome AI 1989 ✓ Homocystinuria AI 1989 ✓ Marfans syndrome
▶ Vertebrae plana	✓ Eosinophilic granuloma

⇨ Remember:	
▶ Multiple enchondromatosis:	Olliers disease
▶ Enchondromas with Hemangiomas:	Maffucis Syndrome
▶ Fallen fragment sign:	Aneurysmal Bone cyst

3

ORTHOPEDICS

⇨ **Limb deformities in:**

► Limb abducted and externally rotated in :	✓ Anterior dislocation Hip
► Limb flexed, adducted and internally rotated in :	✓ Posterior dislocation Hip
► Cubitus varus (Gun stock deformity):	✓ Supracondylar# of humerus
► Cubitus valgus:	✓ # lateral condyle humerus

⇨ **Differentiate limb deformities:**

■ Flexion, adduction, internal rotation:	Posterior dislocation of hip. (FADIR)
■ Flexion, abduction, external rotation:	Anterior dislocation of hip. (FABER)
■ Flexion, adduction, external rotation:	# NOF (FADER)

➲ Bone Tumors (High Yield Facts Commonly Asked)

⇨ **Benign Tumors:**

The common benign bone tumors include:

- **Enchondroma, osteochondroma, chondroblastoma, and** **PGI 2006**
- **Chondromyxoid fibroma, of cartilage origin;** **PGI 2003**
- **Osteoid osteoma and osteoblastoma, of bone origin;** **PGI 2006**
- **Fibroma and desmoplastic fibroma, of fibrous tissue origin;**
- **Hemangioma, of vascular origin;**
- **And giant cell tumor, of unknown origin.**

Malignant Tumors: The most common malignant tumors of bone are **plasma cell tumors.** The four most common malignant non hematopoietic bone tumors are

- **Osteosarcoma,**
- **Chondrosarcoma,**
- **Ewing's sarcoma, and**
- **Malignant fibrous histiocytoma**

Rare malignant tumors include

- **Chordoma** (of notochordal origin), **AI 1998**
- **Malignant giant cell tumor and**
- **Adamantinoma (of unknown origin), and**
- **Hemangioendothelioma (of vascular origin).**

Bone Marker Tests

Urine or blood tests for Bone resorption include:

- **C-telopeptide (C-terminal telopeptide of type 1 collagen (CTx))** - a peptide fragment from the carboxy terminal end of the protein matrix; aids in monitoring antiresorptive therapies, such as bisphosphonates and hormone replacement therapy, in postmenopausal women and people with low bone mass (osteopenia) **MAH 2012**
- **N-telopeptide (N-terminal telopeptide of type 1 collagen (NTx))** - a peptide fragment from the amino terminal end of the protein matrix; it is recommended that the test be performed at baseline before starting osteoporosis therapy and again 3 to 6 months later
- **Deoxypyridinoline (DPD)** - a collagen breakdown product with a ring structure
- **Pyridinium Crosslinks** - a group of collagen breakdown products that includes DPD; used to monitor therapy response; not as specific for bone collagen as the telopeptides
- **Tartrate-resistant acid phosphatase (TRAP) 5b** - 5b is the isoform of TRAP produced by osteoclasts during bone resorption

Bone formation blood tests include:

- **Bone-specific alkaline phosphatase (ALP)** - one of the isoenzymes (types) of ALP; it is associated with osteoblast cell function and thought to have a role in bone mineralization
- **Osteocalcin (bone gla protein)** - a protein formed by osteoblasts; part of the non-collagen portion of the new bone structure;
- **P1NP (Procollagen Type 1 N-Terminal Propeptide)** - formed by osteoblasts; reflects rate of collagen and bone formation;

Importance of bone density

Increased bone density is seen due to:

- ✓ Thick cortex
- ✓ Increased trabeculations
- ✓ Coarse trabeculae **PGI 2011**
- ✓ Periosteal reaction **PGI 2011**
- ✓ Thickened bone
- ✓ Sclerosis
- ✓ Dead bone

Increased Bone Density is seen in

Adults	Children
✷ Myelosclerosis **PGI 2011**	✷ Osteopetrosis
✷ Flourosis	✷ Pyknodysostosis
✷ Osteoblastic metastasis	✷ Lead poisoning

3

ORTHOPEDICS

✷ Lymphoma	✷ Flourosis
✷ Pagets disease	✷ Caffeys disease PGI 2011
✷ Renal osteodystrophy	✷ Hypervitaminosis A
✷ Avascular bony necrosis	✷ Hypervitaminosis D

➲ Tumors According to Location

Epiphyseal ✷✷	Metaphyseal ✷	Diaphyseal✷✷
▶ Chondroblastoma	▶ Chondrosarcoma	▶ Round cell tumors
▶ Osteoclastoma AI 2007	▶ Enchondroma	▶ Ewings sarcoma
PGI 2001	▶ Osteochondroma	▶ Multiple Myeloma
AI 2001	▶ Osteoblastoma	▶ Adamantinoma
	▶ Osteosarcoma	▶ Osteoid osteoma
	▶ Bone cyst	
	▶ Osteomyelitis PGI 2002	

Diaphyseo metaphyseal:

- **Fibrous dysplasia and other fibrous tumors of Bone.**
- **Fibrosarcoma,**
- **Fibroxanthoma,**
- **Chondromyxoid fibroma,**
- **Fibrous cortical defect,**
- **Nonossifying Fibroma.**

Different appearances of bony tumors:

▶ **Onion Skin appearance:**	Ewings sarcoma	**COMED 2007/ JK BOPEE 2011 JKBOPEE 2012**
▶ **Honey-comb appearance:**	Adamantinoma	
▶ **Breech of Cortex:**	Osteoclastoma, Aneurysmal bone cyst	
▶ **Soap bubble appearance:**	**Osteoclastoma**	**MAH 2012**
▶ **Codmans triangle:**	**Osteosarcoma**	
▶ **Sun-ray appearance:**	**Osteosarcoma**	
▶ **Chickenwire pattern:**	Chondroblastoma	**COMED 2K**
▶ **Linear Striations**	**Vertebral Hemangioma**	
▶ **Physalipharous cells**	**Chordoma**	
▶ **Cotton wool/Ground Glass Appearance Fibrous Dysplasia**		**(COMED 06)**

➲ Ewing's Sarcoma***

- Affects children <15 years usually.
- Diaphysial Tumor — PGI 2K
- Common in second decade — COMED 2007
- Onion skin lesions on X ray — COMED 2007, JKBOPEE 2012
- Translocation (t; 11:22)
- Mimics Osteomyelitis — AIIMS 2000
- PAS Positive material (Glycogen) found
- Most radiosensitive bone tumor

➲ Bad Prognostic Indicators in Ewings Sarcoma

- Distant metastasis+
- Size of primary lesion
- Distal tumors have good prognosis
- Fever, anemia, ↑WBC, ↑ESR, ↑LDH — AIIMS 2010
- Abberant p53 expression

➲ Osteosarcoma

- Second most common primary malignant bone marrow.
- Metaphyseal tumor — PGI 2002
- Affects knee joint
- MC site lower end of femur — AIIMS 2000
- Sunburst appearance — AI 2007
- Codmans triangle — AIIMS 2007
- Presents with secondaries in lungs with pneumothorax — AIIMS 1996
- Pulsating bone tumor
- Chemotherapy +limb salvage surgery used for treatment — AI 2004

⇨ Radiological Features of Osteosarcoma

- **Area of irregular destruction in the metaphysis**
- Cortex overlying the lesion is eroded
- **New bone formation** in the mateix of the tumor
- **Periosteal reaction** (the tumor lifts the preiosteum, incites an intense periosteal reaction)
- **Codman's triangle:** a triangular area of subperiosteal new bone is seen at the tumor host cortex junction at the ends of the femur.
- **Sun-ray appearance:** as the periosteum is unable to contain the tumor, the tumor grows into the underlying soft-tissues. ***New bone is laid down along the blood vessels within the tumor growing centrifugally***, giving rise to a Sun-ray appearance on X-ray.

⇨ Osteoclastoma

- Epiphyseal tumor
- Soap bubble appearance — MAH 2012
- Breech of cortex
- Lower end of Femur is most common site

⇨ Chondrosarcoma

- Metaphyseal Tumor
- Dense Punctate Calcifications
- Associated with endosteal scalloping — AI 2002

⇨ Synovial Sarcomas: AIIMS 2009

- The term **"Synovial Sarcoma"** is a **misnomer.** The term originates from the **histological appearance of the cells, which can resemble synovial cells.**
- The tumors <u>do not</u> **arise from synovial tissue**, however. An intra-articular location or even continuity with the joint capsule is extremely rare.
- Plain radiographs frequently show **amorphic calcification** within the tumor.
- Synovial sarcomas can occur across a wide age range.
- Occurs at **extra-articular sites** more often. Seen in sites such as **knee and foot.**
- Synovial sarcomas are relatively common in the distal extremities, including the hand or foot.
- Microscopically, the tumors frequently show **a biphasic growth pattern with "nests of epithelioid cells surrounded by spindle cells".**

➲ Multiple Myeloma❋❋❋

- This malignant neoplasm of marrow cell origin is **the "most common primary malignant neoplasm"** of **bone.❋**
- Myeloma is often encountered in the **late decades of life** and is seen more frequently in **males** than in females. ❋
- The symptoms vary from local pain and discomfort to systemic symptoms of
  - ✓ **Anemia,**
  - ✓ **Fever,**
  - ✓ **Hypercalcemia,** — AI 2010
  - ✓ **Renal failure** related to extensive skeletal involvement and
  - ✓ **Abnormal production of immunoglobulins.❋**
- Myeloma characteristically produces **lytic destruction of bone** with little if any reactive bone formation.
- These lesions are described as **"geographic or punched out"** in appearance.❋ — AIIMS 2000

- **The absence of reactive bone formation** is borne out by the observation that myeloma lesions are often **silent on radionuclide scanning.** ❋
- Pathologic fracture is often the presenting symptom.
- The diagnosis of myeloma is made by **marrow aspiration or the demonstration of abnormal plasma cells at the site of bony destruction.** ❋
- Fifty percent of patients with disseminated disease have **Bence Jones protein in their urine.**
- Serum **electrophoresis demonstrates an abnormal amount of immunoglobulins.** ❋
- Urine electrophoresis is also helpful when the diagnosis is in doubt and may demonstrate abnormal proteins in patients with a normal serum electrophoretic pattern.
- Microscopically, myeloma produces **sheets of plasma cells.** Usually these are well-differentiated cells in which the characteristic arrangements of nuclear chromatin can be recognized with **"Russel Bodies."** ❋

Aneurysmal Bone Cyst

- Aneurysmal bone cyst is **metaphyseal lesion.**
- **Has blood filled spaces**
- **Pulsatile in elderly** — **PGI 2007**
- Aneurysmal bone cyst is **expansile radiolucent** lesion. — **AIIMS 2002**
- Aneurysmal bone cyst may show **"focal cortical destruction, cortical breech".**
- Aneurysmal bone cyst most commonly occurs in Lower end of **HUMERUS**

Unicameral Bone Cyst:

- **Usually a single cavity with connective tissue lining.** — **PGI 2002**
- **Gaint cells seen.**
- **Lytic lesion usually in children.** — **AI 2002**

Chondroblastoma

Chondroblastoma is a **benign cartilaginous tumor.**

Chondroblastoma is **epiphyseal** tumor. — **AIIMS 2005**

Chondroblastoma is characterized by

- **Multi nucleate giant cells,**
- **PAS positive reaction,**
- **"Dense punctuate/stippled or mottled calcification with sclerotic rim."** — **AIIMS 1996**

Most common site is **proximal humerus**

3

ORTHOPEDICS

⇨ Adamantinoma✱✱

- Epithelial tumor from **dental epithelium.**
- Mc sites: **Mandible, Tibia**
- **Diaphysial tumor**
- **Slowly growing, locally invasive benign, cystic lesion.**
- **Occurs in late adolescence/ middle age**
- **"Bubble defect" in anterior tibial cortex** is a feature

⇨ Osteoid Osteoma

- One of the **commonest benign bone tumor.**
- Severe **Pain at night responding to NSAIDS.**
- Mc site: **Femur and tibia**

➲ Most Common Sites of:

Bone secondaries:	Vertebrae	
Multiple Myeloma:	Vertebrae	
Adamantinoma:	Mandible	
Pagets Disease:	Pelvis	JK 2008
Ivory osteoma:	Frontal sinus	
Simple bone cyst:	Upper end of Humerus	
Aneurysmal bone cyst:	Lower end of Humerus	
Osteoclastoma:	Lower end of Femur	
Rhabdomyosarcoma:	Head and neck region	

⇨ Oncogenic osteomalacia

*A syndrome associated with bone pain and muscle weakness, together with the radiologic features of osteomalacia, can occur in patients with mesenchymal tumors such as **benign osteoblastomas, giant cell osteosarcomas, hemangiomas, and occasionally epithelial tumors such as prostate and SCLC (Small cell carcinoma lung)**. Biochemical studies show **hypophosphatemia and subnormal 1, 25-dihydroxyvitamin D levels**. The pathophysiology of this disorder is unclear but appears to involve a hormonally mediated and severe renal phosphate loss as the primary event.*

⇨ Malignancies and Hypercalcemia:

Malignancies can cause hypercalcemia through two non-mutually exclusive mechanisms.

Local osteolytic hypercalcemia is caused by tumor metastatic to bone. Tumor cells may release bone-resorbing factors or so-called **osteoclast-activating factors**, which indirectly lead to bone resorption. Cytokines such as **lymphotoxin and interleukin-1** are potent osteoclast-activating factors.

Humoral hypercalcemia of malignancy is caused by tumor-secreting factors into the circulation that act systemically to increase bone resorption. Such factors may show other **PTH-like actions**, including increasing urinary cAMP and phosphate excretion and decreasing renal calcium excretion. This condition leads to a syndrome with biochemical features closely resembling those of primary hyperparathyroidism.

One such factor commonly associated with many tumors has recently been identified as a polypeptide roughly **twice as large as PTH and homologous in amino acid sequence to the biologically active amino-terminus of PTH. This so-called parathyroid hormone-related peptide** may also be secreted by tumors metastatic to bone, so that humoral and local osteolytic mechanisms may combine to cause hypercalcemia. Some tumors cause hypercalcemia through **excessive synthesis of 1, 25 (OH) 2D, in a manner analogous to that seen in sarcoidosis.**

⇨ Paget's Disease of Bone

- ✓ Also called as **(osteitis deformans)**
- ✓ **Excessive resorption of bone by osteoclasts**, followed by the replacement of normal marrow by vascular, fibrous connective tissue.
- ✓ ***The irregular and often rapid deposition of this new bone, to a great extent still lamellar, results in an increase in the number of prominent, irregular cement lines that give the bone*** its characteristic **"Mosaic" pattern.** **MAH 2012**
- ✓ **Increased generation and overactivity of osteoclasts**
- ✓ **The calcification rate is characteristically increased** in pagetic bone.
- ✓ Bone turnover correlates with the **increased plasma level of bone alkaline phosphatase.**
- ✓ **The increased urinary excretion of small peptides** containing hydroxyproline reflects increased bone resorption. **Pyridinoline (Pyr) and deoxypyridinoline (D-Pyr)**
- ✓ **The pelvic bones are most commonly involved**, followed by the femur, skull, tibia, lumbosacral spine, dorsal spine, clavicles, and ribs; small bones are not as frequently diseased.

⇨ Symptoms of Pagets Disease:

Many patients are **asymptomatic.**

- ***Bone pain*** *is the most common symptom.*
- ***Headaches and hearing loss*** *may occur when Paget's disease affects the skull or spine.*
- ***Somnolence (drowsiness)*** *due to vascular steal syndrome of the skull.*
- ***Nerve compression*** *may occur when Paget's disease affects the skull or spine.*
- ***Somnolence*** *due to vascualr steal syndrome of the skull.*
- ***Paralysis*** *due to vascular steal syndrome of the vertebrae.*
- ***Increased head size, bowing of limb, or curvature of spine*** *may occur may occur in advanced cases.*
- ***Hip pain*** *may occur when Paget's disease affects the pelvis or thigh bone.*
- *Damage to joint cartilage may lead to arthritis.*
- *Teeth may spread intraorally-due to the intra-oral force placed on the anterior teeth.*
- ***Chalkstick fractures.***
- ***Mosaic bone pattern.***
- ***Hypercementosis in teeth*** *may occur.*

- **Angioid streaks** may be present in the retina.
- **Hearing loss** can be due to direct involvement of the ossicles of the inner ear, involvement of bone in the region of the cochlea, or impingement on the eighth cranial nerve in the auditory foramen.
- More serious neurologic complications can result from **overgrowth of bone at the base of the skull (platybasia) and compression of the brainstem.**
- **Compression of the spinal cord can cause paraplegia**, particularly with involvement of the mid-dorsal spine.
- **Pathologic fractures** of vertebrae may also produce spinal cord lesions.

⇨ Complications

- **High-output heart failure**
- **Pathologic fracture**
- **Hyperuricemia and gout**
- **Calcific periarthritis**
- **Sarcoma is the dread complication.** ***(Pagetic osteosarcomas are lytic in appearance on radiographs, in contrast to the sclerotic appearance of radiation-induced osteosarcomas. The tumors are multicentric in about 20% of patients. Fibrosarcomas and chondrosarcomas have also been found)***

⇨ Treatment

- **Osteotomies** are useful in patients with bowing deformities of the tibia.
- Potent bisphosphonates can inhibit bone resorption and are usually well tolerated, **alendronate and** risedronate are used
- **Calcitonin** therapy has largely been replaced by bisphosphonates **High Yield for 2011-2012**

➲ Quick Wrap Up of Pagets Disease of Bone

- Pagets Disease is also called as **Osteitis Deformans.**
- It is because of **extensive osteoclastic activity and disorganised new bone formation.**
- **Commonly** involved bones are: **Pelvis, tibia, skull, spine.** **JK BOPEE**
- **Pelvis being the commonest site.**
- **Serum Calcium and phosphate levels are normal.**
- **Alkaline phosphatase and Osteocalcin levels are increased.**

Pain is the most common presenting feature.

Complications include:

- High output cardiac failure
- Fractures
- Hypercalcemia
- Cranial nerve palsies and spinal stenosis
- Deafness due to otosclerosis
- Steal Syndrome
- Osteosarcoma (dangerous) **UP 2007**

- **Bisphosphonates** are the "Drug of Choice".

Do not Confuse with:

- **Paget's disease of Nipple:** Which is associated with underlying ductal malignancy of breast.
- **Paget's disease of vulva:** Which is not associated with underlying malignancy but can cause vulval cancer.
- **Pagets recurrent fibroid:** A **spindle cell sarcoma** of low potential **occurring in abdominal wall or thighs.**
- **Pagets cells:** upward spread of breast cancer cells into epidermis which are mucin positive.

➲ Fibrous Dysplasia❋❋

- Fibrous dysplasia is a **tumor like lesion.**
- It is **benign** ☛
- It is **developmental in origin** and **hormone dependent.**☛ **MAHE 1998**
- Pathology is replacement of bone by fibrous tissue.
- X ray shows "**Ground glass" appearance and "Chinese lettering of bone"**☛
- Rarely **osteosarcoma** can occur in fibrous dysplasia.☛
- Sexual precocity in girls with polyostotic fibrous dysplasia and cutaneous pigmentation constitutes **"McCune Albright Syndrome".**
- Fibrous dysplasia and McCune-Albright syndrome represent a phenotypic spectrum of disorders caused by **activating mutations in the GNAS1 gene.**

Radiologic Changes

The roentgenographic appearance of the lesions is that of a radiolucent area with a well-delineated, smooth or scalloped border, typically associated with focal thinning of the cortex of the bone

Fibrous dysplasia can cause **bones to become larger** than normal, a feature characteristic of Paget's disease as well.

The **"ground-glass" appearance** is due to the thin spicules of calcified woven bone.

Deformities can include

- ✓ **Coxa vara,**☛
- ✓ **Shepherd's-crook deformity of the femur,**☛ **AMU 2005**
- ✓ **Bowing of the tibia,** ☛
- ✓ **Harrison's grooves, and** ☛
- ✓ **Protrusio acetabuli.**
- ✓ Involvement of facial bones, may create a **leonine appearance (leontiasis ossea).**
- ✓ Fibrous dysplasia of the temporal bones can cause progressive **loss of hearing** and **obliteration of the external ear canal.** ☛
- ✓ Advanced skeletal age in girls is correlated with **sexual precocity** but can occur in boys without sexual precocity. ☛
- ✓ Occasionally, a focus of fibrous dysplasia may undergo cystic degeneration, with an enormous distortion of the shape of the **bone**, and mimic the so-called **aneurysmal bone cyst.**

3

ORTHOPEDICS

➲ Acute Pyogenic Arthritis (SEPTIC)✱✱✱ (AIIMS 2009)

- Joint infection with pyogenic organisms occurs as a result of **hematogenous seeding of the joint,** ☛extension of adjacent osteomyelitis, or penetrating wounds of the joint.
- Hematogenous pyarthrosis is most commonly observed in children under the age of 5 years.
- **S. aureus is the most common etiologic agent**, followed by Haemophilus influenzae, Streptococcus, Gonococcus, and Pneumococcus. ☛
- Acute pyarthrosis is **almost always monarticular.** ☛
- Patients with immune deficiency may present with multiple joint involvement.
- **The hip joint** is the most frequently involved.

Clinical Considerations

The onset of pyogenic arthritis is **acute, with fever, irritability, and pain.**☛

In the early stages of infection, a **limp** may develop, which rapidly progresses to severe pain, preventing ambulation.

On examination, one observes swelling, overlying erythema, and exquisite tenderness to direct palpation. Any attempt at joint motion produces paroxysms of pain.

Laboratory studies demonstrate

- ✓ **Elevated** white blood cell count and an
- ✓ **Elevated** erythrocyte sedimentation rate.
- ✓ Aspiration of the involved joint under sterile conditions reveals a **cloudy, turbid synovial fluid, with a cell count ranging from 50,000 to 200,000 polymorphonuclear neutrophils per cu. cm.**
- ✓ A Gram's stain of the involved joint fluid shows organisms in 50% of cases. The joint fluid is sent for aerobic and anaerobic culture.
- ✓ **Blood cultures** are frequently positive.

Radiographs in the early stages of septic arthritis reveal no bony change.

- ✓ There is distention in the joint capsule secondary to increased pressure within the joint, and the joint may appear abnormally widened.
- ✓ In severe cases, there may be pathologic dislocation of the joint or pathologic separation of the epiphysis. In untreated or inadequately treated cases, destruction of articular cartilage eventually produces joint narrowing.

Treatment

Pyogenic arthritis is an emergency.

When the diagnosis has been established, intravenous antibiotics are administered without awaiting the results of culture.

Septic Arthritis	Transient synovitis
► Less common.	► **Mc cause** of hip pain and limp in children.
► Patient is **sick.**	► Patient is not sick.
► High grade fever **usual.**	► High grade fever unusual.
► Pain is **severe.**	► Pain is not severe.
► ESR, CRP, WBC ↑ (AIIMS 09)	► ESR, CRP, WBC usually normal.

➲ Osteomyelitis

- **Osteomyelitis is the term used to denote infection of bone.** ☛
- **Earliset site of bone involvement is in Metaphysis.** **(AIIMS 09)**
- The majority of bone infections are the result of **Staphylococcus aureus.**☛

The **isolated necrotic bone** within the abscess cavity is called a **sequestrum.** ☛☛☛ **JKBOPEE 2012**

- New bone formation occurring about the periphery of the abscess represents the body's attempt to wall off the infection. This new bone is called **involucrum.** ☛☛
- In some instances, a static abscess cavity remains without further enlargement. This equilibrium between host and organism is known as a **Brodie's abscess in long bones.** **(JIPMER 06)**
- Young children may demonstrate the phenomenon known as **pseudoparalysis.** ☛These children refuse to move the involved limb, mimicking a neurologic deficit.
- **Radiographs:** It takes some time for osteomyelitic lesions to appear on radiographs.
- The lesion of osteomyelitis appears on radiograph in not less than two weeks.
- As a result alternative diagnostic modalities are used to pick up osteomyelitis in the form of **MRI and Bone scans.**
- Most cases of acute osteomyelitis are due to Staph Aureus and MRSA strains are common nowadays.
- It is not advisible to wait for radiological changes to appear in case of acute osteomyelitis and then to start treatment.

⇨ Diagnosis:

- ESR Increased
- CRP Increased
- TLC Increased
- MRI (90% sensitive 95% specific)☛
- Bone scans 60% sensitive and 33% specific)☛
- Blood cultures positive in 65% cases. (Confirmatory) ☛ **(UP 07)**

⇨ Radiographic changes in osteomyelitis:☛ ☛ ☛

- Hazziness
- Loss of density of effected bones
- Subperoosteal reaction
- Bone death and appearance of **(sequestrum)** **JKBOPEE 2012**
- Periosteal new bone formation **(involcrum)**

3

ORTHOPEDICS

⇨ Time related changes in acute osteomyelitis:☛ ☛☛

- **Soft tissue swelling:** Less than a week
- **Periosteal reaction:** after ten days (DNB 91)
- **Lytic changes:** after two weeks

- Early diagnosis of acute **osteomyelitis** is critical because prompt antibiotic therapy may prevent the necrosis of bone.
- The evaluation usually begins with plain radiographs because of their ready availability, although they frequently show no abnormalities during early infection.
- In 95% of cases, the technetium radionuclide scan using **^{99m}Tc diphosphonate is positive within 24 h of the onset of symptoms.** Falsely negative scans usually indicate obstruction of blood flow to the bone. Because the uptake of technetium reflects osteoblastic activity and skeletal vascularity, the bone scan cannot differentiate **osteomyelitis** from fractures, tumors, infarction, or neuropathic osteopathy.
- **Ga citrate- and ^{111}In-labeled leukocyte** or immunoglobulin scans, which have greater specificity for inflammation, may help distinguish infectious from noninfectious processes and indicate inflammatory changes within bones that for other reasons are already abnormal on radiography and technetium scanning.
- **Ultrasound can be used to diagnose osteomyelitis** by the detection of subperiosteal fluid collections, soft tissue abscesses adjacent to bone, and periosteal thickening and elevation.
- **MRI is as sensitive as the bone scan for the diagnosis of acute osteomyelitis** because it is able to detect changes in the water content of marrow. MRI yields better anatomic resolution of epidural abscesses and other soft tissue processes than CT and is currently the imaging technique of choice for vertebral **osteomyelitis.**

- ▶ Most common organism of acute osteomyelitis: **staph aures.** (PGI 97)
- ▶ Most common organism of acute osteomyelitis in **drug addicts: Pseudomonas**☛
- ▶ Most common mode of infection: **hematogeneous**☛
- ▶ Most common site in bone : **metaphysis** ☛ (JIPMER 95)

The blood stasis, resulting from loop like arrangement of blood vessels, is probably responsible for the metaphysis being a favorite site for bacteria to settle. The metaphysis has relatively fewer phagocytic cells than epiphysis and diaphysis allowing infection to occur more easily.

- ▶ Most common site of acute osteomyelitis in **infants :Hip**☛
- ▶ Most common site of acute osteomyelitis in **children: Femur** ☛
- ▶ Most common site in **adults: Thoracolumbar spine**☛

- Osteomyelitis in **sickle cell disease:** Salmonella☛☛
- Osteomyelitis after **foot wound:** Pseudomonas aeruginosa☛
- Osteomyelitis involving **prosthetic joints:** S. aureus☛
- Osteomyelitis involving IV **drug abusers:** S. aureus☛

➲ Garres Sclerosing Osteomyelitis

Rare form of non suppurative osteomyelitis characterized by cortical thickening and marked sclerosis.

No abscess formation is seen.

X ray shows increased bone density and cortical thickening without abscess cavity. Treatment is surgical.

⇨ Post traumatic osteomyelitis

Most commonly due to staph aureus.

E coli,Proteus and pseudomonas are also involved

⇨ Types of Sequestrum

• **Ring Sequestrum:**	• Amputation stumps **MAHE 2005**
• **Tubular Sequestrum:**	• Osteomyelitis (Hematogeneous)
• **Rice grain Sequestrum :**	• Tuberculosis

➲ Skeletal Tuberculosis

- ▶ In bone and joint disease, pathogenesis is related to **reactivation of hematogenous foci** or to spread from adjacent paravertebral lymph nodes. ☛
- ▶ **Weight-bearing joints** (spine, hips, and knees ¾ in that order) are affected most commonly. ☛
- ▶ Spinal tuberculosis **(Pott's disease or tuberculous spondylitis)** often involves two or more adjacent vertebral bodies. ☛
  - ■ **Upper thoracic spine** is the most common site of spinal tuberculosis **in children,**
  - ■ Vertebral tuberculosis is the commonest form of skeletal tuberculosis (50%)
  - ■ Most commonly affects **lower thoracic and thoracolumbar region**
  - ■ **Typical paradiscal lesion** is characterized by destruction of adjacent bone end plates and diminution of intervening disk.
- ▶ The lower thoracic and upper lumbar vertebrae are usually affected in adults. From the anterior superior or inferior angle of the vertebral body, the lesion reaches the adjacent body, also destroying the intervertebral disk.
- ▶ With advanced disease, collapse of vertebral bodies results in **kyphosis (gibbus).**
- ▶ A **paravertebral "cold" abscess** may also form. ☛
- ▶ In the upper spine, this abscess may track to the chest wall as a mass; in the lower spine, it may reach the inguinal ligaments or present as a psoas abscess.
- ▶ **Pathologic Considerations**
- ✓ The histologic appearance of the tuberculous lesion in bone resembles that observed in visceral tuberculosis. Histiocytes, Langhans giant cells, and fibroblastic proliferation are all present.

3

ORTHOPEDICS

- ✓ Caseous necrosis is **less frequently** seen in joint lesions than in pulmonary lesions.
- ✓ The destruction produced by granulomatous inflammation is **characteristically slow.**
- ✓ Within the joint, invasion of bone tends to occur at the margins where synovium is attached to bone, producing a characteristic marginal defect.
- ✓ As destruction proceeds, the joint becomes filled with necrotic products and fragments of articular cartilage, material called rice bodies because of its resemblance to grains of rice.

- **Computed tomography (CT) or magnetic resonance imaging (MRI)** reveals the characteristic lesion and suggests its etiology, although the differential diagnosis includes other infections and tumors.
- **Aspiration of the abscess or bone biopsy confirms the tuberculous etiology**, as cultures are usually positive and histologic findings highly typical.
- **Skeletal tuberculosis responds to chemotherapy**, but severe cases may require surgery.

- **Melon seed bodies** are seen in Tuberculous **Tenosynovitis**
- **Tuberculous Arthritis** leads to **Fibrous ankylosis**
- **Earliest** sign in Potts Disease is **Narrowing of Disk Space** **(CUPGEE 99)**
- **Earliest symptom of Spinal TB is Pain** **(JIPMER 90)**
- **Commonest** vertebrae involved in Pott's disease is **T9-T12** **(PGI 85)**
- **TB in spine starts in Vertebral Body** **(PGI 85)**
- **Spina Ventosa is caused by Myc Tuberculosis (Tuberculous Dactylitis)** **(Comed 08) (Kerala 01)**

Skeletal Actinomycosis:

- **Actinomyces Israeli is the MC organism**
- **Oro cervico facial form is the MC type of skeletal actinomycosis**
- **"Lower jaw" (Mandible) is the commonest site** **PGMEE K 2005**
- **Induration and Sinus Formation are a feature**
- **Pencillin G is the DOC**

Rickets

- Rickets is characterized by **defective mineralization** of bones and cartilage. **PGI 1998**
- Osteomalacia is **defective mineralization** of bones.
- Rickets is **seen before** closure of growth plates.

⇨ Causes

- Nutritional rickets: vit D deficiency, Malabsorption
- Accelerated loss of vit D: Phenytoin, Rifampicin, Barbiturates
- Impaired hydroxylation in liver and Kidney:
- Liver disease, Hypoparathyroidism, Renal failure, Renal Tubular Acidosis
- Vit D Resistant rickets, Fanconis syndrome, Wilsons disease.

⇨ Clinical Features

Failure of calcification of cartilage and osteoid. PGI 1998

Epiphyseal enlargement occurs (thickening of knees, ankles, wrists)

- **Craniotabes** PGI 2003
- **Genu valgum,**
- **Coxa vara**
- **Short stature**
- **Protrubent abdomen**
- **Wide open fontanella** AIIMS 2007
- Enlargement of costochondral junction. **(Ricketic rosary)** AIIMS 2007
- Lateral indentation of chest due to pull of diaphragm on ribs. **(Harrisons groove)**
- **Triradiate pelvis**
- Forward projection of sternum. **(Pectus Carinatum)**
- **Kyphoscoloiosis**

⇨ Radiographic features

- **Thickening and widening of epiphysis** PGI 2003
- **Cupping and fraying of metaphysic** PGI 1998
- **Irregular metaphyseal margins**
- **Flaring of anterior ends of ribs**
- **Bowing of diaphysis**

⇨ Biochemical

- **Serum calcium : Normal or low**
- **Serum phosphate : Low**
- **Alkaline phosphatase : High**
- **PTH : High**

➲ Osteomalacia

- Which means softening of bones
- Is the adult counterpart of rickets & primarily due to deficiency of Vitamin-D.
- This results in failure to replace the turnover of calcium & phosphorus in the organic matrix of bone.
- Aetiology is lack or exposure to sunlight.
- Other causes are a diaterary deficiency of Vit. D, undermutrition, during pregnancy, mal-absorption syndrome or after partial gastrectomy. Other conditions that may cause osteomalacia include:

✓ Hereditary or acquired disorders of vitamin D metabolism

✓ Kidney failure and acidosis

✓ Liver disease

✓ Phosphate depletion associated with not enough phosphates in the diet

✓ Side effects of medications used to treat seizures

Spontaneous fractures occur usuallyin spine, & may result in kyphosis Investigations

Radiological:

- **Diffuse rarefaction of bones (osteolytic)**
- **Looser's zone (pseudo-fractures)**
- **Triradiate pelvis in females**
- **Protrusio-acetabuli: the acetabuli: the acetabulum protrudint in to the pelvis.**

Serum Calcium & phosphate levels are low & alkaline phosphatise is high.

⇨ Fracture NOF (Neck of Femur)

- Fracture NOF is the **most common** site of fracture in elderly.☛
- Velocity of trauma in most cases is **trivial**. (Low velocity trauma)
- Most common patients are **elderly females** with predisposing causes like

✓ **Osteoporosis,**

✓ **Osteomalacia,**

✓ **Diabetes,**

✓ **Stroke patients,**

✓ **Alcoholics,**

✓ **Caissons disease,**

✓ **Steroid therapy**

- Limb is shortened, adducted and externally rotated.
- Pain around hip with **flexion, adduction and external rotation** is suggestive of Intracapsular Fracture NOF.
- **(Telescopic Test is done)**☛☛
- Tenderness of hip on palpation with painful movements at hip joint is a feature.

⇨ Classification of Fracture Neck of Femur (# NOF)

- **Intracapsular:** Subcapital, Transcervical☚
- **Extracapsular:** Basal, Pertrochanteric☚

⇨ Avascular necrosis is seen in

▶ Head of femur	ICS 2005
▶ Scaphoid	PGI 2004
▶ Talus	PGI 2011

[99mTc] pertechnetate or [99mTc] diphosphonate scintigraphy may be useful in avascular necrosis

➲ Avascular Necrosis

✓ also called osteonecrosis.

✓ is a disease resulting from the temprorary or permanent loss of the blood suply to an area of bone.

✓ The head of the femur is a common site.

⇨ Risk factors include:

- Alcoholism,
- Excessive steroid used,
- Post trauma
- Caisson disease (decompression sickness),
- Vascular compression,
- Hypertension, vasculitis, thrombosis, damage from radiation.
- Sickle cell anemia,
- Gaucher's Disease.
- In some cases it is idiopathic (no cause is found).
- Rheumatoid arthritis.

➲ Sickle Cell Disease:

Sickle cell disease is associated with several musculoskeletal abnormalities

- Children under the age of 5 may develop diffuse swelling, tenderness, and warmth of the hands and feet lasting from 1 to 3 weeks. The condition, referred to as **sickle cell dactylitis or hand-foot syndrome** has also been observed in sickle cell disease and sickle cell thalassemia. Dactylitis is believed to result from infarction of the bone marrow and cortical bone leading to periostitis and soft tissue swelling. Radiographs show **periosteal elevation, subperiosteal new bone formation, and areas of radiolucency and increased density involving the metacarpals, metatarsals, and proximal phalanges.**
- Sickle cell crisis is often associated with **periarticular pain and joint effusions.**

3

ORTHOPEDICS

- Patients with sickle cell disease may also develop **osteomyelitis**, which commonly involves the **long tubular bones.** These patients are particularly susceptible to bacterial infections, especially **Salmonella infections**, which are found in more than half of cases. Radiographs of the involved site show **periosteal elevation initially**, followed by disruption of the cortex.
- Sickle cell disease is also associated with **bone infarction resulting from thrombosis** secondary to the sickling of red cells.
- **Avascular necrosis of the head of the femur** is seen.
- It also occurs in the humeral head and less commonly in the distal femur, tibial condyles, distal radius, vertebral bodies, and other juxtaarticular sites.
- **Septic arthritis is occasionally encountered in sickle cell disease.** Multiple joints may be infected. Joint infection may result from hematogenous spread or from spread of contiguous osteomyelitis.
- Microorganisms identified include **staphylococcus, Streptococcus, Escherichia coli, and Salmonella.**
- **The latter is not seen as frequently in septic arthritis as it is in osteomyelitis.**
- **The bone marrow hyperplasia in sickle cell disease results in widening of the medullary cavities, thinning of the cortices, and coarse trabeculations and central cupping of the vertebral bodies.**

⇨ Sesamoid Bones

- ► **Sesamoid: Seed Like**
- ► **Sesamoid bones have no periosteum**☛

- ► **Patella is the largest sesamoid bone**☛
- ► **Fabella is a sesamoid bone in lateral head of gastrocneumus**☛
- ► **It can be split into two or three bones as well Fabella bipartite or tripartite respectively**☛
- ► **Riders bone is a sesamoid bone in adductor longus.**☛

➲ Osteogenesis Imperfecta (OI)

OI is also called as **Brittle bone disease** or **"Lobstein syndrome"** **KCET 2012**

- ► Basic defect is in **Collagen Type 1.**☛ ☛ **UP 2007**
- ► It is transmitted either as AD or AR Inheritance.
- ► **Type 1 OI** is the **most common type.**
- ► OI is inherited as **autosomal dominant trait** <u>**mostly**</u>.☛ **PGI 2003**
- ► **"Blue sclera"** is present in several types of OI but not all.☛ **PGI 2003**
- ► **Grey sclera** is a feature as well.

Other ocular features of OI are:☛

- ► **Saturn ring, Arcus juvenilis, Hypermetropia and Retinal Detachment are seen.**☛
- ► The sclera is **normal** in some types of OI.

- Feature of OI is **generalized osteopenia** with recurrent fractures and skeletal deformity. Fracture healing however is normal. Fracture in utero may be seen. Laxity of joint ligaments leads to **hypermobility.**
- Some people have associated" **dentogenesis imperfecta"**: small fragile and discoloured teeth.
- **Dermis** may be abnormally thin and skin is susceptible to easy bruising
- **Hearing loss** due to involvement of inner and middle ear bones may produce deafness.
- **Wormian bones** are a feature.
- **"Pop corn calcification" and "whorls of radiodensities"** are a radiographic feature.
- Treatment is largely **supportive**

Osteopetrosis:

Osteopetrosis is also called as

- **Albers Schonberg disease** or
- **Marble bone disease**

- It is characterized by
  - ✓ **Anemia,**
  - ✓ **Hepatoslpeenomegaly,**
  - ✓ **Infections, and**
  - ✓ **Pathological fractures.**
- There is **osteoclast dysfunction.**
- Radiographically there is **increased opacity** of bones.
- **Endobones (bone within a bone)** is seen.

Osteoporosis

Osteoporosis is defined as a **reduction of bone mass (or density)** or the presence of a fragility fracture. This reduction in bone tissue is accompanied by deterioration in the architecture of the skeleton, leading to a markedly increased risk of fracture.

Bone loss begins before menses cease in women and in the third to fifth decades in men. Once the menopause is established, the rate of bone loss is accelerated several-fold in women. During the first 5 to 10 years of the menopause, **trabecular bone is lost faster than cortical bone.**

Estrogen deficiency may increase local production of bone-resorbing cytokines such as interleukin-1 (IL-1), IL-6, and tumor necrosis factor. Once the period of rapid postmenopausal bone loss ends, bone loss continues at a more gradual rate throughout life. The osteopenia that results from normal aging, which occurs in both women and men, has been termed type II or "senile" osteoporosis.

Endocrine disorders such as **hyperthyroidism, hyperparathyroidism, hypercortisolism, and growth hormone deficiency** can cause osteoporosis.

Several noninvasive techniques are now available for estimating skeletal mass or density.

These include

- Dual-energy x-ray absorptiometry (DXA),
- Single-energy x ray absorptiometry (SXA),
- Quantitative computed tomography (CT), and
- Ultrasound.

The diagnosis of Osteoporosis is made when a patient has characteristic osteoporotic fracture. In absence of such a fracture, evaluation of osteoporosis is done by T score measurement based on bone mass

■ T score >-1	Normal*
■ T score Between-1 and -2.5	Osteopenia*
■ T Score <-2.5	Osteoporosis*

⇨ **Major factors for osteoporosis:**

- Low cacium intake
- Sedentary lifestyle
- Cigarrate smoking
- Excessive alcohol
- Excessive caffeine
- Medications (corticosteroids, thyroxine)
- Female gender
- Early menopause
- Slender build
- Positive family history

Drugs Causing Osteoporosis

- → Glucocorticoids
- → Anticonvulsants
- → Cytotoxic drugs
- → Cyclosporine
- → Lithium
- → Heparin
- → GnRH analouges
- → Almunium
- → Throxine in increased doses

⇨ **Glucocorticoid-induced osteoporosis is by:**

- **Inhibition of osteoblast function** and potential increase in osteoblast apoptosis, resulting in impaired synthesis of new bone; ☚ ☚
- **Stimulation of bone resorption**, probably as a secondary effect;☚
- **Impairment of the absorption of calcium** across the intestine, probably by a vitamin D-independent effect; ☚
- **Increase of urinary calcium loss**☚ and induction of some degree of secondary hyperparathyroidism;
- **Reduction of adrenal androgens** ☚and suppression of ovarian and testicular secretion of estrogens and androgens; and
- **Potential induction of glucocorticoid myopathy**, ☚which may exacerbate effects on skeletal and calcium homeostasis, as well as increase the risk of falls.

Treatment of Osteoporosis:

- Bisphosphonates
  - Etidronate
  - Zoledronate
  - Tiludronate
  - Pamidronate
  - Alendronate
  - Risedronate
- Selective Estrogen Receptor Modulator (SERM) eg: Raloxifene
- Parathormone (PTH)
- Cinacalcet: *Activator of calcium sensing receptor in the parathyroid gland (augments feedback inhibition of PTH by Ca^{++})*
- Calcitonin: *Acts by inhibition of osteoclastic activity*
- Strontium Ranelate: *Blocks osteoclast differentiation/promote their apoptosis—inhibitsbone resorption, Promote bone formation*
- Donesumab: *Monoclonal antibody against RANK ligand effective against osteoporosis.*
- Plicamycin
- Gallium nitrate
- Calcium as dietary supplement — AIPGME 2012

⇨ **Remember electrolyte disturbances in related disorders: ❋ ❋ ❋**

Primary Hyperparathyroidism☚ ☚	↑Ca	↓Po4	↑PTH
Sec Hyperparathyroidism☚ ☚	↓Ca	↓Po4	↑PTH
Malabsorption	↓Ca	↓Po4	↑PTH
Renal Failure☚	↓Ca	↑Po4	↑PTH
Paget's Disease☚	Ca(N)	Po4(N)	

RHEUMATOID ARTHRITIS (RA)

I PROVIDE THIS TOPIC IN DETAIL AS LOTS OF QUESTIONS ARE ASKED FROM HERE.

- **Rheumatoid arthritis (RA)** is a **chronic multisystem disease** of unknown cause.
- Disease of synovium. (Synovial membrane) **UP 1988**
- **Disease starts in synovium** **AI 1995**
- **Synovium is the part affected most** **TN 2003**

The characteristic feature of RA is **persistent inflammatory synovitis**, usually involving peripheral joints in a **symmetric distribution.** **UP 1988**

Familial, immunological and infective causes are implicated. **PGI 1988**

Women are affected approximately three times more often than men. **PGI 2001**

The **class II major histocompatibility complex** allele **HLA-DR4.** and related alleles are known to be major genetic risk factors for RA.

Microvascular injury and an increase in the number of synovial lining cells appear to be the **earliest lesions in rheumatoid synovitis.** **AI 1995**

RA most often causes symmetric arthritis with characteristic involvement of certain specific joints such as the **proximal interphalangeal and metacarpophalangeal joints.** **PGI 2001**

The distal interphalangeal joints are rarely involved. Synovitis of the wrist joints is a nearly uniform feature of RA and may lead to limitation of motion, deformity, and **median nerve entrapment (carpal tunnel syndrome).** ☛

Synovitis of the elbow joint often leads to flexion contractures that may develop early in the disease. The knee joint is commonly involved with synovial hypertrophy, chronic effusion, and frequently ligamentous laxity. Pain and swelling behind the knee may be caused by extension of inflamed synovium into the popliteal space **(Baker's cyst).** ☛☛

On occasion, inflammation from the synovial joints and bursae of the upper cervical spine leads to **atlantoaxial subluxation.** This usually presents as pain in the occiput but on rare occasions may lead to compression of the spinal cord.

Characteristic changes of the hand include

- (1) **Radial deviation at the wrist with ulnar deviation of the digits**, often with palmar subluxation of the proximal phalanges (**"Z" deformity**); ☛☛
- (2) Hyperextension of the proximal interphalangeal joints, with compensatory flexion of the distal interphalangeal joints (**swan-neck deformity**); ☛ **COMED 2005**
- (3) Flexion contracture of the proximal interphalangeal joints and extension of the distal interphalangeal joints (**boutonniere deformity**); and ☛ **COMED 2005**
- (4) Hyperextension of the first interphalangeal joint and flexion of the first metacarpophalangeal joint with a consequent loss of thumb mobility and pinch. ☛
- **Trigger finger** also occurs. **PGI 1998**

⇨ CRITERIA FOR CLASSIFICATION OF RHEUMATOID ARTHRITIS

Any 4 criteria must be present to diagnose rheumatoid arthritis; criteria 1 through 4 must have been present for >= 6 week.

- **Morning stiffness for >= 1 h**
- **Arthritis of >= 3 joint areas**
- **Arthritis of hand joints (wrist, metacarpophalangeal or proximal interphalangeal joints)**
- **Symmetric arthritis**
- **Rheumatoid nodules (Pathogonomic)** AIIMS 2005
- **Serum rheumatoid factor, by a method positive in < 5% of normal control subjects**
- **RHEUMATOID FACTOR is "IgM directed against IgG"** AI 2011
- **Aggregates of immune complexes within polymorphonuclear leukocytes are often seen in rheumatoid synovial fluid and have been termed "RA cells" or "ragocytes."**
- **Radiographic changes (hand X-ray changes typical of rheumatoid arthritis that must include erosions or unequivocal bony decalcification)**

- **Extra-articular Manifestations** As a rule, these manifestations occur in individuals with **high titers of autoantibodies to the Fc component of immunoglobulin G (rheumatoid factors).** TN 2003
- **Rheumatoid nodules** develop in 20 to 30% of persons with RA.
- Clinical weakness and atrophy of skeletal muscle are common. **Muscle atrophy** may be evident within weeks of the onset of RA.
- **Rheumatoid vasculitis** Neurovascular disease presenting either as a mild **distal sensory neuropathy or as mononeuritis multiplex** may be the only sign of vasculitis. **Cutaneous vasculitis** usually presents as crops of small brown spots in the nail beds, nail folds, and digital pulp. Larger ischemic ulcers, especially in the lower extremity, may also develop. Myocardial infarction secondary to rheumatoid vasculitis has been reported, as has vasculitic involvement of lungs, bowel, liver, spleen, pancreas, lymph nodes, and testes. Renal vasculitis is rare.
- Pleuropulmonary manifestations, which are more commonly observed in men, include **pleural disease, interstitial fibrosis, pleuropulmonary nodules, pneumonitis, and arteritis**
- Clinically apparent heart disease attributed to the rheumatoid process is rare, but evidence of **asymptomatic pericarditis** is found at **autopsy in 50% of cases.** PGI 1997
- RA tends to spare the central nervous system directly, although vasculitis can cause peripheral neuropathy. Neurologic manifestations may also result from **atlantoaxial or midcervical spine subluxations.**

- Nerve entrapment secondary to proliferative synovitis or joint deformities may produce **neuropathies of median, ulnar, radial (interosseous branch), or anterior tibial nerves.**
- The rheumatoid process involves the eye in fewer than 1% of patients. Affected individuals usually have long-standing disease and nodules. The two principal manifestations are **episcleritis**, which is usually mild and transient, and **scleritis**, which involves the deeper layers of the eye and is a more serious inflammatory condition. Histologically, the lesion is similar to a **rheumatoid nodule** and may result in thinning and **perforation of the globe (scleromalacia perforans).**

- **Felty's syndrome** consists of chronic RA, splenomegaly, neutropenia, and, on occasion, anemia and thrombocytopenia.
- **Osteoporosis** secondary to rheumatoid involvement is common and may be aggravated by glucocorticoid therapy.
- RA in the Elderly **Aggressive disease** is largely restricted to those patients with **high titers of rheumatoid factor**. By contrast, elderly patients who develop RA without elevated titers of rheumatoid factor (seronegative disease) generally have less severe, often self-limited disease.

The **presence of rheumatoid factor does not establish the diagnosis of RA** as the predictive value of the presence of rheumatoid factor in determining a diagnosis of RA is poor. **Thus fewer than one-third of unselected patients with a positive test for rheumatoid factor will be found to have RA.** Therefore, the rheumatoid factor test is **not useful as a screening procedure.**

A number of additional autoantibodies may be found in patients with RA, including

- **Antibodies to filaggrin ❋**
- **Antibodies to citrulline ❋**
- **Antibodies to calpastatin ❋**
- **Antibodies to components of the spliceosome (RA-33), and an unknown antigen, Sa. ❋**

⇨ Goals of therapy of RA are:

- Relief of pain
- Reduction of inflammation
- Protection of articular surfaces
- Maintainence of function
- Control of systemic involvement

- **First Aspirin and NSAIDs are used.☚**
- **Second line involves use of low dose glucocorticoids☚**
- **Third line involves use of DMARDS (Disease modifying Anti rheumatic drugs) Methotrexate, Gold Compounds, Pencillamine, Hydroxychloroquine and sulfasalazine☚**
- **Fourth line is use of TNF alpha blockers. (Infliximab and Etarnacept)☚**
- **Fifth line is use of Immunosupressants and Cytotoxic drugs.☚**

⇨ CPPD Deposition Disease

Clinical manifestations of CPPD deposition include:

- The **knee is the joint most frequently affected** in CPPD arthropathy. Other sites include the wrist, shoulder, ankle, elbow, and hands. Rarely, the temporomandibular joint and ligamentum flavum of the spinal canal are involved.
- Clinical and radiographic evidence indicates that CPPD deposition is **polyarticular in at least two-thirds of patients**
- If radiographs reveal punctate and/or linear radiodense deposits in fibrocartilaginous joint menisci or articular hyaline cartilage **(chondrocalcinosis)**, the diagnostic certainty of CPPD is further enhanced.
- Definitive diagnosis requires **demonstration of typical crystals** in synovial fluid or articular tissue
- Acute attacks of CPPD arthritis may be precipitated by **trauma, arthroscopy, or hyaluronate injections.** Rapid diminution of serum calcium concentration, as may occur in severe medical illness or after surgery (especially parathyroidectomy), can also lead to **pseudogout** attacks.
- Polarization microscopy usually reveals **rhomboid crystals with weak positive birefringence.** PGI 2000

TREATMENT

Treatment by **joint aspiration and NSAIDs, or colchicine**, or intra-articular glucocorticoid injection may result in return to prior status in 10 days or less.

Uncontrolled studies suggest that **radioactive synovectomy (with yttrium 90).**

Patients with progressive destructive large-joint arthropathy usually require **joint replacement.**

- ✓ **Deposition of Calcium Pyrophosphate crystals.☚**
- ✓ **Crystals are Rhomboid in shape☚**
- ✓ **Thery are positively Birefrigent.☚**
- ✓ **Usually large joints affected.**

⇨ Gout

- ✓ **Metatarsopharyngeal joints involved,**
- ✓ **Usually great Toe (Podagra)☚**
- ✓ **Assymetric joint involvement usually☚**
- ✓ **Negatively birefrigent crystals seen☚**
- ✓ **NSAIDS, colchicines, Allopurinol used in treatment.**

⇨ Psoriatic Arthritis

- ▶ **Distal Interphalyngeal Joints usually involved.** **TN 2003**
- ▶ **Rheumatoid-like polyarthritis:**
- ▶ **Asymmetrical oligoarthritis: typically affects hands and feet he**
- ▶ **Sacroilitishe**
- ▶ **DIP joint disease he**
- ▶ **Arthritis mutilans (severe deformity fingers/hand, 'telescoping fingers') he**

▶ PIP joint involvement	RA, OA, Psoriatic arthritis
▶ PIP and DIP	OA, Psoriatic arthritis
▶ PIP and DIP and MCP and wrist	Psoriatic arthritis UP 2007

➲ Ankylosing Spondylitis

Typically a young man who presents with lower back pain and stiffness.

HLA 27 association AI 1989

- Stiffness is usually worse in morning and improves with activity☛
- **Enthesopathy** is characteristic. **PGI 1997**
- **Bamboo spine** **TN 1989**
- **Squaring of vertebrae**
- **Pain improves with exercise.** **KERALA 2003**
- peripheral arthritis (25%, more common if female) h

Other features - **the 'A's** ☛

- ▶ **Apical fibrosis**
- ▶ **Anterior uveitis**
- ▶ **Aortic regurgitation**
- ▶ **Achilles tendonitis**
- ▶ **AV node block**
- ▶ **Amyloidosis**
- ▶ **And cauda equina syndrome**

X-rays are often normal early in disease, later changes include:

- **Sacroiliitis: subchondral erosions, sclerosis❋**
- **Squaring of lumbar vertebrae❋**
- **'Bamboo spine' (late and uncommon)❋he❋ JIPI❋**

Important Points not to be forgotten:

- ➨ **Strongest HLA B27 association**
- ➨ Primary site of pathology in Ankylosing spondylitis is site of **ligamentous attachment to bone (enthesis).** Calcification of ligaments can occur.
- ➨ **Sacroiliits is one of the earliest manifestations of AS,** with features of both enthesitis & synovitis.
- ➨ Initial symptom is usually dull pain, insidious in onset, felt deep in lower lumbar or gluteal region accompanied by low-back morning stiffness that improves with activity & returns following periods of inactivity.
- ➨ **Bamboo spine & squaring of vertebrae** can be found in spine in case of AS.
- ➨ "Schober test" is a **useful measure of flexion of lumber spine, which may reveal decreased spinal mobility, an important feature of AS.**
- ➨ Most serious complication of the spinal disease is **spinal fracture,** Cervical spine is most commonly involved.

➲ Osteoarthritis (OA):

- Involves hip, knee usually — AI 1997
- Disease of elderly and obese usually
- Does not affect MCP joints. — Kerala 1996
- **Fibrillation of cartilage** is the earliest change seen.
- Herbendens nodes **(DIP)** involved — AI 2005
- Bouchard's nodes seen **(PIP)** involved
- Ankylosis occurs — PGI 2003
- Radiological features:
- ✓ **Osteophyte formation** — UPSC 2002
- ✓ **Subchondral sclerosis**
- ✓ **Cyst formation occurs**

- ✓ **Epiphyseal widening** is a feature of Rickets
- ✓ **Epiphyseal dysgenesis** is a feature of Hypothyroidism
- ✓ **Epiphyseal enlargement** is a feature of Juvenile Rheumatoid arthritis.

➲ Hemophilic Arthropathy

- Hemophilia is a **sex-linked recessive genetic disorder** characterized by the **absence or deficiency of factor VIII (hemophilia A, or classic hemophilia)** or **factor IX (hemophilia B, or Christmas disease)**
- **Hemophilia A is more common type.**
- **Spontaneous hemarthrosis is a common problem** with both types of hemophilia and can lead to a chronic deforming arthritis.
- The frequency and severity of hemarthrosis are **related to the degree of clotting factor deficiency.**
- Hemarthrosis becomes evident after 1 year of age, when the child begins to walk and run.
- In order of frequency, the joints most commonly affected are the **knees,** ankles, elbows, shoulders, and hips. Small joints of the hands and feet are occasionally involved.
- **Squaring of patella** is a feature. — COMED 03
- In the initial stage of arthropathy, hemarthrosis produces a **warm, tensely swollen, and painful joint.** Widening of the femoral intercondylar notch, enlargement of the proximal radius, and squaring of the distal end of the patella are seen.
- The patient holds the affected joint in flexion and guards against any movement.
- Blood in the joint remains liquid because of the absence of intrinsic clotting factors and the absence of tissue thromboplastin in the synovium.

- The blood in the joint space is resorbed over a period of a week or longer, depending on the size of the hemarthrosis.
- **Recurrent hemarthrosis leads to the development of a chronic arthritis.**
- **Bleeding into muscle and soft tissue** also causes musculoskeletal disorders.
- When bleeding involves periosteum or bone, a pseudotumor forms. These occur distal to the elbows or knees in children and improve with treatment of the hemophilia

⇨ Orthopedic importance of knee joint

- **Most common site of Septic arthritis.** **SGPGI 2005**
- **Most common site of Syphilitic arthritis.**
- **Most common site of Gonococcal arthritis.**
- **Most common site of Pseudo gout.**
- **Most common site of Hemophilic arthritis.**
- **Most common site of Osteochondritis dessicans.**

➲ Important Points About Ligaments of Knee Joint

- ✓ Swelling of the knee after trauma usually denotes the presence of a significant injury. The tests described **(anterior drawer and Lachman test)** are classic for an injury to the **anterior cruciate ligament.**
- ✓ **The lateral collateral ligament** if disrupted, would allow the leg to be bent inward to a greater extent than normally possible **(varus test).**
- ✓ **The medial collateral ligament** when injured, would produce the opposite findings: the leg could be bent outward more than the normal leg **(valgus test).**
- ✓ **The medial meniscus** when injured, produces loose intraarticular bodies and locking of the knee.
- ✓ **The posterior cruciate ligament** is much less commonly injured than the anterior cruciate.

⇨ Dial test/Tibial lateral rotation test

Designed to show loss of the posterolateral support structures of the knee.

Patient may be placed supine or prone. The examiner flexes the knee to 30°, extends the foot over the side of table and stabilizes the femur on the table. The examiner then laterally rotates the tibia and femur and compares the amount of rotation with that on good side. The test is then repeated with the knee flexed to 90°. If the tibia rotates less at 90° than at 30° an isolated posterolateral (popliteus corner) injury is more likely. If the knee rotates more at 90°, injury to both ***popliteus corner and posterior cruciate injury*** are more likely.

➲ Menisci: AIIMS 2009 Important Topic for Examinations

The peripheral edges of the menisci are convex, fixed, and attached to the inner surface of the knee joint capsule, except where the popliteus is interposed laterally; these peripheral edges also are attached loosely to the borders of the tibial plateaus by the coronary ligaments.

The inner edges are concave, thin, and unattached. The menisci are largely avascular except near their peripheral attachment to the coronary ligaments.

The inferior surface of each meniscus is flat, whereas the superior surface is concave, corresponding to the contour of the underlying tibial plateau and superimposed femoral condyle.

The medial meniscus is a C-shaped structure larger in radius than the lateral meniscus, with the posterior horn being wider than the anterior.

The medial meniscus is much larger in diameter, is thinner in its periphery and narrower in body, and does not attach to either cruciate ligament. It is loosely attached to the medial capsular ligaments.

The lateral meniscus is **more circular** in form, covering up to two-thirds of the articular surface of the underlying tibial plateau.

The lateral meniscus is smaller in diameter, thicker in periphery, wider in body, and more mobile than the medial meniscus.

The lateral meniscus, because it is **firmly attached to the popliteus muscle and to the ligament of Wrisberg or of Humphry**, follows the lateral femoral condyle during rotation and therefore is less likely to be injured.

Vascular supply to the medial and lateral menisci originates predominantly from the lateral and medial genicular vessels.

⇨ X ray Appearances of Different Types of Arthritis:

► Osteophytes	► Osteoarthritis
► Syndesmophytes	► Ankylosing spondylitis
► Bamboo spine	► Ankylosing spondylitis
► Pencil in cup deformity	► Psoriatic arthritis
► Calcification of articular cartilage	► Pseudogout
► Erosions with ↓Joint space	► Rheumatoid Arthritis
► Arthritis mutilans	► Psoriatic arthritis
► Piano key sign	► Rhematoid arthritis KCET 2012
► Sausage digits	► Psoriasis

3

ORTHOPEDICS

⇨ Volkmans Ischemic contracture (Features) (P)

- ▶ Pallor
- ▶ Pain (Most important sign) COMED 2008
- ▶ Paralysis
- ▶ Parasthesias
- ▶ Pulsenessnes☛

1. **Median nerve mostly involved**☛
2. **Deformity:** Flexion of wrist, Extension of Fingers at MCP, Flexion at IP, Pronation of forearm
3. **Seddons area of Affection** is infarct of muscles in the form of an ellipsoid where the axis is in the line of anterior interosseous artery and central line in middle of forearm called sedons area
4. **Flexor digitorum profundus and Flexor Pollicis Longus** are muscles damaged. AIIMS 1992

- ▶ **Garres operation**☛
- ▶ **Maxpages operation**☛
- ▶ **Tendon transfer and**☛
- ▶ **Muscle transplant are treatment options**☛

⇨ The Reflex Sympathetic Dystrophy Syndrome (RSDS)✱✱✱

- ▶ The reflex sympathetic dystrophy syndrome (RSDS) is now referred to as **complex regional pain syndrome, type 1**, by the new Classification of the International Association for the Study of Pain.
- ▶ It is characterized by
  - — **Pain and swelling,**
  - — **Usually of a distal extremity, accompanied by vasomotor instability,**
  - — **Trophic skin changes, and**
  - — **The rapid development of bony demineralization**☛ ☛
- ▶ **A precipitating event** can be identified in at least two-thirds of cases. These events include
  - ✓ **Trauma, such as fractures and crush injuries;**
  - ✓ **Myocardial infarction;**
  - ✓ **Strokes;**
  - ✓ **Peripheral nerve injury;**
  - ✓ **Use of certain drugs, including barbiturates, anti-tuberculous drugs, and, more recently, cyclosporine** administered to patients undergoing renal transplantation.
- ▶ The pathogenesis of RSDS is thought to involve **abnormal activity of the sympathetic nervous system** following a precipitating event☛

⇨ **Remember**

- **Iliotibial tract syndrome:** Synovium deep to ilio tibial tract is inflamed where it rubs on lateral femoral condyle. Common in marathon runners.
- **Medial shelf syndrome:** Synovial fold above medial meniscus is inflamed
- **Fat pad syndrome:** Tenderness deep to patellar tendon may be caused by fat caught in Tibiofemoral joint.

➲ Scoliosis

⇨ Associated with Congenital Scoliosis — AIIMS 2009

- ✓ Hemivertebrae
- ✓ Wedge vertebrae
- ✓ Block vertebrae
- ✓ Unsegmented bar

Classification of Congenital Scoliosis

Failure of formation:

Partial failure of formation (wedge vertebra)

Complete failure of formation (hemivertebra)

Failure of segmentation:

Unilateral failure of segmentation (unilateral unsegmented bar)

Bilateral failure of segmentation (block vertebra)

Associations — AI 2010

- **Hemivertebrae**
- **Wedge vertebrae**
- **Block vertebrae**
- **Unsegmented bar**

- ▶ **Turn Buckle cast Scoliosis**☛
- ▶ **Rissers cast Scoliosis**☛
- ▶ **Milwaukees brace Scoliosis** ☛ — PGMEE 2005
- ▶ **Boston brace Scoliosis**☛ — DNB 04

Cobbs angle is measured in <u>scoliosis</u> — SGPI 2004

3

ORTHOPEDICS

⇨ Important Diseases

▶ **Burtons Disease**	Combination of scurvy and Rickets❋	
Less formation of osteoid matrix occurs in scurvy		**AI 2010**
▶ **Engelmann Disease**	Progressive Diaphseal Dysplasia❋	**(MP 02)**
▶ **Trevor's Disease**	Dysplasia Epiphysis Hemimelica❋	**(NIMS 96)**
▶ **Caffey's disease**	Osteomyelitis of Jaw❋	**(NIMS 96)**
▶ **De Queirvans Disease**	Tenovaginitis of APL and EPB (Tendon)❋	
▶ **Blount's disease**	Tibia vara	**PGI 2000**

➲ Scurvy

In the synthesis of collagen, ascorbic acid is required as a cofactor for prolyl hydroxylase and lysyl hydroxylase. These two enzymes are responsible for the hydroxylation of the proline and lysine amino acids in collagen. Hydroxyproline and hydroxylysine are important for stabilizing collagen by cross-linking the propeptides in collagen.

Defective collagen fibrillogenesis "impairs osteoid formation in bone" in scurvy.

Musculoskeletal abnormalities include –

Osteolysis,

Joint space loss,

Osteonecrosis,

Osteopenia, and/or periosteal proliferation.

Trabecular and cortical osteoporosis.

Children experience severe lower limb pain related to subperiosteal bleeding. **AIIMS 2009**

⇨ Important Tests Frequently Asked

▶ Barlow's Test☛☛	CDH	**(PGI 99)**
▶ **Ortaloni's Test☛**	**CDH**	**KCET 2012**
▶ Galleazzi test	CDH	
▶ Allis test	CDH	
▶ Harts test	CDH	
▶ Thomas Test☛	Fixed Flexion Deformity	**(TN 03)**
▶ Allens Test☛	Palmar arch integrity	**(SGPI 04)**
▶ Gaenslen's Test☛	Sciatica	
▶ **Mc Murray's Test☛**	**Menisci**	**MAH 2012**
▶ Anterior Drawer Test	Ant Cruciate Ligament	
▶ Lachman's Test ☛	Ant Cruciate Ligament	**(Karnataka 03)**
▶ Pivot Shift Test☛	Ant Cruciate Ligament	**(AIIMS 02)**
▶ Posterior Drawer Test☛	Post Cruciate Ligament	

▶ **Apprehension test/sign** ☛	Anterior Shoulder Joint Dislocation	**(UP 07)**
▶ **Genslens test**	Sacroiliac joint pain	
▶ **Phalens Test** ☛	Carpal tunnel Syndrome	**(JIPMER 92)**
▶ **Finkilsteins Test** ☛	De Queirvans Disease	
▶ **Adsons test**	Thoracic outlet syndrome	
▶ **Wringing test**	Lateral epicondylitis	
▶ **Cozens test**	Lateral epicondylitis	
▶ **Lift off test**	Subscapularis	**AI 2010**

⇨ Tests for Shoulder

Anterior Shoulder Dislocation:

- **Dugas test** - Pt. Seated and instructed to place hand on opposite shoulder and touch elbow to chest – (+) pain and inability to perform indicates dislocation.
- **Callaways test** - Measure girth of affected shoulder and compare to unaffected – (+) increased girth indicates dislocation.
- **Bryant's sign** - Look for lowering of Axillary fold – (+) dislocation on low side
- **Hamilton ruler test** - Dislocated shoulder ruler placed on lateral epicondyle of humerus can touch acromion simultaneously.

⇨ A Ruptured Disk

- Refers to a tear or break in the laminae of the **annulus fibrosus** through which the gel like **nucleus pulposus entrudes.**
- This condition occurs more often on the **posterior portions of the disks** particularly in the lumbar portion of the back where the disk may dislocate, or slip.
- A "Slipped disk" leads to severe, intense pain in the lower back and extremities and the displaced disk compresses the lower spinal nerves.

➲ Disk Prolapse

The nerve root affected is usually the one which leaves the spinal canal **below the next vertebra.** This is because the root at the level of the prolapsed disk leaves the canal in the upper half of the foramen. Thus the nerve root involved and disk prolapsed between L4 and L5 is L5, although it is the L4 root which exits the canal at this level.

- **Commonest site for disc prolapsed in lumbar regions is L4 - L5**
- **Commonest site for disc prolapsed in cervical region is C5 - C6.**

Stages of disk prolapsed in chronological order are

- **Stage of degeneration**
- **Stage of protrusion.**
- **Stage of extrusion.**
- **Stage of sequestration.**

3

ORTHOPEDICS

⇨ Newer Topics

➲ An Overuse Syndrome

It is a syndrome that can affect almost all of your body parts. It is caused by overusing something. Repetitive or misappropriate use of a body part can hasten or worsen the injury.

Numerous human body disorders are now classed as **Occupational overuse syndrome**, including:

- Common Calluses
- Housemaid's knee or prepatellar bursitis
- Tennis elbow
- Repetitive Strain Injury (RSI)

It is necessary to ***distinguish the symptoms of OOS from the normal pains of living***, such as muscle soreness after unaccustomed exercise or activity. OOS pains must also be distinguished from the pain of arthritis or some other condition. The early symptoms of OOS include:

- Muscle discomfort
- Fatigue
- Aches and pains
- Soreness
- Hot and cold feelings
- Muscle tightness
- Numbness and tingling
- Stiffness
- Muscle weakness

➲ Soft Tissue Sarcomas

⇨ Soft Tissues Include

- ✓ **Muscles,**
- ✓ **Tendons,**
- ✓ **Fat,**
- ✓ **Fibrous tissue,**
- ✓ **Synovial tissue,**
- ✓ **Vessels, and Nerves.**

High yield for 2011-2012

- Approximately 60% of soft tissue sarcomas arise in the extremities, with the **lower extremities** involved three times as often as the upper extremities..
- Thirty percent **arise in the trunk, the retroperitoneum** accounting for 40% of all trunk lesions.
- The remaining 10% arise in the **head and neck.**
- **Malignant transformation of a benign soft tissue tumor is extremely rare**, *with the exception that malignant peripheral nerve sheath tumors (neurofibrosarcoma, malignant schwannoma) can arise from neurofibromas in patients with neurofibromatosis.*

- Sarcomas in bone or soft tissues occur in patients who are treated with radiation therapy. The tumor nearly always arises in the irradiated field. The risk increases with time.
- **Viruses** Kaposi's sarcoma (KS) in patients with HIV type 1, classic KS, and KS in HIV-negative homosexual men is caused by human herpes virus (HHV8)
- **Immunologic Factors** Congenital or acquired immunodeficiency, including therapeutic immunosuppression, increases risk of sarcoma.
- Ninety percent of synovial sarcomas contain a characteristic chromosomal translocation t(X;18) (p11;q11) involving a nuclear transcription factor on chromosome 18 called *SYT* and two breakpoints on X.

➲ Achondroplasia High Yield for 2011-2012

- ✓ is inherited as an **autosomal dominant trait,**
- ✓ Although most cases are sporadic and due to new **fibroblast growth factor receptor 3 (FGFR3)** mutations
- ✓ The appearance of **short limbs,** particularly the proximal portions, **with a normal trunk** is characteristically accompanied by a large head, a saddle nose, and an exaggerated lumbar lordosis.
- ✓ The length of the spine is almost always normal. Features of the disorder are usually recognizable at birth.
- ✓ Formation and maturation of the secondary ossification centers and articular cartilage are not disturbed. Appositional growth at the metaphysis continues, with resulting flare in this region of the bone; intramembranous bone formation at the periosteum is normal

In several types of the so-called **craniosynostosis syndromes**

- **Pfeiffer,**
- **Crouzon,**
- **Jackson-Weiss, and**
- **Apert syndromes),** mutations have been identified in the ***FGFR1*** **or** ***FGFR2*** **genes.**

➲ Enchondromatosis (Dyschondroplasia, Ollier's disease) High Yield for 2011-2012

- ✓ **Disorder of the growth plate** in which the hypertrophic cartilage is not resorbed and ossified normally. It results in masses of cartilage with disorderly arrangement of the chondrocytes showing variable proliferative and hypertrophic changes.
- ✓ These masses are located in the metaphyses in clo se association with the growth plate in children but may be diaphyseal in teenagers and young adults. The disorder is usually recognized in childhood by the appearance of deformities or retardation in growth. The most common sites of involvement are the ends of long bones, usually in the region where rate of growth is most marked.
- ✓ The pelvis is often involved, but ribs, sternum, and skull are seldom affected. There is a tendency toward unilateral involvement.
- ✓ **Chondrosarcoma develops occasionally** in the enchondromata.
- ✓ The association of **enchondromatosis and cavernous hemangiomata in the soft tissues including the skin is known as *Maffucci's syndrome*.**
- ✓ Both Ollier's disease and Maffuci's syndrome have been associated with other primary malignancies as diverse as **granulosa cell tumor of the ovary and cerebral gliomas.**

➲ Multiple Exostoses (Diaphyseal Aclasis or Osteochondromatosis) High Yield for 2011-2012

- **Disorder of the metaphysis,** transmitted in an **autosomal dominant manner**, in which areas of the growth plate become displaced, presumably by growing through a defect in the perichondrium, or so-called ring of Ranvier. The spongiosa forms within the mass as vessels invade the cartilage.
- The lesions may be **solitary or multiple and are usually located in the metaphyseal areas of long bones, with the apex of the exostosis directed toward the diaphysis.**
- Often the lesions produce no symptoms, but occasionally, interference with the function of a joint or tendon or compression of nerves may result. Dwarfism may occur. The metacarpals may be shortened, resembling those seen in Albright's hereditary osteodystrophy.
- Multiple exostoses are sometimes seen in patients with pseudohypoparathyroidism.
- An exostosis may suddenly begin to enlarge long after growth should have ceased, and rarely, chondrosarcomas may develop from the cartilage cap of an exostosis.

⇨ Pyknodysostosis

- Pyknodysostosis is an **autosomal recessive form of osteosclerosis** that superficially resembles osteopetrosis.
- It is a **form of short-limbed dwarfism associated with bone fragility** and a tendency to fracture with minimal trauma.
- Life span is usually **normal.**
- In addition to a generalized **increase in bone density**, features include
  - **Short stature;**
  - **Separated cranial sutures;**
  - **Hypoplasia of the mandible;**
  - **Kyphoscoliosis and deformities of the trunk;**
  - **Persistence of deciduous teeth;**
  - **Progressive acroosteolysis of the terminal phalanges;**
  - **High, arched palate;**
  - **Proptosis;**
  - **Blue sclerae;**
  - **A pointed, beaked nose.**
- Patients usually present because of frequent fractures.
- *(remember the clinical presentation)* ☛ ☛

⇨ Osteomyelosclerosis

- In osteomyelosclerosis, **the marrow cells are replaced by diffuse fibroplasia,** occasionally accompanied by **osseous metaplasia and increased skeletal density on roentgenograms.**
- It is a **myeloproliferative disorder** and is characteristically accompanied by **extramedullary hematopoiesis.**
- **Hyperostosis corticalis generalisata (van Buchem's disease)** is characterized by **osteosclerosis of the skull (base and calvaria), lower jaw, clavicles, and ribs and thickening of the diaphyseal cortices of the long and short bones.** Alkaline phosphatase levels in the serum are elevated, and the disorder may be due to increased formation of bone of normal structure. The major manifestations are due to neural compression and consist of optic atrophy, facial paralysis, and perception deafness.
- **In hyperostosis generalisata with pachydermia** the sclerosis is due to increased formation of subperiosteal spongy bone and involves the epiphyses, metaphyses, and diaphyses. Pain, swelling of joints, and thickening of the skin of the lower arms are common.

➲ Progressive Diaphyseal Dysplasia

- **Camurati-Engelmann Disease** **MP 2002**
- This is an **autosomal dominant** disorder
- **Symmetric thickening and increased diameter of the diaphyses of long bones** occurs, particularly in the femur, tibia, fibula, radius, and ulna.
- **Pain over affected areas,** fatigue, abnormal gait, and muscle wasting are the major manifestations.
- **Serum alkaline phosphatase levels may be elevated**, and, on occasion, hypocalcemia and hyperphosphatemia may be found.
- Other abnormalities include **anemia, leukopenia, and an elevated erythrocyte sedimentation rate.**

➲ Melorheostosis

- This rare, sporadic condition usually begins in childhood and is characterized by a slowly **progressive linear hyperostosis** in one or more bones of one limb,
- Usually in a lower extremity.
- All segments of the bone may be involved, with sclerotic areas that have a **"Candle Dripping Wax"** or **"flowing" distribution.** **JK 2009**
- The involved limb is often extremely painful.

⇨ Osteopoikilosis

Osteopoikilosis is characterized by **dense spots of trabecular bone <1 cm in diameter**, usually of uniform density, located in the epiphyses and adjacent parts of the metaphyses.

All bones may be involved **except the skull, ribs, and vertebrae.**

3

ORTHOPEDICS

⇨ Stickler Syndrome

- Stickler syndrome is an inherited disorder of connective tissues characterized by **a typical facies with midface hypoplasia, high myopia with early onset, progressive hearing loss and arthropathy.** ☛☛
- The joint problems include both **generalized joint hypermobility** and **early degenerative joint disease.** ☛
- **Retinal detachment** is a serious complication of the syndrome.
- Mutations in the **COL2A1 gene** of type II collagen have been demonstrated in some families.

⇨ Iselin's Disease

Iselin's disease is apophysitis at the insertion of **peroneus brevis at the base of the fifth metatarsal.**

➲ Stress Fractures

- Stress fractures are undisplaced fatigue fractures, which develop as a result of **repeated loading**. The lower limbs are most frequently affected.
- **The metatarsals (march fractures) and the tibia being the most frequently involved** bones.☛☛
- **March fracture involves 2, 3 metatarsals most commonly.** **PGI 2000, KCET 2012**
- Younger children and even toddlers can present with stress fractures but they are more common in adolescents where the proximal third of the tibia is the most frequent site.
- Symptoms of localized pain develop insidiously and are usually relieved by rest.
- Treatment involves **protection from further trauma, which sometimes involves immobilization and always involves abstinence from the causative stress,**☛ usually running. Once symptoms have resolved a gradual return to activity can be begun.

⇨ Chronic Recurrent Multifocal Osteomylelitis (CRMO) and SAPHO Syndrome

The **SAPHO syndrome** is an inflammatory disorder of unknown etiology characterized by

- ✓ **Synovitis,**
- ✓ **Acne,**
- ✓ **Pustulosis,**
- ✓ **Hyperostosis and**
- ✓ **Osteitis.** ❋❋

CRMO, which is characterized **by multifocal osteitic lesions** is thought to be part of the same spectrum of disease. The etiology is unknown❋

⇨ Adolescent Hallus Valgus

- ✓ Hallux valgus or 'bunions' in adolescents is **usually familial** rather than the result of **poor footwear.**
- ✓ There is often an associated bunionette of the fifth toe and patients often have a characteristically broad forefoot with varus of the first metatarsal (metatarsus primus varus).
- ✓ Surgery is best deferred until skeletal maturity is reached.
- ✓ Surgical treatment gives good results for symptomatic feet with a painful bunion but caution should be exercised in the pain free patient who may be disappointed if surgery leaves a better looking but painful foot.

➲ Enthesitis Related Arthritis

Enthesitis is defined as **inflammation of the insertion of tendons into bones.☛** This new diagnostic group is intended to define those with disease related to the HLA antigen B27, and avoids the term juvenile spondyloarthropathy; inaccurate because of the rarity of spinal involvement in children.

Enthesitis related arthritis is defined as arthritis and enthesitis; or arthritis; or enthesitis with at least two of the following features:

1. **Sacroiliac joint tenderness and/or inflammatory spinal pain;** ☛
2. **Presence of HLA B27;** ☛ AIIMS 1997
3. **Family history in at least one first or second degree relative of medically confirmed HLA B27 associated disease;** ☛
4. **Anterior uveitis that is usually associated with pain, redness, or photophobia;** ☛
5. **Onset of arthritis in a boy after 8 years of age.**

➲ Ehlers-Danlos Syndrome

- Ehlers-Danlos syndrome (EDS) consists of a **group of disorders of connective tissue** characterized by:
- **Joint hypermobility plus fragility and laxity of the skin.**☛
- These conditions are characterized by abnormalities in collagen genes resulting in the **production of abnormal collagen and consequent tissue fragility.** ☛
- EDS has **soft, hyperextensible skin, 'cigarette paper' scars, easy bruising and marked hypermobility.** EDS type II is similar to type I but less severe.☛ PGI 2001
- Also seen is serious involvement with a **high incidence of rupture of the arteries, the colon or the pregnant uterus.** Management of EDS consists of patient education and support, with genetic counseling for the more severe forms.

➲ Pigmented Villonodular Synovitis

is characterized by the **slowly progressive, exuberant, benign proliferation of synovial tissue,**☛ usually involving a single joint. The most common age of onset is in the third decade, and women are affected slightly more often than men PGMEE 2003

- The synovium has a **brownish color and numerous large, finger-like villi** ☛that fuse to form **pedunculated nodules.** ☛
- There is marked **hyperplasia of synovial cells** in the stroma of the villi. ☛
- **Hemosiderin granules** and lipids are found in the cytoplasm of macrophages and in the interstitial tissue.☛
- **Multinucleated giant cells** may be present. The proliferative synovium grows into the subsynovial tissue and invades adjacent cartilage and bone.☛

The clinical picture of **pigmented villonodular synovitis** is characterized by the **insidious onset of swelling and pain in one joint, most commonly the knee.**

Other joints affected include the hips, ankles, calcaneocuboid joints, elbows, and small joints of the fingers or toes. The disease may also involve the **common flexor sheath of the hand or fingers.** Less commonly, tendon sheaths in the wrist, ankle, or foot may be involved. Radiographs may show

- ✓ **Joint space narrowing,**
- ✓ **Erosions, and**
- ✓ **Subchondral cysts.** The joint fluid contains blood and is dark red or almost black in color. **Lipid-containing macrophages** may be present in the fluid. The joint fluid may be clear if hemorrhages have not occurred.

The treatment of **pigmented villonodular synovitis** is **complete synovectomy.** ☛

➲ Synovial Chondromatosis

- is a disorder characterized by **multiple focal metaplastic growths of normal-appearing cartilage in the synovium or tendon sheath.** ☛Segments of cartilage break loose and continue to grow as **loose bodies.**
  SGPGI 2005
- When calcification and ossification of loose bodies occur, the disorder is referred to as **synovial osteochondromatosis.**☛
- The disorder is **usually monarticular** ☛and affects **young to middle-aged individuals.** The knee is most often involved, followed by hip, elbow, and shoulder.
- Symptoms are pain, swelling, and decreased motion of the joint.
- Radiographs may show several rounded calcifications within the joint cavity.
- **Treatment is synovectomy;**☛ however, the tumor may recur.

➲ De Quervain Syndrome

- Also known as **washerwoman's sprain** or **mother's wrist**
- is a **tendinosis of the sheath or tunnel that surrounds two tendons** that control movement of the thumb. **(extensor pollicis brevis and abductor pollicis longus muscles)**
- De Quervain is potentially **more common in women;** the speculative rationale for this is that women have a greater styloid process angle of the radius.
- Symptoms are **pain, tenderness, and swelling over the thumb side of the wrist, and difficulty gripping.**
- **Finkelstein's test** is used to diagnose de Quervain syndrome in people who have wrist pain.

⇨ Dupuytren's Contracture

- **Is palmar fibromatosis**
- Is a **fixed flexion contracture of the hand** where the fingers bend towards the palm and cannot be fully extended (straightened).
- It is named after Baron Guillaume Dupuytren, the surgeon who described an operation to correct the affliction.
- Dupuytren's contracture is caused by underlying contractures of the **palmar aponeurosis (or palmar fascia).**
- The **ring finger and little finger** are the fingers **most commonly affected.**
- The middle finger may be affected in advanced cases, but the index finger and the thumb are nearly always spared.
- Dupuytren's contracture progresses slowly and is **usually painless.**
- The palmar aponeurosis becomes hyperplastic and undergoes contracture.
- Incidence increases after the age of 40; at this age men are affected more often than women.

Dupuytren's disease primarily affects:

- *People of Scandinavian or Northern European ancestry*
- *Men rather than women*
- *People over the age of 40*
- *People with a family history*
- *People with liver cirrhosis*

➲ Klippel-Feil Syndrome

Klippel-Feil syndrome is a **congenital fusion of the cervical vertebrae**

Cardio respiratory, Genitourinary, and Auditory systems are frequently involved

Klippel-Feil syndrome gene locus is on **long arm of chromosome 8.**

The "classic features" of Klippel-Feil syndrome are

Short neck,
Low posterior hair line
Limited range of neck motion.

Conditions "Commonly Associated" with Klippel- Feil Syndrome"

- Scoliosis
- Renal Abnormalities
- Cardiovascular Anomalies (Ventricular septal defects; most common)
- Deafness
- Synkinesis (Mirror Movements)
- Respiratory Anomalies (Failure of lobe formation, Ectopic lungs, Restriction of lung function by shortened trunk, scoliosis, rib fusion, or deformed costovertebral joints
- Sprengel Deformity.

➲ Brown Tumors

✓ **Brown tumors** are tumors of bone that arise as a result of **excess osteoclastic activity**, such as **Hyperparathyroidism**, and consist of ***fibrous tissue, woven bone and supporting vasculature, but no matrix.***

✓ They are **radiolucent on X-ray.**

✓ The osteoclasts consume the trabecular bone that osteoblasts lay down and this front of reparative bone deposition followed by addition resorption can expand beyond the usual shape of the bone, involving the periosteum and causing bone pain.

✓ The characteristic brown coloration results from **"Hemosiderin" deposition into the osteolytic cysts.**

Madelung Deformity

- This wrist deformity results from an **unexplained premature growth arrest of the ulnar aspect**
- Continued normal growth of the ulnar physis and the radial and dorsal aspects of the distal radial physis leads to progressive deformity.
- The **distal ulna becomes more prominent** and the distal radial articular surface becomes angulated towards the ulna.
- Madelung's deformity **usually occurs in girls** and is most often bilateral.
- The condition is usually sporadic but may be inherited as part of dyschondrosteosis **(Leri-Weill disease)**, and has been associated with a variety of conditions including **Hurler's syndrome, Turner's syndrome, multiple hereditary exostoses and Ollier's disease.** Damage to the growth plate from trauma or infection can also give rise to Madelung-like deformities.
- Most patients do not present until adolescence when deformity and discomfort with activity are often marked.
- Treatment strategies for these patients include corrective radial osteotomy and ulnar shortening or other procedures to remove or stabilize the distal ulna, which is frequently the site of pain and wrist degeneration **of the distal radial physis (or growth plate).**

Chondromalacia Patellae

- It is due to an **irritation of the undersurface of the sesamoid bone patella.**
- The undersurface of the patella is covered with a layer of smooth cartilage. This cartilage normally glides effortlessly across the knee during bending of the joint.
- However, in some individuals, **the patella tends to rub against one side of the knee joint, and the cartilage surface become irritated, and knee pain is the result.**
- The pain of chondromalacia patellae is **typically felt after prolonged sitting, like for a movie, and so is also called "movie sign" or "theater sign".**
- The condition may result from acute **injury to the patella or from chronic friction between the patella and the groove in the femur** through which it passes during motion of the knee.
- Pain at the front of the knee due to overuse can be addressed with a basic program consisting of RICE
  - ✓ Rest,
  - ✓ Ice,
  - ✓ Compression,
  - ✓ Elevation,
  - ✓ Anti-inflammatory medications,

Example: *A teenage girl complains of pain in knee on climbing stairs and on getting up after sitting for a long time.*

High Yield for 2011-2012

➲ ITBS (Ilio Tibial Tract Syndrome)

- It is one of the leading causes of **lateral knee pain in runners.**
- The iliotibial band is a **superficial thickening of tissue on the outside of the thigh**, extending from the outside of the pelvis, over the hip and knee, and inserting just below the knee.
- The band is **crucial to stabilizing the knee during running, moving from behind the femur to the front while walking.**
- The continual rubbing of the band over the **lateral femoral epicondyle**, combined with the repeated flexion and extension of the knee during running may cause the area to become inflamed.

High Yield for 2011-2012

➲ Congenital Talipes Equinovarus (CTEV; Congenital Club Foot)

- Congenital talipes equinovarus is a **common foot abnormality**
- It is **twice as common in boys,**
- **Bilateral in up to 50%**, and has a **familial predisposition.**
- Clinically the hindfoot is in **equinus and varus** (inversion) and the **heel is difficult to feel.**
- The **forefoot is adducted and plantarflexed** on the hindfoot giving a cavus or high arched appearance, and there is a deep transverse skin crease on the medial border of the foot.
- **Internal tibial torsion is present** and the foot and calf are often smaller than the opposite side.
- The navicular is medially displaced on the head of the talus.

➲ Congenital Vertical Talus

- ✓ This is a rigid foot deformity that presents clinically as a **'rocker bottom'** foot.
- ✓ In about 50% the condition is associated with other congenital neuromuscular and genetic disorders like neural tube defects and arthrogryposis.

➲ Breaststroker's Knee

Competitive breaststrokers can develop medial knee pain along the medial collateral ligament.
Rest and avoidance of the technique is helpful.

⇨ Blount's disease

- ✓ It is a **growth disorder of the tibia** (that causes the lower leg to angle inward, resembling a bowleg.
- ✓ It is also known as **"tibia vara"**.
- ✓ Blount's disease occurs in **young children and adolescents.**
- ✓ The cause is unknown but is thought to be due to the **effects of weight on the growth plate.**
- ✓ The inner part of the tibia, just below the knee, fails to develop normally, causing **angulation of the bone.**
- ✓ Unlike bowlegs, which tend to straighten as the child develops, Blount's disease is **progressive** and the condition worsens. It can cause severe bowing of the legs and can affect one or both legs.
- ✓ This condition is more common among children of African ancestry. It is also **associated with obesity, short stature, and early walking.**

High Yield for 2011-2012

3

ORTHOPEDICS

⇨ Cauda Equina Syndrome

- Is a serious neurologic condition in which there is acute loss of function of the **lumbar plexus, neurologic elements (nerve roots) of the spinal canal below the conus of the spinal cord.**
- After the conus, the canal contains a mass of nerves **(the cauda equina or "horse-tail")** that branches off the lower end of the spinal cord and contains the nerve roots from L1-5 and S1-5. The nerve roots from L4-S4 join in the sacral plexus which affects the sciatic nerve, which travels caudally (toward the feet). **Causes:**
- Direct trauma from lumbar puncture.
- Burst fractures resulting in posterior migration of fragments of the vertebral body,
- Severe disk herniations,
- Spinal anesthesia involving trauma from catheters and high local anesthetic concentrations around the cauda equina.
- Penetrating trauma such as knife wounds or ballistic trauma.
- Lumbar spinal stenosis.

Spinal inflammatory conditions such as

- Paget disease,
- Chronic inflammatory demyelinating polyneuropathy
- Ankylosing spondylitis.

Signs

- Signs include weakness of the muscles of the lower extremeties innervated by the compressed roots (often paraplegia),
- Sphincter weaknesses causing urinary retention and post-void residual incontinence
- Also, there may be decreased anal tone and consequent fecal incontinence;
- Sexual Dysfunction;
- Saddle Anesthesia;
- Bilateral leg pain and weakness; and
- Bilateral absence of ankle reflexes.
- Pain may, however, be wholly absent; the patient may complain only of lack of bladder control and of saddle-anesthesia, and may walk into the consulting-room.

Diagnosis is usually confirmed by an **MRI scan or CT scan**, depending on availability.

➲ Thromboembolism after Orthopedic Surgeries

"A patient after hip replacement developes severe chest pain and CVS collapse MOST Probably has Pulmonary embolism"

Thromboembolic disease is one of the **most common serious complications** arising from total hip arthroplasty.

Total hip arthroplasty without routine prophylaxis increases chances of pulmonary embolism tremendously.

Venous thrombosis occurred after total hip replacement in 50% of patients, and fatal pulmonary emboli occurred in 2%.

Spinal and epidural anesthesia carry a lower risk of deep vein thrombosis and pulmonary embolism than general anesthesia.

Thromboembolism **can occur in vessels in the pelvis, thigh, and calf.** Of all thromboses, 80 to 90% occur in the operated limb.

The **clinical diagnosis** of deep vein thrombosis usually is made on the basis of

- **Pain and tenderness in the calf and thigh,**
- **Positive Homan sign,**
- **Unilateral swelling and erythema of the leg,**
- **Low-grade fever and**
- **Rapid pulse.**

In at least 50% of patients, the diagnosis is not clinically apparent, however.

The clinical diagnosis of pulmonary embolism is based on symptoms of

- ✓ **Chest pain (especially if pleuritic in nature),**
- ✓ **Evaluation by electrocardiogram and**
- ✓ **Chest radiographs, and**
- ✓ **Determination of arterial blood gas levels.**

- **Most** pulmonary emboli are **not clinically apparent.**
- **Venography** is considered the most sensitive and specific test for the detection of calf and thigh thromboses. It does not reliably detect pelvic vein thrombosis.
- **B-mode or duplex Doppler ultrasound** venography is accuracte in detection of femoral thrombosis, but it is not
- As helpful in diagnosis of calf and pelvic thrombi.
- The diagnosis of pulmonary embolism usually is **confirmed by radionuclide perfusion lung scanning**. It is noninvasive and can be done at the bedside with portable equipment.
- **Pulmonary angiography** is invasive and carries higher risks, but is required occasionally when perfusion lung scanning is equivocal.
- It also is generally agreed that pharmacological prophylaxis should be used in almost all patients.
- The most commonly used agents are **Warfarin, Low-molecular-weight heparin (LMWH), Fondaparinux, and Aspirin.**

Neurogenic Arthropathy

The disorder develops in a setting of impaired pain perception and position sense, and can cause a rapidly destructive osteoarthritis-like arthropathy.

The problems appear to be due to unfelt minor injury, without the normal response of pain, causing resting of, and natural splinting (by muscle contraction or shifting position) of the affected joints.

The most commonly encountered setting is diabetic foot disease. Can occur in a wide variety of other conditions, including

- **Tabes dorsalis (syphilis),**
- **Syringomyelia,**
- **Arnold-Chiari malformation,**
- **Meningomyelocele,**
- **Leprosy,**
- **Tumors of peripheral nerve or spinal cord,**
- **Vertebral disease with damage to peripheral nerves,**
- **Amyloidosis, and**
- **Familial hereditary neuropathies.**

The joints affected are those that have lost pain innervation, possibly in association with palsies of nearby muscles.

➲ Causes of Loose Bodies in Knee Joint are

- ➲ Hemarthrosis.
- ➲ Tuberculosis.
- ➲ Rheumatoid arthritis.
- ➲ Osteoarthritis.
- ➲ Syphilis.
- ➲ Arbroscent lipoma.
- ➲ Traumatic synovitis.
- ➲ Meniscal Tear.
- ➲ Osteochondritis desiccans.
- ➲ Introduced foreign body.
- ➲ Secondary carcinoma.
- ➲ Synovial chondritis.

➲ Musculoskeletal Manifestations in Syndromes Commonly Asked:

Down syndrome, or trisomy 21, is the most common autosomal chromosome abnormality. The incidence increases as maternal age increases. The classic features are hypotonia, upslanting palpebral fissures, epicanthal folds, excess nuchal skin, an enlarged tongue, **clinodactyly of the fifth fingers, and a single transverse palmar crease.**

Edwards syndrome or trisomy 18, has features of small palpebral fissures, low-set ears, low birth weight, **microcephaly, rocker-bottom feet, cleft lip**, hypotonia, and **clenched hands.**

Fetal alcohol syndrome is characterized by **growth retardation, small palpebral fissures, smooth philtrum, a thin upper lip, microcephaly, and a short nose**. Features often go unnoticed in the newborn period, although sometimes tremulousness and irritability occur.

Marfan syndrome is associated with **increased stature, thin limbs, scoliosis, joint hypermobility,** and ocular manifestations. Features often go unnoticed in the newborn period.

Turner syndrome has features of prominent low-set ears, excess nuchal skin, **broad chest,** epicanthal folds, lymphedema of hands and feet, and **short stature.**

➲ Bone Scan High Yield for 2011-2012

is a nuclear scanning test that identifies

- ✓ New areas of bone growth or breakdown.
- ✓ Find cancer that has metastasized to the bones, and
- ✓ Monitor (infection and trauma) to bones

- ➢ **Technetium-99m** is used as a radioactive tracer that medical equipment can detect in the body.
- ➢ It is well suited to the role because it emits readily detectable 140 keV gamma rays
- ➢ The "short" half life of the isotope (in terms of human-activity and metabolism allows for scanning procedures which collect data rapidly, but keep total patient radiation exposure low.

For a bone scan, a radioactive tracer substance is injected into a vein in the arm. The tracer then travels through the bloodstream and into the bones. This process may take several hours. A special camera (gamma) takes pictures of the tracer in the bones. This helps show cell activity and function in the bones.

Areas that absorb little or no amount of tracer appear as dark or "cold" spots, which may indicate a lack of blood supply to the bone (bone infarction) or the presence of certain types of cancer.

***Areas of rapid bone growth or repair absorb increased amounts of the tracer and show up as bright or "hot" spots** in the pictures. Hot spots may indicate problems such as arthritis, the presence of a tumor, a*

➲ Common Nuclear Medicine Therapies Include:

- **131I-sodium iodide** for hyperthyroidism and thyroid cancer,
- **Yttrium-90-**ibritumomab tiuxetan and Iodine-131-tositumomab for refractory Lymphoma,
- **^{131}I-MIBG** (metaiodobenzylguanidine) for neuroendocrine tumors, and
- Palliative bone pain treatment with Samarium-153 or Strontium-89.

➲ SPECT:

- Single photon emission computed tomography (SPECT) is a nuclear medicine imaging technique using gamma rays.
- To acquire SPECT images, the **gamma camera is rotated around the patient.**
- Projections are acquired at defined points during the rotation, typically every 3-6 degrees. In most cases, **a full 360 degree rotation is used to obtain an optimal reconstruction.**
- The time taken to obtain each projection is also variable, but 15-20 seconds is typical.
- This gives a total scan time of **15-20 minutes.**

Isotope	Symbol	Z	$T_{1/2}$	Decay
✓ Fluorine-18	^{18}F	9	109.77 m	➠ β^+
✓ Gallium-67	^{67}Ga	31	3.26 d	➠ ec
✓ Krypton-81m	^{81m}Kr	36	13.1 s	➠ IT
✓ Rubidium-82	^{82}Rb	37	1.27 m	➠ β^+
✓ Technetium-99m	^{99m}Tc	43	6.01 h	➠ IT
✓ Indium-111	^{111}In	49	2.80 d	➠ ec
✓ Iodine-123	^{123}I	53	13.3 h	➠ ec
✓ Xenon-133	^{133}Xe	54	5.24 d	➠ β^-
✓ Thallium-201	^{201}Tl	81	3.04 d	➠ ec
✓ Yttrium-90	^{90}Y	39	2.67 d	➠ β^-
✓ Iodine-131	^{131}I	53	8.02 d	➠ β^-

➲ Clinical Oriented Problems

Kindly Look Into Highlighted Text and Don't look at the answers initially.

High Yield Questions for 2011/2012 (AIIMS/AIPGE/ PGI)

➔ A 15 year old boy was treated for retinoblastoma at the age of 1 year presented with pain and swelling around the knee, X-ray showed some typical appearance. Most likely diagnosis is: **Osteosarcoma** (MP 2008)

- **High Yield for 2011-2012**
- **MAH 2012**

➔ A 46-year-old woman presents with chronic widespread musculoskeletal pain, fatigue, and frequent headaches. She states that her musculoskeletal pain improves slightly with exercise. On examination, painful trigger points are produced by palpitation of the trapezius and lateral epicondyle of the elbow. Signs of inflammation are absent and laboratory studies are within normal. Most likely diagnosis is: **fibromyalgia**

- **(High Yield for 2011-2012)**

➔ A 30-year-old woman consults a physician because of a painless, pea-like lesion on the back of her wrist. She finds the lesion annoying and disfiguring, and so has it removed by a surgeon. Grossly, the lesion is white and translucent, and oozes gelatinous material when cut. Most likely diagnosis is: **Ganglion cyst**

- **(High Yield for 2011-2012)**

➔ A 17-year-old girl is brought to the emergency department with a 2-day history of a painful and swollen right big toe. She also has had a fever, with temperatures up to 38.9 C (102 F), at home for 2 days. Her parents decided to bring her to the hospital tonight because she hasbeen unable to sleep due to the pain. On physical examination, her temperature is 101.8 F (38.8 C). Her first metatarsal joint of the right foot is markedly swollen and very painful to touch. An aspirated fluid from the joint reveals a white blood count of 55,000/mm_3. The most likely diagnosis is: **Septic arthritis**

- **(High Yield for 2011-2012)**

➔ A 72 -year-old man from comes for a follow up visit. The man was a farmer and has been healthy for most of his life Gamma-glutamyl transpeptidase level and total calcium level are within normal limits. Upon further questioning, the man denies any abdominal pain, nausea, vomiting, or other gastrointestinal symptoms. His Serum levels show

Serum alanine aminotransferase (ALT) 15 U/L

Serum alkaline phosphatase 770 U/L

Serum aspartate aminotransferase (AST) 26 U/L

Total serum bilirubin 0.8 mg/dL

But his systemic examination shows slightly diminished hearing and a mild, chronic bilateral tinnitus. The most likely diagnosis is: **Osteitis deformans**

- **(High Yield for 2011-2012)**

* A **benign growth** of **hyaline cartilage** lying in the **medullary cavity** of a bone arising from **ectopic cartilaginous rests in the phalanges and metacarpals** and Radiographically, producing a **lucent defect** with well-defined margins and surrounding sclerotic reactive bone are most likely : **Enchondromas**
* **(High Yield for 2011-2012)**

➔ **A 12 year old** has a **solitary lesion** in his left femur which is exquisitely painful. Pain is described as a persistent discomfort unrelated to activity or rest and is often worse at night. Curiously, **pain is relieved for several hours by the use of Non steroidal anti-inflammatory drugs.** The lesion is composed of a central nidus of closely packed trabeculae **of woven bone**.

Most likely lesion is: **Osteoid osteoma**

* **(High Yield for 2011-2012)**

➔ **A 15 year old** has a lesion in the **metaphyseal end of his distal femur**. Areas of **lytic bone destruction mixed with areas of reactive and tumor bone formations are seen.** This tumor rapidly permeates through the **overlying cortex** into the subperiosteal space and produces a **characteristic appearance of trabecular bone** oriented at right angles to the underlying cortical surface.

Most likely tumor is: **Osteosarcoma**

* **(High Yield for 2011-2012)**

➔ **A girl** presents with complaints of **local pain and swelling in her femur**. There is **fever, leukocytosis, and an increased erythrocyte sedimentation rate**. The radiographic appearance shows the lesion to be **occurring in the diaphysis with periosteal elevation** is seen because of permeation of the cortex by tumor with Varying degrees of bone destruction and varying degrees of reactive new bone formation create a wide range of radiographic appearances. Microscopically, the tumor is composed of **uniform round cells gathered in nests or cords and separated by thin fibrous septa**. The Tumor is **positive for glycogen on periodic acid-Schiff.**

Most likely cause is: **Ewing sarcoma**

* **(High Yield for 2011-2012)**

➔ **A 72 year old** has pain and **discomfort in addition to fever, anemia hypercalcemia, and renal failure** related to extensive skeletal involvement and the abnormal production of immunoglobulins.

The lesions would be characteristic of : **Myeloma**

* **(High Yield for 2011-2012)**

(I Provide Classic Examples of Orthopedic Problems. Try To Make Diagnosis Initially Without Looking At Answers.)

➲ Clinical Scenarios

▶ *An itching, squeezing pain sensation after amputation that an amputated limb is still attached and functioning with intensly painful sensations*	**Phantom limb pain❋**
▶ *Complex and progressive disease with pain swelling and changes in skin __without__ demonstrable nerve lesions after injury*	**Reflex Sympathetic Dystrophy/Sudecks Atrophy❋**
▶ *Complex and progressive disease with pain swelling and changes in skin __with__ demonstrable nerve lesions after injury*	**Causalgia❋❋**
▶ *A 13 year old boy with a hot, tender swelling arising from diaphysis of bone with characteristic feature of onion skinning.*	**Ewings Sarcoma** **JKBOPEE 2012**
▶ *An obese boy in 2nd decade presents with Pain and with limited Flexion, Abduction and femoral head seen downwards and Posteriorly*	**Slippped Femoral Epiphysis ❋**
▶ *A 10 year old boy with Pain and limp. X ray shows distorted femoral neck and Head*	**Perthes Disease❋**
▶ *An elderly boy after trauma presents with expansile osteolytic and cystic bony lesion with thin wall*	**Aneurysmal Bone Cyst❋**
▶ *An elderly man Presents to orthopedic clinic with Pain in bones On X ray **cortical widening** of bones. **Molten wax" or "Candle Dripping Wax" Appearance** of bones is noted*	**Melorheostosis❋**
▶ *A male presents with triad of Lytic bony lesions on skull,diabetes Insipidus and Exomphalos*	**Hand Schuller Christian Disease❋**

▶ *An infant presents with failure to thrive, Pancytopenia. Bones are brittle and fracture easily. Defect is found in Osteoclasts*	**Infantile Osteopetrosis ❋**
▶ *A two year old presents with multiple fractures in different stages of healing brought by over concerned parents*	**Battered Baby Syndrome❋**
▶ *A six year old with b/l symmetrical fractures and blue sclera. Bones are osteopenic and brittle*	**Osteogenesis Imperfecta❋**
▶ *An athelete after trauma and haematoma formation at elbow comes to you with hard calcific mass found in the muscle Belly*	**Myositis ossificans❋** **(AI 88)**
▶ *A patient with multiple injuries on day 2 develops Tacchycardia, Taccypnea, ↓PO_2 and rash.*	Fat embolism ❋ **(UPSC 95)**
▶ *A patient after hip replacement develops chest pain and CVS collapse.*	**Pulmonary Thromboembolism** **AI 2010**

➲ Important Questions Repeated and Frequently Asked

- **Tarsal tunnel syndrome** occurs in Rheumatoid arthritid. AIIMS 2009
- **Crescent fracture** is fracture of iliac bone with sacroiliac disruption. AIIMS 2009
- **JERK test** is used in testing posterior gleno humeral instability. AIIMS 2009
- **Velpau Sling and Swathe bandage** is used for: Acromiocalvicular dislocation. AIIMS 2008
- **Watson jones operation** is done for: **Unstable hip** AIIMS 2008
- **Remember Watson jones tendodesis is done for ankle joint. (Lateral instability of ankle)**
- **Rissers localization cast** is used for: Scoliosis AIIMS 2008
- Differentiation between RA and SLE on x ray is because of **erosion** in case of RA AIIMS 2008
- Staging of bone tumors is done by **Enneking staging.** AIIMS 2007
- **Kanavel sign** is present in **Tenosynovitis.** AIIMS 2007

■ **Winging of scapula** is due to injury of :	**Long thoracic nerve**	**UPSC 2007**
■ **Disruption of myelin** with intact axons is:	**Neuropraxia**	**UP 2007**
■ **Mc nerve** involved **in supracondylar # humerus** is :	**Median nerve**	**UP 2007**
■ **Bohlers angle** refers to which bone:	**Calcaneum**	**AI 2007**
■ **Meralgia parasthetica** involves :	**Lateral cutaneous nerve of thigh**	**AI 2007**
■ <u>**Tardy ulnar palsy**</u> is due to	<u>**Lateral**</u> **condylar #**	**PGI 2002**
■ <u>**Gun stock deformity**</u> involves	<u>**Supracondylar**</u> **#**	**PGI 06**
■ **Surgical neck of humerus** is related to	**Axillary nerve**	**COMED 2007**
■ **Anterior dislocation** of shoulder injures :	**Axillary nerve**	**UPSC 2007**
■ **Apprehension test** involves	**Shoulder joint**	**UP 2007**
■ **Bennets fracture** involves :	**First metacarpal**	**COMED 2007**
■ **Carpal tunnel syndrome** is tested by:	**BP cuff test, Phallens test**	**MAHE 2007**
■ **Cobbs angle** is measured in	<u>**Scoliosis**</u>	**SGPI 2004**
■ **# spine** is most commonly due to	**Flexion injury**	**AI 2007**
■ **Burst #** spine is due to	**Compression force**	**AI 2007**
■ **Most common type of #**	**Dens is type II**	**COMED 2007**
■ **Hinge # skull** is most common in	**Motorcyclists**	**MAHE 2007**
■ **Electric bulb sign** is seen in	<u>**Posterior**</u> **dislocation hip**	**AIPGE 2006**
■ **Modified Allens test** is used for	**Radial artery**	**SGPI 2004**
■ **Thomas test** is used for	**Fixed flexion deformity**	**TN 2003**
■ **Mutations of type I collagen results in**	**Osteogenesis imperfecta**	**UP 2007**

3

ORTHOPEDICS

NOTES

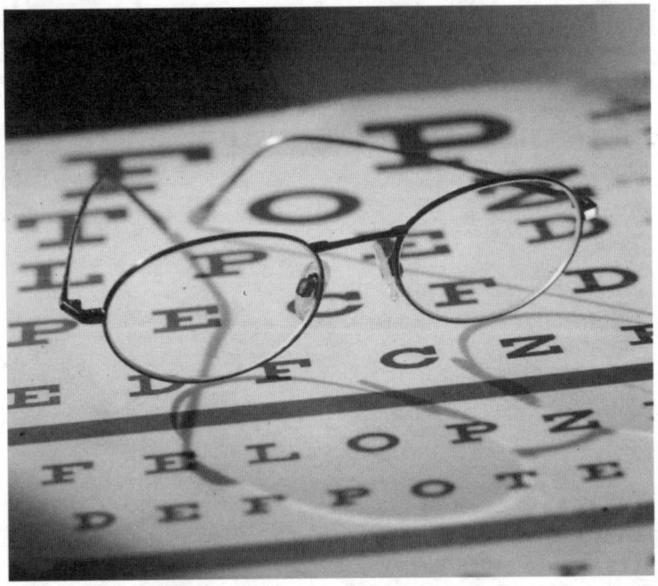

OPHTHALMOLOGY

➲ Anatomy and Important Dimensions of Eye

▶ Diameter of Macula:	✓ 5.5 mm	
▶ Diameter of Fovea:	✓ 1.5 mm	
▶ Diameter of optic disk:	✓ 1.5 mm	JK 2001
▶ Diameter of Foveola:	✓ 0.35 mm	

▶ Antero posterior Length of eye ball	✓ 24 mm	UP 1997
▶ Height of eye ball:	✓ 23 mm	
▶ Vertical Length of eye ball:	✓ 23 mm	
▶ Circumference of eye ball:	✓ 70 mm	
▶ Depth of anterior chamber:	✓ 2-3 mm	AI 1992
▶ Volume of eye ball:	✓ 6.5 ml	
▶ Volume of vitreous	✓ 4 ml	JK 2001
▶ Volume of Orbit	✓ 30 cc.	JK 2007

Thickness of Lens is 3.5 -5 mm

➲ Muscles of Eye and their Innervations: Special High Yield Points for 2011/2012

- The "**Extorter**" of Eye Ball is **Inferior Oblique and Inferior Rectus.**
- The "**Intorter**" of Eye ball is **Superior Oblique and Superior Rectus.** PGI 2004, AIIMS 1995
- Action of Superior oblique is **Abduction, Intorsion and depression.** PGI 1997
- Dilator Pupillae dilates pupil and is supplied by **Sympathetics.**
- Sphincter Pupillae constricts pupil and is supplied by **Parasympathetics.**
- LR_6SO_4
  - Lateral Rectus is supplied by **6th Cranial Nerve** (Abducent)
  - Superior Oblique is supplied by **4th Cranial Nerve** (Trochlear) AIIMS 2004
  - Rest other ocular muscles are supplied by **3rd Cranial Nerve** (Occulomotor)
  - Levator palpabrae superioris is supplied by 3rd caranial nerve. MAHE 2005
  - Muscle attached to posterior tarsal margin: **Mullers muscle** KERALA 1994

Third nerve gets affected in a variety of syndromes of Mid Brain such as: PGI 1988

- **Benedicts Syndrome**
- **Claudes Syndrome**
- **Webers Syndrome**
- **Nothangels Syndrome**

Trigeminal nerve (Fifth Cranial nerve) is involved in **afferent pathway of corneal reflex**

4

OPHTHALMOLOGY

➲ Muscles in Ophthalmology

VOLUNTARY extraoccular muscles:

- Four recti
- Two obliqui
- Levator palpabrae superioris

INVOLUNTARY extraoccular muscles:

- Superior tarsal
- Inferior tarsal
- Orbitalis

⇨ Glands of Eye

- **Zeis glands:** Large sebaceous glands
- **Molls glands:** Sweat glands
- **Meibomian glands:** Tarsal glands

⇨ Vascularity of Eye is by

STRUCTURE	BLOOD SUPPLY
Uveal tract	Ciliary arteries
Covjunctive	Palpaberal branches of nasal and lacrimal arteries
Cornea	Avascular
Sclera	Avascular
Lens	Avascular
Optic nerve	Ophthalmic artey

➲ Gems about Pupil

- Sphincter pupillae is a circular "**constrictor muscle**" innervated by **Parasympathetic** Nervous system.
- Dilator Pupillae is a "**radial dilator**" innervated by **Sympathetic** Nervous system.
- Pupillary inequality is called "**Anisocoria**".
- **III Nerve lesion causes dilated pupil, Ptosis.** **AIIMS 2011**
- **Horners syndrome causes constricted pupil.**
- **Argyl Robertson Pupil:** Small pupils, irregular in shape which don't react to light but react to accommodation. (**ARP: Accomdation Reflex present**) **TN 1999**
- **Marcus Gunn Pupil (Pupillary Escape):** Illumination of one eye normally produces constriction. In case light source is swung from eye to eye, affected pupil may **"paradoxically" dilate. (Marcus Gunn Pupil) (Defect anterior to optic chiasma)** **MAHE 2005**
- **Aides Pupil:** Is dysfunction of constrictor muscle and hence does not respond to light or to accommodation**(Tonic pupil)**

⇨ Absolute Afferent Pupillary Defect

An absolute afferent pupillary defect **(Amaurotic pupil)** is caused by a **complete optic nerve lesion** and is characterized by:

- The **involved eye is completely blind** (i.e., no light perception).
- Both pupils are **equal in size.**
- When the affected eye is stimulated by light neither pupil reacts but when the normal eye is stimulated both pupils react normally.
- The **near reflex is normal** in both eyes.

⇨ Relative Afferent Pupillary Defect

Also called as (Marcus Gunn pupil) is caused by an **incomplete optic nerve lesion** or severe retinal disease. Thus the pupils respond weakly to stimulation of the diseased eye and briskly to that of the normal eye. The difference between the pupillary reactions of the two eyes is highlighted by the **swinging-flashlight test** in which a light source is alternatively switched from one eye to the other and back, thus stimulating each eye in rapid succession.

- When the normal eye is stimulated both pupils constrict.
- Then when the light **is swung to the diseased eye, both pupils dilate instead of constricting.**
- When the normal eye is stimulated, both pupils constrict.

➲ Marcus Gunn Jaw winking Syndrome

- Usually unilateral.
- Abnormal regeneration like in Freys syndrome. That a **branch of the mandibular division of the fifth cranial nerve is misdirected** to the levator muscle.
- Retraction of the ptotic lid in conjunction with stimulation of the ipsilateral pterygoid muscles by **chewing, sucking, opening the mouth or contralateral jaw movement.**
- Less common stimuli to winking include jaw protrusion, smiling, swallowing and clenching of teeth.
- **Treatment is with** Surgery if jaw-winking or ptosis represents a significant functional or cosmetic problem.

➲ Cornea

- **The cornea is quite unlike most tissues in that it is perfectly transparent.**
- **The epithelium** consists of a thin layer of **non-keratinized stratified squamous**, PGI 2001
- Corneal epithelium is **very thin** (only a few cells thick).
- Corneal epithelium lies flat against the underlying substantia propria.
- There is absence **of connective tissue** papillae
- **The Basement membrane** between corneal epithelium and substantia propria is exceptionally thick and is called **Bowman's membrane**.
- **The substantia propria** of the cornea is mostly collagen and ground substance, with fibroblasts as the most common cell type. AIIMS 1986
- Collagen of the cornea is organized into extremely **regular layers**. All the collagen fibers in one layer arranged in parallel, and alternating layers run in different directions. AIIMS 1986

- Corneal connective tissue has no blood vessels.
- Even though cells of the cornea are not very active metabolically, they still need oxygen and nutrients.
- As long as the cornea is in direct contact with air, oxygen can be absorbed directly. **AI 96**
- Nutrients can diffuse into cornea from aqueous humor. **(Avascular coat)** **PGI 1999**
- Cells of corneal connective tissue are limited to fibroblasts.
- **There is** no immune-system component; hence the relative ease with which corneal tissue can be transplanted without need for careful tissue typing.
- **Descemet's membrane:** Is a thick basal lamina made of elastic fibers over endothelium.
- **Corneal endothelium:** Is simple squamous epithelium present below Descmets membrane. Corneal epithelium contains **free nerve endings**. Since pain seems to be the only sensation of cornea.

⇨ Layers of Retina

- Retinal pigment epithelium (RPE)
- Layer of rod and cone cells outer segments
- Outer limiting membrane
- Outer nuclear layer
- Outer plexiform layer
- Inner nuclear layer
- Inner plexiform layer
- Ganglion cell layer MOST RESISTANT TO RADIATION **AIIMS 2011**
- Nerve fiber layer
- Internal limiting membrane

⇨ The "Medial Longitudinal Fasciculus" **AIIMS 2008**

The Medial longitudinal fasciculus (MLF) connects the

- ✓ **Oculomotor (III),**
- ✓ **Trochlear (IV), and**
- ✓ **Abducens (VI) nuclei** and
- ✓ Is essential for **conjugate gaze.** **SGPI 2005**

"A lesion in the MLF will result in the inability to medially rotate(adduct) the ipsilateral eye on attempted lateral gaze." (Intranuclear opthalmoplegia INO) **AIIMS 2002**

However, a lesion of the motor fibers of the right oculomotor nerve would also lead to the same symptoms. The way to truly distinguish between an INO from a lesion of the medial rectus muscle or a lesion of the motor fibers of CN III is to determine whether the patient can converge her eyes. If the innervation of the medial rectus muscle is interrupted, the patient will not be able to move the ipsilateral eye medially for either conjugate or dysconjugate (convergence) movements. **However, if the lesion is in the MLF, this would only affect conjugate movement, and not convergence.**

➲ Important Membranes in Ophthalmology

❐ Bowmans Membrane	"Anterior" limiting membrane of Cornea
❐ Descements Membrane	"Posterior" limiting membrane of Cornea
❐ Bruchs Membrane	Pigment membrane in Retina
❐ Elschings Membrane	Astroglial membrane covering Optic Disk

➲ Important Glands in Ophthalmology

➨ Glands of Zeis :	✓ Sebaceous glands☛☛
➨ Glands of Moll:	✓ Modified sweat glands☛☛
➨ Glands of Krause and Wolfring:	✓ Accessory Lacrimal glands☛☛

⇨ Structures Passing Through "Inferior Orbital Fissure"

Structures passing through "Inferior orbital fissure": ☛☛☛

- Maxillary division of Trigeminal nerve
- Infraorbital artery
- Zygomatic nerve
- Branches of inferior ophthalmic vein

⇨ Annulus of Zinn

"The Annulus of Zinn", also known as the "Annular tendon" or "Common Tendinous Ring" is a ring of fibrous tissue surrounding the optic nerve at its entrance at the apex of the orbit. It is the origin for five of the six extraocular muscles. JKBOPEE

Annulus of Zinn (Annulus communis tendinis) is seen to transmit: ☛☛ (NAO)

- Occulomotor nerve
- Nasociliary nerve
- Abducent nerve.

⇨ Superior Orbital Fissure

Structures passing through "Superior Orbital Fissure" are:

Live Free To See NO Insult At All.

- Lacrimal Nerve
- Frontal Nerve
- Trochlear Nerve
- Superior Ophthalmic Vein
- Nasociliary Nerve
- Inferior Ophthalamic Vein
- Abducent Nerve

Structures passing through "**Optic Canal**":

- **Optic nerve and ophthalmic artery**

"Optic Nerve Glioma"

- Causes **gradual, painless loss of vision,**
- A tumor of **ist decade of life**

Associated with:

- **Optic atrophy,**
- **Pappilodema,**
- **Neurofibromatosis.**

Embryology of Eye (Very Important Topic for Pg Examinations)

The Eyes are derived from

- **The neuroectoderm of the forebrain**
- **The surface ectoderm of the head**
- **The mesoderm between the above layers**
- **Neural crest cells**

- The **neuroectoderm** of the forebrain differentiates into the
- **Retina,** **MAH 2012**
- **The posterior layers of the iris, and the optic nerve plus**
- **Ciliary epithelium,** **PGI 2011**
- **Sphincter puppilae and** **PGI 2011**
- **Dilator puppilae** **PGI 2011**
- The **surface ectoderm** forms the lens of the eye and the corneal epithelium. The mesoderm between the neuroectoderm and surface ectoderm gives rise to the fibrous and vascular coats of the eye. Mesenchyme is derived from mesoderm.
- **Neural crest cells** migrate into the mesenchyme from the neural crest and differentiate into the choroid, sclera, and corneal endothelium. Homeobox-containing genes, including the **transcription regulator Pax6, fibroblast growth factors**, and other inducing factors play an important role in the molecular development of the eye.
- Eye development is first evident at the **beginning of the fourth week.**
- **Optic grooves** appear in the neural folds at the cranial end of the embryo. As the neural folds fuse to form the forebrain, the optic grooves evaginate to form hollow diverticula-**optic vesicles**-that project from the wall of the forebrain into the adjacent mesenchyme The cavities of the optic vesicles are continuous with the cavity of the forebrain. Formation of the optic vesicles is induced by the mesenchyme adjacent to the developing brain, probably through a chemical mediator. As the optic vesicles grow, their distal ends expand and their connections with the forebrain constrict to form hollow optic stalks.

- **The optic vesicles** soon come in contact with the **surface ectoderm**. Concurrently, the surface ectoderm adjacent to the vesicles thickens to form lens placodes, the primordia of the lenses Formation of lens placodes is induced by the optic vesicles after the surface ectoderm has been conditioned by the underlying mesenchyme. An inductive message passes from the optic vesicles, stimulating the surface ectodermal cells to form the lens primordia. The lens placodes invaginate as they sink deep to the surface ectoderm, forming **lens pits.** The edges of the pits approach each other and fuse to form spherical lens vesicles which soon lose their connection with the surface ectoderm. Development of the lenses from the lens vesicles is described after formation of the eyeball is discussed.
- As the lens vesicles are developing, the **optic vesicles invaginate to form double-walled optic cups.** The opening of each cup is large at first, but its rim infolds around the lens By this stage, the lens vesicles have lost their connection with the surface ectoderm and have entered the cavities of the optic cups. Linear grooves-retinal fissures (optic fissures)-develop on the ventral surface of the optic cups and along the optic stalks the fissures contain vascular mesenchyme from which the hyaloid blood vessels develop. The hyaloid artery, a branch of the ophthalmic artery, supplies the inner layer of the optic cup, the lens vesicle, and the mesenchyme in the cavity of the optic cup. The hyaloid vein returns blood from these structures. As the edges of the retinal fissure fuse, the **hyaloid vessels** are enclosed within the primordial optic nerve **Distal parts of the hyaloid vessels eventually degenerate, but proximal parts persist as the central artery and vein of the retina.**

Development of the Retina

The retina develops from the walls of the optic cup, an outgrowth of the forebrain The outer, thinner layer of the optic cup becomes the retinal pigment epithelium (pigmented layer of retina), and the inner, thicker layer differentiates into the neural retina (neural layer of retina).

Congenital Anomalies of the Eye

- **Coloboma of the Retina**
- This defect is characterized by a localized gap in the retina, usually inferior to the optic disk. The defect is bilateral in most cases. A typical coloboma of the retina results from defective closure of the retinal fissure.
- **Coloboma of the Iris:** Coloboma is a defect in the inferior sector of the iris or a notch in the pupillary margin, giving the pupil a keyhole appearance
- **Congenital Detachment of the Retina**
- **Cyclopia:** In this very rare anomaly, the eyes are partially or completely fused, forming a single median eye enclosed in a single orbit There is usually a tubular nose (proboscis) superior to the eye.
- **Microphthalmia:** The eye may be very small with other ocular defects or it may be a normal-appearing rudimentary eye. The affected side of the face is underdeveloped and the orbit is small. Microphthalmia may be associated with other congenital anomalies (e.g., trisomy 13). Most cases of simple microphthalmia are caused by infectious agents (e.g., rubella virus, Toxoplasma gondii, and herpes simplex virus) that cross the placental membrane during the late embryonic and early fetal periods.
- **Anophthalmia:** denotes congenital absence of the eye, which is rare. The eyelids form, but no eyeball develops.

4

OPHTHALMOLOGY

Mesoderm	Surface Ectoderm	Neuroectoderm
Sclera Choroid Corneal stroma and endothelium AIIMS 09, AIIMS 08 Iris stroma and endothelium Blood vessels Muscles **except iris muscles** **But only** smooth muscles **of iris are derived from mesoderm. COMED 2006** Part of vitreous	Corneal epithelium Conjuctival epithelium AIIMS 2006 Lens AIIMS 2006 Lacrimal and tarsal glands **L2 C2**	Epithelium of iris and ciliary body AIIMS 03 Muscles of iris (constrictor pupillae and dilator pupillae) **Retinal pigment epithelium** **Optic vesicle** **Optic nerve** Part of vitreous

Important Mile Stones in Development of Eye

Eye of new borne is "**Hypermetropic**" by 2-3D	AIIMS 1996
Myelination of optic nerve is **complete at birth.**	
Orbit is **divergent.**	
At 6 weeks **Fixation reflex** is apparent.	
At 2-4 months is **critical period** for development of fixation reflex.	AI 1995
During **Ist 6 months** binocular single vision develops.	
Binocular vision has important role in **depth perception.**	
At **6-8 months depth perception** develops.	

Angles of Eye

— **Alpha angle**: Between visual axis and optical axis.	AI 1988
— **Kappa angle**: Between puppilary axis and visual axis.	AI 1988
— **Visual angle**: angle subtended by object at nodal point of lens.	COMED 2006

Ophthalmological Tests

Direct Ophthalmoscopy	Indirect Ophthalmoscopy
Condensing lens **not required**	Condensing lens **required**
Examination **close** to patient	Examination at a **distance**
Image is **virtual and erect**	**Image is real and inverted** MAH 2012
Magnification is **15 times**	Magnification is **5 times** PGI 1997
Stereopsis **absent**	Stereopsis **present**
Area of field in focus **is 2 disc diopters**	Area of field in focus **is 8 disk diopters**
Examination through hazy media **not possible**	Examination through **hazy media possible**
Illumination **not so bright**	Illumination **bright**
	Is done for **examination of periphery of retina** up to orra seratta. PGI 2002

✓	**Keratometry:** Measures **Curvature** of Cornea	PGI 1999
✓	**Pachymetry: Thickness** of cornea	
✓	**Campimetry:** Measures field of vision	
✓	**Electronystatogram:** Graph of movement of eye:	AMC 1999
✓	**Anomoloscope** detects **color blindness**	DNB 1990
✓	**Retinoscopy: objective assessment of refractive state of eye.**	COMED 2008

Remember:

✓	**Tonometry** measures IOP.	
✓	**Tonography** measures rate of fall in IOP from which facility of aqeous outflow is measured	
✓	**Gonioscopy measures angle of anterior chamber**	PGI 1997
✓	**Best type tonometry is applanation tonometry**	MAHE 2005
✓	**Arden ratio is seen in EOG**	AI 2010

⇨ Macular Function is Tested by

▶	**Indirect slit lamp biomicroscopy**	
▶	**Photo stress test**	
▶	**Two point discrimination test (Card Board test)**	MAHE 2005
▶	**Amsler grid test**	PGI 2K
▶	**Maddox rod test**	MAHE 2005
▶	**Entopic view test**	
▶	**LASER interferometry.**	

⇨ Visual Tests Done in Infants

▶	**Visual evoked potentials**	
▶	**Teller acuity tests**	
▶	**Cardiff acuity tests**	
▶	**Visual acuity by Landolts rings**	MAH 2002

▶	**Swinging flash light test** tests: pupil.	COMED 2008
▶	**Snellens chart tests:** vision.	KERALA 1994
▶	**Retinoscopy** detects errors of refraction.	CUPGEE 1996

4

OPHTHALMOLOGY

⇨ Hirschberg and Kappa Tests

The Hirschberg Test
Is done while the child is binocularly viewing the examiner's transilluminator/penlight in primary gaze. The transilluminator/penlight is held at about 50 cm from the child and held just underneath the examiner's observing eye. The examiner observes the location of the corneal reflexes relative the center of the pupil. A nasal displacement is signified by a (+) sign and a temporal displacement is signified by a (-) sign. The amount of displacement is recorded in the distance, in millimeters, away from center. A normal location will likely be either centered, or +0.5 mm nasally displaced. JK BOPEE 2012
Kappa Test
Is a test of monocular fixation and is done while the child is monocularly viewing the examiner's transilluminator/penlight. The transilluminator/penlight is maintained at 50 cm away. The purpose of this test is to determine the visual axis of each eye. The examiner observes the location of the corneal reflexes relative the center of the pupil in the right eye and then in the left eye. A nasal displacement is signified by a (+) sign and a temporal displacement is signified by a (-) sign, with the amount quantified in millimeters away from center. Again, a normal location will likely be either centered, or +0.5 mm nasally displaced.

➲ Electroretinography: High Yield for 2011-2012 AIPGME

The electroretinogram (ERG) is the record of an action potential produced by the retina when it is stimulated by light of adequate intensity.

The normal ERG is **biphasic.**

- ❒ **The a-wave** is the initial fast negative deflection directly generated by photoreceptors.
- ❒ **The b-wave** is the next slower positive deflection with larger amplitude. Although it is generated from fluxes of potassium ions within and surrounding Müller cells. The b-wave consists of b-1 and b-2 Subcomponents. **The former probably represents both rod and cone activity and the latter mainly cone activity.**

Normal ERG:

1. Scotopic ERG
2. Photopic ERG

Multifocal ERG

Multifocal ERG is a method of producingtopographical maps of retinal function. The stimulus is scaled for variation in photoreceptor density across the retina.

Interpretation: As there is much variation in EOG amplitude in normal subjects, the result is calculated by dividing the maximal height of the potential in the light (Light peak) by the minimal height of the potential in the dark (dark trough). This is expressed as a ratio **(Arden ratio)** or as a percentage. The normal value is over 1.85 or 185%.

Visual Evoked Potential:

The visual evoked potential (VEP) is a recording of electrical activity of the visual cortex created by stimulation of the retina. The main indications are monitoring of visual function in babies and the investigation of optic neuropathy, particularly when associated with

This Farnsworth Munsell 100 Hue test is an easy-to-administer but highly effective method for measuring any individual's color vision.

The test consists of four trays containing a total of 85 removable color reference caps (incremental hue variation) spanning the visible spectrum. Color vision abnormalities and aptitude are detected by the ability of the test subject to place the color caps in order of hue. The Farnsworth-Munsell 100 Hue Test itself is used to separate persons with normal color vision into classes of superior, average and low color discrimination and to measure the zones of color confusion of color defective people.

Some examples of its use are:

- Examination of inspectors of color goods, color graders and color matchers.
- Testing for type and degree of color defectiveness.
- Detection of poor color vision in sales people.
- Selection of applicants for vocational training.
- Design of specialized tests for color vision.
- Measurement of effects of medical treatments.
- Independent control on validity of other color vision tests.

The Farnsworth-Munsell Dichotomous D-15 Test is an abridged version of the 100 Hue Test that is intended for screening color vision defects only. It can be used to detect color vision defects such as red-green and blue-yellow deficiencies as opposed to color acuity. Contains a reference cap and 15 numbered disks with all different hues.

Important Points about Lid

- **"Recurrent" chlazion is predisposed to sebaceous cell carcinoma.** **AIIMS 2006**
- **"Basal cell carcinoma" is the most common type of lid carcinoma.** **AIIMS 1996**
- **Adhesion of margins of two lids is called ankyloblepharon.** **MANIPAL 2006**

Congenital Chronic Dacrocystitis

- Failure of nasolacrimal duct to open into inferior meatus of nose leads to dacrocystitis.
- Presents with **epiphora (Abnormal Tear Overflow)** **AI 2002**
- **And regurgitation of pus.**
  - **Congenital blockage**
  - **Presence of epithelial debris**
  - **Membranous occlusion at its upper end near lacrimal sac**
  - **Complete non-canalization**
  - **Rarely bony occlusion**

Treatment options for congenital NLD obstruction are:

- **Massage over the lacrimal sac area and topical antibiotics**
- **Lacrimal syringing (irrigation) with normal saline and antibiotic solution**
- **Probing of NLD with Bowman's probe**
- **Intubations with silicone tube**
- **Daxeyoxyaroehinoaromy (DCR)**
- **Conjuctivocystorhinostomy.** **PGI 2005**

4

OPHTHALMOLOGY

➲ Field Defects

"Visual Field Defects"

The main points for the exam are:

- **Left homonymous hemianopia means visual field defect to the left, i.e., lesion of right optic tract** **DNB 2011**
- Homonymous quadrantanopias: **PITS** (Parietal-Inferior, Temporal-Superior)
- Incongruous defects = optic tract lesion; congruous defects= optic radiation lesion or occipital cortex

Homonymous Hemianopia

- **Incongruous defects: lesion of optic tract** **SGPI 2005**
- **Congruous defects: lesion of optic radiation or occipital cortex**
- **Macula sparing: lesion of occipital cortex**

Homonymous Quadrantanopias

- Superior: Lesion of temporal lobe **PGI 2003, PGI 2002**
- Inferior: Lesion of parietal lobe
- Mnemonic = PITS (Parietal-Inferior, Temporal-Superior)

Bitemporal Hemianopia **AIIMS 2002**

- Lesion of **optic chiasm**
- **Upper quadrant defect** > **lower quadrant defect** = **inferior chiasmal compression**, commonly a pituitary tumor
- **Lower quadrant defect** > **upper quadrant defect** = **superior chiasmal compression**, commonly a craniopharyngioma

➲ Cranial Nerve II (OPTIC nerve)

- ❒ It is the nerve of **Vision.**
- ❒ It is **not a true nerve** but basically a **diverticulum of the brain** or a tract of the C.N.S.
- ❒ It is **covered by the meninges** and hence any infection can spread directly to the brain.
- ❒ The Optic nerve has **no neurilemma** sheath and once damaged it **cannot regenerate.**
- ❒ It leaves the Orbit through the **Optic Canal.**

<u>The complete Optic Pathway has</u>: **PGI 2002**

1) A receptor
2) A pathway to the Thalamus
3) A nucleus in the Thalamus
4) A radiation from the thalamus to the Cortex
5) A sensory area in the Cortex

The receptors are the **rods and cones of the retina** and the thalamic nucleus for vision is the **lateral geniculate body.**

Functionally, the **retina** is composed of 3 elements i.e. three neurones carry the impulses in the retina "Itself", these are:

1. The receptor cells (the rods and cones)
2. The bipolar nerve cells
3. The ganglion cells

- The **rods and cones** synapse with the bipolar cells (in the retina).
- The **bipolar cells** synapse with the ganglion cells (in the retina also).
- The **axons of the ganglion cells** from the **OPTIC NERVE** which contains nasal and temporal fibers.
- The optic nerves pass to the **OPTIC CHIASMA** (which lies immediately in front of the pituitary gland).
- **The nasal fibers of the optic nerve cross to the opposite side while the temporal fibers remain on the same side.**
- The part of the visual pathway which passes backwards from the chiasma is called the **OPTIC TRACT**.
- Each optic tract carries **«temporal» fibers of its «own» side and «nasal» fibers from the «opposite» side.**
- Most of the fibers of the optic tract end in the **lateral geniculate body** while some fibers leave the optic tract to end in the **superior colliculus** of the midbrain and in the **pretectal nucleus.**

- The fibers of the optic tract which reach the superior Colliculus and the pretectal nucleus are concerned with the light reflex (i.e., narrowing of the pupil in response to excess light) while those fibers of the optic tract which reach the **lateral geniculate body** from part of the visual pathway which will reach the visual cortex.
- **The OPTIC RADIATION (or the geniculo-calcarine tract)** [The pathway from the lateral geniculate body to the visual area of the cortex]
- **The lateral geniculate body (L.G.B.) is the thalamic centre for vision.**
- The axons of the cells of the L.G.B. form the **«optic radiation»** which passes in the internal capsule to reach to the **«striate area» or the Area 17 or the Visual Area in the occipital lobe.**
- **The optic radiation has** fibers running downwards and forwards.
- **THE VISUAL AREA**

  The **«Visual Area»** surrounds the calcarine fissure on the medial surface of the occipital lobe. It is formed of the **cuneus** and the **lingual gyrus.**

4

OPHTHALMOLOGY

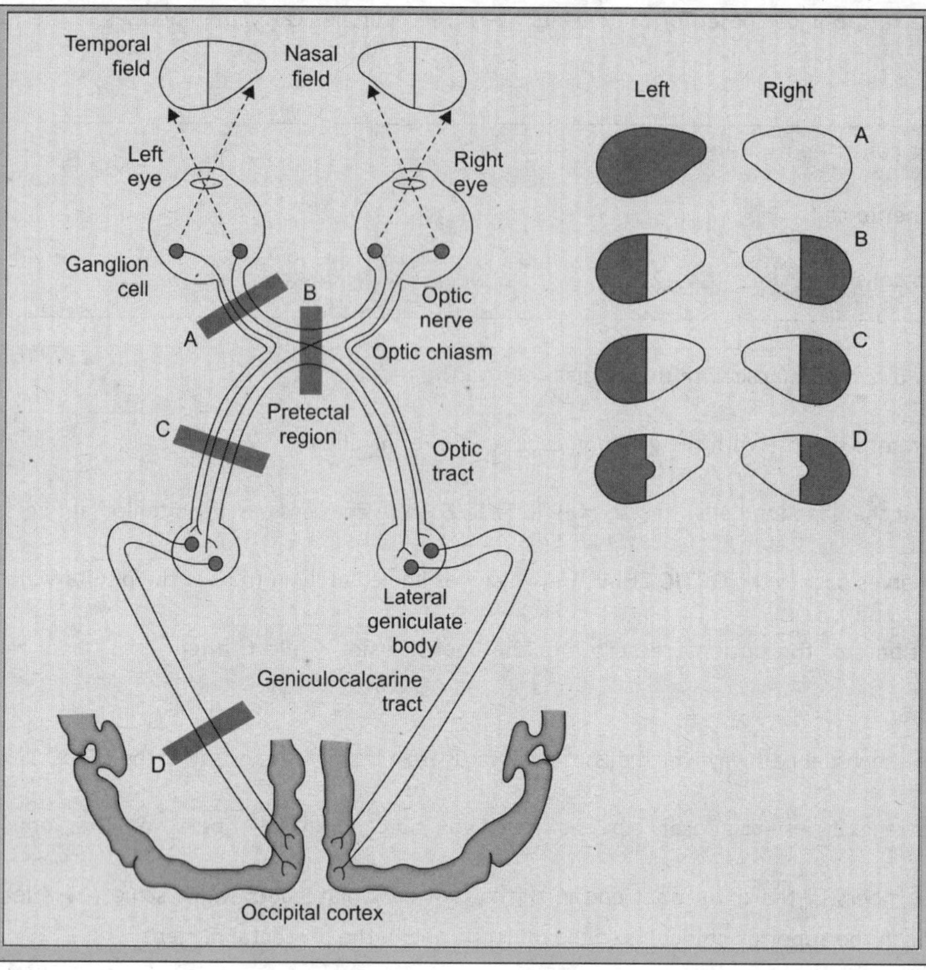

A.	Destruction to one **optic nerve → blindness** in the corresponding eye
B.	Lesion to the middle part of the optic **chiasma** is produced usually from a rumour of the pituitary gland (which lies very close to the optic chiasma). The nasal fibers of the optic nerve which decussate in the chiasma are destroyed and visual impulses from the nasal halves of each retina cannot pass to the optic tract; this means that there will be a **defect in the temporal field of each eye** (a condition called **Bitemporal hemianopia**); in this case the left eye does not see images in the left ½ if its field and the right
C.	eye does not see images in the right ½ of its field **AIIMS 2006, PGI 2001**
D.	A lesion of the optic tract interrupts fibers from one half of each retina. If the left tract is destroyed, visual function will be lost in the left halves of both retinas. In this case there is blindness for objects in the right ½ of each field of vision; this condition is called right homonymous hemianopia. In spite of the fact that one optic tract may be completely interrupted, vision is sometimes preserved in small area (the area of the macula) which is the centre of fixation of the eye. **DNB 2011**
E.	A lesion which destroys the **left optic radiation → right homonymous hemianopia** (as in case of lesion of the left optic tract) **PGI 1997**

- Destruction of area 17 causes blindness.
- Destruction of area 18: Patient can see but cannot recognize what he sees. This is called as "Mind blindness"
- Destruction of area 19: Patient may be able to recognize objects but cannot recall their meaning. This is called "Word Blindness".

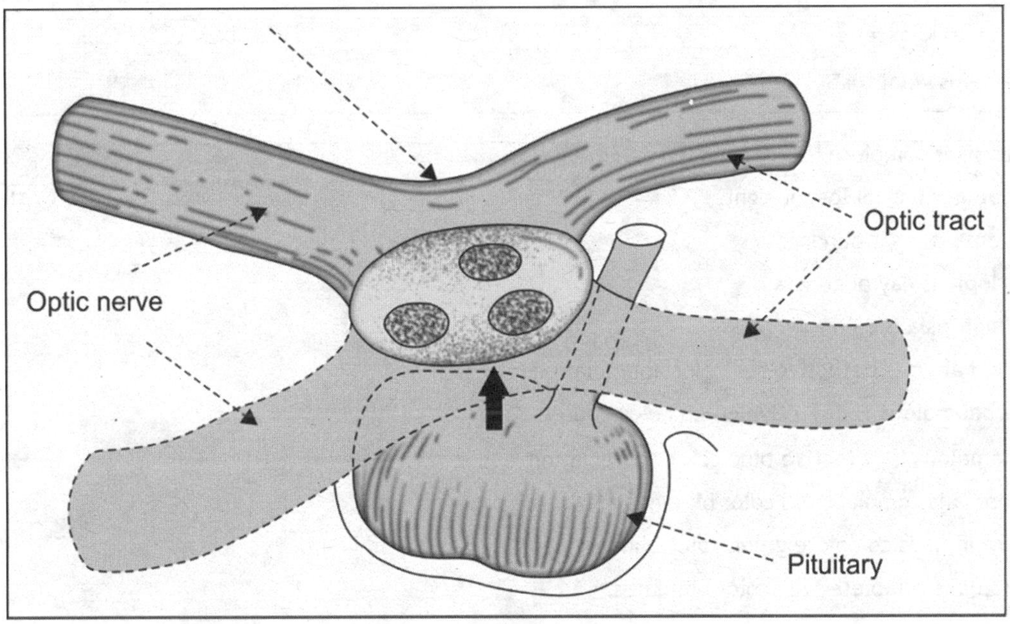

Fig: The pituitary tumor compressing the optic chiasma

Lesion	Clinical Outcome
❒ Lesions of optic nerve	✓ Complete ipsilateral blindness
❒ Saggital (Central) lesions of chiasma e.g. a pituitary tumor	✓ Bilateral hemianopia
❒ Lesions of temporal lobe	✓ Superior quadrantic hemianopia "Pie in sky"
❒ Lesion of parietal lobe	✓ Inferior quadrantic hemianopia " Pie on floor"
❒ Lesions of occipital lobe	✓ Homonymous hemianopia usually sparing of the macula.

⇨ An Optic Nerve Injury May Result in

a) Loss of vision in that eye.

b) Dilatation of pupil.

c) Loss of light reflex.

The afferent pathway for light pupillary reflex is: **Optic nerve**

4

OPHTHALMOLOGY

➲ VISION:

⇨ Color Vision is Tested by

► Ishihara plates	PGI 2007
► Hardy rand Rattler plates	PGI 2007
► Edridge green lantern test	
► City university test	
► Fansworth Munsell 199 hue test	
► Nagels anamoloscope	
► Holmgreens wool test	

✓ **Amaurosis** is complete loss of sight	
✓ **Amblyopia** is partial loss of sight.	AIIMS 1997
✓ **Nyctalopia** is night blindness	
✓ **Hamarlopia** is day blindness	
✓ **Achromatopsia** is color blindness	
✓ **Protanomalous** is **defective** red color appreciation	
✓ **Dueteranomalous** is **defective** green color appreciation	
✓ **Tritanomalous** is **defective** blue color appreciation	
✓ **Protanopia** is complete red color blindness.	AI 2002
✓ **Deuteronopia** is complete green color blindness.	
✓ **Tritanopia** is complete blue color blindness.	

⇨ Amaurosis

This term refers to a "**transient ischemic attack of the retina.**"
❒ Because neural tissue has a <u>**high rate of metabolism**</u>, interruption of blood flow to the retina for more than a few seconds results in **transient monocular blindness**, a term used interchangeably with amaurosis fugax. ☛☛
❒ Patients describe a rapid fading of vision like a **curtain descending**, sometimes affecting only a portion of the visual field. ☛☛ CMC 2001
❒ Amaurosis fugax usually **occurs from an embolus** that becomes stuck within a retinal arteriole
❒ **Ophthalmoscopy** reveals zones of **whitened, edematous retina** following the distribution of branch retinal arterioles. ☛☛
❒ Complete occlusion of the central retinal artery produces arrest of blood flow and a milky retina with a **cherry-red fovea.**
❒ Emboli are composed of either **cholesterol (Hollenhorst Plaque)**, ☛☛ calcium, or platelet-fibrin debris. JK BOPEE
❒ The most common source is an atherosclerotic plaque in the **carotid artery or aorta**, although emboli can also arise from the heart, especially in patients with diseased valves, atrial fibrillation, or wall motion abnormalities.

- Retinal arterial occlusion also occurs rarely in association with **retinal migraine, lupus erythematosus, anticardiolipin antibodies, anticoagulant deficiency states (protein S, protein C, and antithrombin III deficiency), pregnancy, intravenous drug abuse, blood dyscrasias, dysproteinemias, and temporal arteritis.**
- Amaurosis fugax **warns of a patient at high-risk for stroke.**
- Marked systemic hypertension causes sclerosis of retinal arterioles, splinter hemorrhages, **focal infarcts of the nerve fiber layer (cotton-wool spots),** and **leakage of lipid and fluid (hard exudate)** into the macula. In hypertensive crisis, sudden visual loss can result from vasospasm of retinal arterioles and consequent retinal ischemia. In addition, acute hypertension may produce visual loss from ischemic swelling of the optic disk.

⇨ Hard Exudates

Are yellow spots seen in the retina, usually in the posterior pole near the macula **PGI 2009**

They are lipid break-down products that are left behind after localized edema resolves. These can be seen in any conditions that are associated with chronic vascular leakage, such as:

- **Diabetic retinopathy**
- **Hypertensive retinopathy**
- **Coat's disease**
- **Capillary hemangioma of the retina (Von Hippel-Lindau Disease)**
- **Choroidal neovascularization**
- **Retinal arterial macroaneurysm**
- **Retinal vein occlusion, angiomas**

⇨ Optic Reflexes

1. The Light Reflex

(Constriction of the pupil in response to excess light)

This is a "**protective**" reflex: **the pupil becomes narrow to prevent excess light from injuring the rods and cones in the retina.**

Types: There are 2 types of light reflex – **Direct** and **Indirect**

Direct Pupillary Reflex:

Light falls on the RIGHT eye → constriction of the RIGHT pupil.

In direct Pupillary Reflex: (Consensual light reflex)

Light falls on the RIGHT eye → constriction of the LEFT pupil.

⇨ Pathway of the Light Reflex

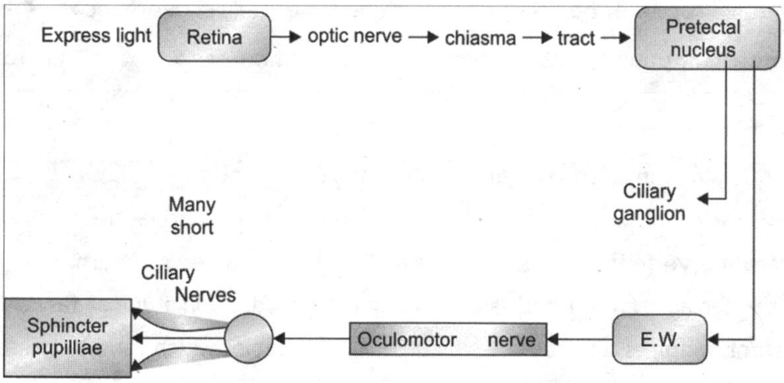

- Excess light → RETINA → optic nerve → optic chasma → optic tract PGI 1999
- Some fibers leave the optic tract to reach the **PRETECTAL NUCLEUS** (which is part of the superior colliculus in Man). Each pretectal nucleus sends fibers to the Edinger-Westphal (E.W.) part of the oculomotor nucleus of the two sides. PGI 2001
- Edinger- Westphal part of the oculomotor [III] nucleus of the **Rt and Lt.** sides → (preganglionic fibers) in the oculomotor [III] nerves (of both sides) → the cilliary ganglia (on both sides).
- Each ciliary ganglion → (postganglionic fibers) in the short ciliary nerves →sphincter pupiliae muscle → constriction of the pupil.

Accommodation:

An object placed 6 meters or more from the eye considered a "far" object and light rays falling on the eye from it are parallel and are brought to focus on the retina. This is vision "**at rest**".

A "near" object is placed nearer than 6 metres from the eye (e.g. a book). Light rays falling on the eye from a near object are divergent. In order to bring them to focus on the retina the **LENS MUST INCREASE ITS THICKNESS** to have a stronger refractive power. This is called accommodation. In order for the lens to increase its thickness, the ciliary muscle must contract; contraction of the ciliary muscle → **relaxation of the suspensory ligament of the lens** → thicker and more powerful lens.

⇨ Pathway of Accomodation

Light from a near object → RETINA → optic nerve → optic chiasma → optic tract → Lateral geniculate body (L.G. B.) → optic radiation → AREA 17 of the occipital cortex.

The first picture which falls on the eye does not fall in focus on the retina so the first picture which reaches the visual cortex is blurred (not seen clearly). Area 17 now sends signal to area 19.

In order to make the picture fall on the retina area 19 sends signal to the **superior colliculus** (in the midbrain) **(by way of the occipito-tectal tract)**. The superior colliculus then sends orders to **Edinger-Westphal nucleus** of the third nerve → **contractions of the ciliary muscle → relaxation of the suspensory ligament → thicker and more powerful lens → picture NOW falls in focus on the retina** can be seen clearly when it reaches the visual area.

Why does a student who studies for a long time become tired?

This is because he is contracting 3 sets of his muscles:

- **Contracting the ciliary muscle of both eyes (i.e. accommodation).**
- **Contracting the medial rectus of both eyes at the same time (i.e., convergence).**
- **Contracting the constrictor pupillae of both eyes (to prevent spherical aberration) and to see clearly.**

⇨ Corneal Reflex

Light touching of the cornea or conjunctiva results in blinking of the eyelids. AI 2006

On touching the cornea **afferent impulses from the cornea or conjunctiva** travel through the **ophthalmic division of the trigeminal nerve** to the sensory nucleus of the trigeminal nerve. Internuncial neurons connect with the motor nucleus of the facial nerve on both sides through the medial longitudinal fasciculus. The **facial nerve which carries the efferent impulses** supplies the orbicularis oculi muscle, which causes closure of the eyelids.

Remember:

- **Rods are more sensitive to light.**
- **Cones**, on the other hand, are sensitive to specific wavelengths of light allowing you to **discern colors**

The Fovea is a small shallow depression in the central region of the eye located such that

- Most of the incident light collected by the cornea and lens is focused onto this region
- Most of the inner layers of the retina are markedly reduced or absent and what dominates is a layer of photoreceptors
- Retinal vessels are also absent in the region of the fovea
- Is most sensitive part of eye AIIMS 1992

Disorders of Cranial Nerves Related to Eye

The Third (Oculomotor) Nerve Palsy

It supplies all extraocular muscles except the superior oblique and the lateral rectus AI 2002

Complete paralysis results in:

- **External ophthalmoplegia:** In a **complete lesion** inability to move the eye upward, inward and downward. PGI 2003
- **External Squint:** the eye is deviated laterally and downwards due to the unopposed action of the lateral rectus and superior oblique.
- **Diplopia:** A person sees double.
- **Ptosis:** drooping of the upper eyelids due to paralysis of levator palpabrea superioris. AIIMS 2011
- **Dilated non-reactive pupil** due to paralysis of the sphincter pupillae.
- The **pupil also shows no reaction to light** (direct or consensual), or to accommodation.
- **Puppilary sparing** is seen in Diabetes mellitus. AIIMS 1995

The Fourth (Trochlear) Nerve Palsy

- There is weakness or paralysis of the **superior oblique muscle which normally moves the eye downwards and inwards.** PGI 1999
- **Result:** defective depression of the adducted eye. The patient is unable to look at his shoulder.
- **Symptom Presentation: DIPLOPIA** (double vision), **when looking downwards** e.g. when reading or descending the stairs. The head may tilt to the opposite side to minimize the diplopia

The Sixth (Abducent) Nerve Palsy

The sixth nerve supplies the **lateral rectus which normally rotates the eye laterally.**

Its paralysis causes: AIIMS 08

- **Internal Squint:** The eyeball is turned inwards due to unopposed adduction of the medial rectus.
- **Diplopia,** which is maximum on **looking outwards.**
- **Limitation of abduction** of the corresponding eye.

⇨ Arygyll Robertson Pupil

This Consists of:

- Constriction of the pupil (meiosis), which fails to dilate completely with mydriatics.
- Irregularity of the pupil.
- Absence of light reflex, but normal accommodation reflex. This combination is diagnostic of the condition.
- It is especially seen in Syphilis of the Nervous System (NEURO SYPHILIS). ☚☚

⇨ Adie's Tonic Pupil

- The pupil is dilated in one eye.
- Loss of light reflex (direct and consensual). ☚☚
- The condition is benign and is seen in healthy individuals (mostly females).

⇨ Horner's Syndrome☚☚

This results from paralysis of the sympathetic fibers at any site along its long course in the head, in the neck or mediastium as a result, e.g, of neoplasm or trauma. It consists of:

- **Ptosis**, which is partial - the lid may be slightly raised voluntarily. **PGI 2000**
- **Enopthalmos** **AI 1996**
- **Miosis**: fixed construction i.e. does not dilate on shading the eye. **AI 1998**
- **Anhydrosis:** Loss of sweating on ipsilateral half of head and face when the lesion is proximal to sympathetic fiber separation along the external carotid.
- Loss of the ciliospinal reflex.

Causes:

- Brainstem (Vascular-syringobulbia).☚☚
- Cervical cord (Glioma- syringobulbia).☚☚
- Damage to C8, T1.☚☚
- Cervical sympathetic chain damage by: pancoast tumor of lung.☚☚

⇨ Remember Important Points about Nerves Supplying Eye

- The sixth cranial nerve innervates the lateral rectus muscle.
- Palsy of Abducens nerve produces horizontal diplopia, worse on gaze to the side of the lesion.
- Foville's syndrome following "Dorsal pontine injury" (VI, VII) CN
  - ✓ Includes lateral gaze palsy, VI,
  - ✓ Ipsilateral facial palsy, and VII,
  - ✓ Contralateral hemiparesis incurred by damage to descending corticospinal fibers.
- **Millard-Gubler syndrome** following **"Ventral pontine injury"** is similar, except for the eye findings. There is lateral rectus weakness only, instead of gaze palsy, because the abducens fascicle is injured rather than the nucleus.
- **Infarct, tumor, hemorrhage, vascular malformation, and multiple sclerosis are the most common etiologies of brainstem abducens palsy.**

- ► In the cavernous sinus, the nerve can be affected by carotid aneurysm, carotid cavernous fistula, tumor (pituitary adenoma, meningioma, nasopharyngeal carcinoma), herpes infection, and Tolosa-Hunt syndrome.
- ► **Unilateral or bilateral abducens palsy is a classic sign of raised intracranial pressure.**

Oculomotor Nerve: The third cranial nerve innervates the medial, inferior, and superior recti; inferior oblique; levator palpebrae superioris; and the iris sphincter.

Total palsy of the oculomotor nerve causes **ptosis, a dilated pupil, and leaves the eye "down and out"** because of the unopposed action of the lateral rectus and superior oblique **AIIMS 2012, AIPGME 2011**

Injury to structures surrounding fascicles of the oculomotor nerve descending through the midbrain has given rise to a number of classic eponymic designations.

- ► **Nothnagel's Syndrome**, injury to the superior cerebellar peduncle causes **ipsilateral oculomotor palsy and contralateral cerebellar ataxia.**
- ❒ **Benedikt's Syndrome**, injury to the red nucleus results in **ipsilateral oculomotor palsy and contralateral tremor, chorea, and athetosis.**
- ❒ **Claude's Syndrome** incorporates features of **both the aforementioned syndromes**, by injury to both the red nucleus and the superior cerebellar peduncle.
- ❒ **Weber's Syndrome**, injury to the cerebral peduncle causes **ipsilateral oculomotor palsy with contralateral hemiparesis.** **UPSC 1995**

Trochlear Nerve: The fourth cranial nerve originates in the midbrain, just caudal to the oculomotor nerve complex.

- ► Fibers exit the brainstem dorsally and cross to innervate the contralateral superior oblique.
- ► The principal actions of this muscle are to **depress and to intort the globe.**
- ► **Supplies superior oblique muscle.**
- ► A palsy therefore results **in hypertropia and excyclotorsion.**
- ► The **"head tilt test"** is a cardinal diagnostic feature.

➲ Eye Lid Tumors

Basal cell, squamous cell, or meibomian gland carcinoma should be suspected for any **"nonhealing, ulcerative lesion" of the eyelids.**

Basal cell Carcinoma:

- ► **It is the most common tumor of eye lid.** ☛☛
- ► **Lower lid is the most common site.**

Found in association with

- ► **Xeroderma pigmentosa,** ☛☛
- ► **Gorlin Goltz syndrome**☛☛

⇨ Ptosis

"Ptosis": Drooping of upper eye lids	**AI 1995**
Tylosis: hypertrophy and drooping of eye lids.	**AIIMS 1986**

4

OPHTHALMOLOGY

- **Blepharoptosis** This is an abnormal drooping of the eyelid. Unilateral or bilateral ptosis can be congenital, from dysgenesis of the levator palpebrae superioris, or from abnormal insertion of its aponeurosis into the eyelid.
- **Mechanical Ptosis** This occurs in many **elderly patients from stretching and redundancy of eyelid skin and subcutaneous fat (dermatochalasis).** The extra weight of these sagging tissues causes the lid to droop. Enlargement or deformation of the eyelid from infection, tumor, trauma, or inflammation also results in ptosis on a purely mechanical basis.
- **Aponeurotic Ptosis** This is an **acquired dehiscence or stretching of the aponeurotic tendon, which connects the levator muscle to the tarsal plate of the eyelid.** It occurs commonly in older patients, presumably from **loss of connective tissue elasticity**. Aponeurotic ptosis is also a frequent sequela of eyelid swelling from infection or blunt trauma to the orbit, cataract surgery, or hard contact lens usage.
- **Myogenic Ptosis** The causes of myogenic ptosis include **myasthenia gravis** and a number of rare myopathies that manifest with ptosis.
- **In the Kearns-Sayre variant**, retinal pigmentary changes and abnormalities of cardiac conduction develop. Peripheral muscle biopsy shows characteristic "ragged-red fibers."
- **Oculopharyngeal dystrophy** is a distinct autosomal dominant disease with onset in middle age, characterized by ptosis, limited eye movements, and trouble swallowing.
- **Myotonic dystrophy**, another autosomal dominant disorder, causes ptosis, ophthalmoparesis, cataract, and pigmentary retinopathy. Patients have muscle wasting, myotonia, frontal balding, and cardiac abnormalities.
- **Neurogenic Ptosis** This results from a lesion affecting the innervation to either of the two muscles that open the eyelid: Muller's muscle or the levator palpebrae superioris.
- **In Horner's syndrome**, the eye with ptosis has a smaller pupil and the eye movements are full.
- **Patient with non retractable ptosis gets corrected due to action like mimicking, chewing in marcus gunn jaw winking syndrome.** **AI 2010**
- **In an oculomotor nerve palsy**, the eye with the ptosis has a larger, or a normal, pupil. If the pupil is normal but there is limitation of adduction, elevation, and depression, a pupil-sparing oculomotor nerve palsy is likely **AIIMS 1997**
- **Corrected by Blaskowicks operation.** **Delhi 1991**

⇨ Horner's Syndrome **AIIMS 08**

- **Ptosis,** **JK BOPEE 2011**
- **Miosis,**
- **Anhydrosis,**
- **Loss of ciliospinal reflex**
- **Treated by Fansella servat operation.** **AI 2003**

Additional Signs :

- Slight elevation of the inferior eyelid
- The pupillary reactions are normal to both light and accomodation.
- The pupil is slow to dilate
- Keterochrornia (ipsilateral iris is of lighter color) in congenital Homer's syndrome
- Anhydrosis not always

Cavernous Sinus Thrombosis: Features

Infection from nose, sinuses, orbits or pharynx with high fever, chills and

- **Ptosis**
- **Proptosis**
- **Chemosis**
- **Loss of accommodation and loss of puppilary reflex**
- **Dilated pupil**
- **Diplopia**
- **Engorged retinal veins**

Dermoid cyst:	✓ Located subcutaneously along embryonic lines of closure.
Capillary hemangioma:	✓ Most common tumor of orbit and periorbital areas in **childhood.**
Orbital pseudotumor:	✓ Enlargement of extraoccular muscles
Cavernous hemangioma:	✓ Most common benign orbital tumor. Most common in second to fifth decade

Refractive Errors

Myopia

- Myopia is **short sightedness.**
- Rays of light focused **in front** of retina **PGI 2006**
- **Big eye ball is seen. PGI 1983**
- Corrected by **concave lens.**
- **Deep** anterior chamber.
- Patient squeezes eyes to see distant things clearly.
- ✓ **Myopic crescents (on temporal side)**
- ✓ **Foster fuchs spots**
- ✓ **Cystoid degeneration**
- ✓ **Lattice and snail track degeneration. AIIMS 98**
- ✓ **Peripheral retinal degeneration. AIIMS 1993**
- ✓ **Posterior staphyloma**

➲ Surgeries for Myopia

— Radial keratotomy (SMALL DEGREE)	JK 2006
— Photo refractive keratotomy	
— Automated lamellar keratectomy	
— Soft Contact lens	APPG 2006
— LASIK	Manipal 2006
— LASEK	
— Intracorneal rings	
— Clear lens extraction	

⇨ Hypermetropia

- ▶ Is **long sightedness.**
- ▶ Rays of light focused **behind retina.**
- ▶ Corrected by **convex lens.**
- ▶ **Shallow** anterior chamber.
- ▶ Eye ball and cornea are **small.**

Presbyopia:	
❐ Not an error of refraction.	
❐ Weakness of ciliary muscles, ligaments	
❐ Loss of elasticity of lens capsule.	PGI 1983
❐ Condition of **physiological insufficency of accomdation.**	PGI 2004
❐ **Loss of power of accommodation is seen.**	CUPGEE 1996
❐ Physiological change appropriate for age.	
❐ Treatment is **convex lens.**	PGI 2002

⇨ Astigmatism

▶ Is **spherical abbertion**	PGI 1985
▶ Due to **irregular curvature of cornea**	SRMC 2002
▶ Corrected by **convex lens**	

⇨ Aphakia

Is absence of crystalline lens	
❐ Eye becomes **hypermetropic.**	
❐ **Accommodation is lost.**	
✓ **Deep anterior chamber,**	
✓ **Jet black pupil,**	
✓ **Iridodenesis,**	
✓ **Purkinjes image test show only two test images.**	
❐ **Post chamber IOL** is the treatment of choice.	AI 1998
❐ **Spectacles are prescribed to patient of aphakia after 6 weeks of surgery.**	AP 1994

✓	↑inter pupillary distance: **Hypertelorism**
✓	↓inter pupillary distance: **Hypotelorism**
✓	↑inter canthal distance: **Telecanthus**
✓	**Convergent squint (esotropia)** is due to 6 th nerve palsy
✓	**Divergent squint (exotropia)** is due to 3 rd nerve palsy
✓	**In paralytic squint** primary deviation <secondary deviation
✓	**Inconcomitant squint primary deviation = secondary deviation**

⇨ Nystagmus

Congenital Nystagmus

- Is defined as conjugate, spontaneous and involuntary ocular ossilations that appear at birth or during the first three months of life which later on persists throughout the life.
- Oscillations are usually horizontal in direction but may be primarily vertical, torsional, or anycombination of these three.
- Infantile nystagmus often is associated with other ocular conditions that impair visual acuity andoccasionally can herald life-threatening conditions.
- Causes: The cause of congenital nystagmus is not known.
- In terms of genetics, there appears to be different hereditary types of congenital nystagmusincluding, autosomal, X-linked, dominant and recessive.

Some common causes are:

- ▶ **Congenital cataract,**
- ▶ **Congenital toxoplasmosis,**
- ▶ **Macular hypoplasia,**
- ▶ **Aniridia,**
- ▶ **Albinism,**
- ▶ **Optic nerve hypoplasia and**
- ▶ **Leber's congenital amaurosis.**

Pathophysiology:

A defect in motor control of visual fuxationor an abnormal development of fixation of the brainwithout any detectable central nervous system abnormalities, as well as instability of the neuralintegrator responsible for gaze holder may underlie the pathology. Idiopathic congenital nystagmuscan increase during fixation and decreases in non-visual tasks.

✓	**Down beat Nystagmus** is seen in: cerebellar/ brain stem lesions, multiple sclerosis, alcohol, anticonvulsants and lithium intoxication. **PGI 1988**
✓	**Upbeat Nystagmus** is seen in **pontine lesions**
✓	**Vestibular Nystagmus** is seen in **Meniers disease, Vestibular lesions**
✓	**Rotatory Nystagmus: Miners Nystagmus** **JIPMER 1988**

Anisokenia: Difference in **image size. (USE CONTACT LENS)**	**Kerala 1997**
Anisometropia: Difference in **refraction of two eyes.**	**SGPGI 2005**
Anisocoria: Difference in **pupil size of two eyes.**	

Conjuctiva

- **Conjunctivitis** is an inflammatory response of the conjunctival vessels to a variety of insults.
- **Chemical conjunctivitis** caused by instillation of silver nitrate drops is the most common cause of conjunctivitis in the **first 24 hours of life.**
- **Neisseria gonorrhea and Chlamydia trachomatis** are common infectious causes acquired by passage through the birth canal. Chlamydia is the most common cause of infectious ophthalmia neonatorum. Bacteria, such as **Haemophilus, Streptococcus, Staphylococcus,** or **Pneumococcus,** usually cause acute purulent conjunctivitis. Viruses (adenovirus, enterovirus) may cause an isolated conjunctivitis or one associated with an exanthem. **Adenovirus causes epidemic conjunctivitis.** **DNB 2011**
- **Allergic conjunctivitis** usually develops after the neonatal period. Clinically, tearing, conjunctival injection, lid edema, and discharge are characteristic. Pain, photophobia, and decreased vision are rare and indicate corneal disease.
- **Gonococcal conjunctivitis** is purulent and **can occur at birth or after 5 days of age if the patient has received topical antibiotic prophylaxis at birth.**

Conjuctivitis and Most Frequently asked Questions

— **Hemorrhagic Conjunctivitis:** Enterovirus adenovirus coxsackie virus	**DNB 2011**
— **Acute puruluent conjunctivitis** Staph.aureus	
— **Phylentecular conjunctivitis:** Tuberculosis, staph aureus	**AI 2003**
— **Giant papillary conjunctivitis:** Contact lens	**APPG 2006**
— **Acute membranous conjunctivitis:** Cornye bacterium diptheriae, streptococcus hemolyticus	
— **Acute follicular conjunctivitis:** Chlamydia trachomatis	
— **Epidemic kerato conjunctivitis/ Pharyngo Conjuctival fever:** Adeno virus	
— **Granulomatous conjunctivitis:** Granulomatous diseases.	
— **Angular conjunctivitis:** Moraxella	**PGI 2000**

Phylenticular Conjunctivitis

► Type IV hypersensitivity reaction.	**AI 2003**
► Due to staph aureus (MC) and tuberculous protein.	
► Koeppes nodule,	
► Busaca nodules are manifestations.	
► MC allergic manifestation is Koppes nodule	**AIIMS 2001**
► Phylecten is hence due to endogeneous causes. (Papules at limbus)	**AIPGME 2011/12**
► Doc: Topical steroids	

⇨ Inclusion Conjunctivitis

Inclusion conjunctivitis is caused by **chiarnydia trachomatis (serotypes D-K).**

Chlamydial inclusion conjunctivitis:

- Is generally spread by **sexual transmission**
- The modes of transmission are **orogenital activities** and hand to eye spread of infective genital secretions.
- A common mode of transmission is through the **water in swimming pools**; thus the disease may occur in local epidemics (swimming pool conjunctivitis). It is also transmitted from the mother to the newborn.
- Effective Treatment: azithromycin or doxycycline.

"Shield Ulcer" of the Cornea in Vernal conjunctivitis — **MAH 2012**

The cornea may be affected as well in vernal conjunctivitis. An indolent superficial ulcer develops with opaque edges and plaque formation through deposition of mucus and cells. Here one sees a **partially healed shield ulcer** with ring-like superficial opacification and some remaining debris.

Vernal shield ulcers develop in the upper regions of the cornea. **The base of the ulcer is composed of abnormal mucus, fibrin and serum, deposited as a gray plaque. Friction secondary to the roughened superior conjunctiva erodes the corneal epithelium.**

⇨ Spring Catarrh

▶ **Recurrent, bilateral conjuctivitis**	
▶ **Horner Trantas spots on bulbar conjunctiva**	PGI 2003
▶ **More common in <u>summer</u> not spring.**	
▶ **Burning and itching are common.**	
▶ **Cobble stone appearance of palpebral conjunctiva.**	AIIMS 1997
▶ **Pseudogerentoxon with cupid bow appearance.**	
▶ **Papillary hypertrophy,**	PGI 2003
▶ **Type 1 Hypersensitivity**	PGI 2005
▶ **Maxweell lyon sign (stringy, ropy discharge)**	PGI 2001
▶ **Shield ulcer**	
▶ **DOC: steroids**	

⇨ Trachoma

- Trachoma is a **chronic Keratoconjuctivitis** affecting conjunctiva and cornea simultaneously.
- It is caused by **Chlamydia Trachomatis 11 Serotypes (A-K).**
- It is one of the leading causes of preventable blindness.
- **Unhygienic conditions** predispose.
- Incubation period of trachoma varies **from 5-21 days**
- Trachoma is characterized by presence of follicles which contain Histiocytes, lymphocytes and large multinucleated cells called **"Leber cells".**

4

OPHTHALMOLOGY

- Trachoma is characterized by presence of **Limbal follicles or "Herberts Pits"** formed on the cornea near the limbus. **PGI 2000**
- **Conjuctival scarring** may be present in the form of irregular or stellate present in sulcus subtarsalis called "Artls line." **PGI 2002**
- "Pannus": infiltration of cornea with vascularization is a feature.
- **SAFE strategy Surgery, antibiotics, facial cleanliness, environmental improvement.** **AI 2003**
- DOC: Tetracycline **AIIMS 1990**

⇨ **SAFE' Strategy for Trachoma**

It Includes

Surgery- first component of the strategy for correction of trichiasis and entropion

Antibiotics – **Azithromycin, Tetracycline eye ointment.**

Face washing -breaks the cycle of reinfection and prevents transmission of disease.

Environmental Improvement - Poverty and poor living conditions contribute to high rates of blinding trachoma.

Environmental improvement includes.

- **Availability of improved water supplies**
- **Improved household sanitation, particularly safe disposal of feces.**

Pinguecula:

- Is a **small, raised conjunctival nodule** at the temporal or nasal limbus. In adults such lesions are extremely common and have little significance, unless they become inflamed **(pingueculitis).**
- Is hyaline infiltration and elastatoic degeneration.

Pterygium:

- Resembles a pinguecula but has <u>crossed</u> **the limbus to encroach upon the corneal surface.** Removal is justified when symptoms of irritation or blurring develop, but recurrence is a common problem.
- **It is elastatoic degeneration with proliferation of vascularized granulation tissue.** **AIIMS 2008**
- **Stocker's line is seen.** **JK 2008**

- Wing shaped fold of conjunctiva encroaching upon cornea from either side.
- Usually present on nasal side.
- Degenerative and hyperplastic condition of conjunctiva.
- Corneal epithelium, Bowmans layer, superficial stroma are destroyed.

Complications:

- ✓ **Infection**
- ✓ **Cystic degeneration**
- ✓ **Neoplastic change to epithelioma**
- ✓ **Fibrosarcoma, malignant melanoma**

Mitomycin, thiotepa and ß irradiation are used for treatment

⇨ Glaucoma

- Aqueous humor is produced by **Ciliary processes**. At the rate of 2 μl/min.
- Aqueous humor has **less protein** than plasma.
- It **maintains IOP. (Intra ocular pressure)** AI 1988
- It provides **substrates and removes metabolites from cornea.**
- It flows from posterior chamber to anterior chamber.
- **Carbonic anhydrase** is important in aqueous humor production.
- **Conventional outflow** is main pathway and uveoscleral outflow is minor pathway.

⇨ "Congenital Glaucoma"

- **Boys effected** more AI 1988
- Bilateral
- Blepharospasm
- **Big, (Bupthalmos) "ox eyes", Large cornea** PGI 1998
- Blue eyes.
- Presents as photophobia. TN 2003
- Hazy frosted glass cornea due to edema with Habbs striae. **"Habbs striae are due to breaks in descements membrane where corneal opacities appear as lines with double contours."** PGI 2004
- Lens flattened anterio posteriorly.
- Deep anterior chamber.
- **Goniotomy** or **Trabeculotomy** is used for treatment
- **Trabeculectomy** is considered in case of failure of above procedures.
- **Trabeculotomy and trabeculectomy (Combined)** is preferential method of choice. AIIMS 03
- **"Hereditary glaucoma" is due to optineurin abnormality** AIIMS 2003

⇨ "Secondary" Congenital Glaucoma is associated with

- Aniridia
- Neurofibromatosis
- Sturge Weber syndrome
- Rubella
- Mesodermal dysgenesis.

Megalocornea:

- Defined as **diameter of cornea >11.7 mm at birth or >13 mm at age 2 years.**
- Cornea usually clear with normal thickness and vision.
- **Usually bilateral** and **non progressive**
- Associated with **Marfans syndrome.**

4

OPHTHALMOLOGY

4

OPHTHALMOLOGY

⇨ Primary Open Angle Glaucoma

❒ Mostly asymptomatic or **progressive painless** loss of vision.	PGI 2004
❒ Difficulty in near work and frequent change of presbyopic glasses.	
❒ Mild headache or eye ache.	
❒ **Optineurin gene** and **MYOC gene** are implicated in pathogenesis.	AIIMS 03
❒ **Classical Triad is: ↑IOP, classic Field defects, Cupping of optic disk**	

⇨ Visual Field Defects in Glaucoma are

► **Barring of blind spot. (Early)**	PGI 83
► **Paracentral scotoma in Bjerrums area or arcuate area.**	
► **Seidels scotoma.**	
► **Arcuate or bjerrums scotoma.**	
► **Roennes nasal step.**	
► **Tubular vision.**	
► **Total blindness.**	

⇨ Optic Disk Changes in Glaucoma are

❒ Oval cup, Asymmetric cup or Large cup
❒ Splinter hemorrhages
❒ Pallor of cup
❒ Atrophy of retinal nerve fiber layer
❒ Pallor of disk.
❒ **Bayonetting sign, Lamellar dot sign**

Ist line treatment is: **Timolol**	**COMED 2008**
Argon LASER Trabeculoplasty is done in open angle glaucoma	**COMED 2008**

➲ Angle Closure Glaucoma:

⇨ Predisposing Factors

❒ **Shallow anterior chamber**	PGI 2005
❒ **Anterior dislocation of iris- lens diaphragm**	
❒ **Small corneal diameter**	
❒ **Hypermetropia**	

✓ More common in females	
✓ Dilatation of pupil in dim light.	
✓ Atropine, mydriatics worsen the condition	
✓ May present as painful red eye with headache, nausea vomiting	PGI 1999

⇨ Features (In Increasing Order of Severity and Progression)

- Narrow angle, shallow anterior chamber
- IOP ↑ with pupil dilated
- **Sudden onset severe pain in eye** with nausea, vomiting, progressive loss of vision, photophobia, lacrimation.
- **Pupil is semi dilated, vertically oval and fixed.** PGI 2007
- It is **non reactive** to light and accommodation
- Eye becomes **painful, irritable and completely blind**
- **In acute congestive stage of PACG pilocarpine is the "initial DOC".**
- **Laser iridotomy** and **surgical iridectomy** are procedures of choice. SGPGI 2005
- The **fellow eye** requires **prophylactic peripheral iridotomy and surgical iridectomy.**
- **PPP** (Painful, Pilocarpine, Peripheral iridotomy)

⇨ Neo Vascular Glaucoma

Usually associated with neovascularization of Iris **(Rubeosis iridis).** Seen in association with: PGI 1999

- Diabetic retinopathy
- Eales disease
- CRVO
- Sickle cell retinopathy
- CRAO
- Intraocular tumors
- Intraocular inflammation.
- Treated by **Pan Retinal Photocoagulation** AIIMS 2006

➲ Steroid Induced Glaucoma

The steroid **most likely** among the choices to cause steroid induced glaucoma on topical application is **Betamethasone.**

5-6% of people on Betamethasone develop increased IOP after 4-6 weeks.

This condition is more in people with:

- **Primary open angle glaucoma**
- **Ist degree relative**
- **Diabetes Mellitus**
- **High Myopes**

Drugs used in treatment of glaucoma:

Acetazolamide is a carbonic anhydrase inhibitor used in treating glaucoma.

Mannitol is also used as an IV Solution used in treating glaucoma.

Other drugs used in glaucoma are:

- **Topical Pilocarpine 2%**
- **Topical Timolol**

4

OPHTHALMOLOGY

- Topical Dorzolamide
- Topical Brinzolamide.
- Atropine is contraindicated in glaucoma.

Pigmentary glaucoma

- Is a form of **open angle glaucoma** with **AD pattern of inheritance** with **pigment disruption of iris and deposition in anterior chamber.**
- Corneal pigmentation **(Krukenbergs spindle)** is a feature

⇨ Neovascular Glaucoma (NVG) is seen in

- Diabetic retinopathy
- Central retinal venous occlusion
- Sickle cell retinopathy
- Eale's disease
- Chronic intraocular inflammations
- Intraocular tumors
- Long standing retinal detachment
- Central retinal artery occlusion.

High Yield for 2011, 2012

⇨ Treatment of Acute Congestive Glaucoma

Is essentially surgical. However, medical therapy instituted as an emergency and temporary measure before the eye is ready for operation. Different modalities are:

Medical Therapy:

- **IV systemic hyperosmotic agent (Mannitol)**
- **Carbonic anhydrase inhibitor (Acetazolamide)**
- **Analgesics and antiemetics**
- **Pilocarpine eye drops**
- **Beta blocker eye drops (Timolol)**
- **Corticosteroid eye drops**

Surgical Treatment:

- **Peripheral iridotomy**
- **Filtration surgery:**
  - ✓ Full thickness fustula (Elliot's sclerocorneal trephining; Punch sclerectomy; Scheie's thermosclerostomey and iridencleisis)
  - ✓ Pertial thickness fistula (Trabeculectomy)
  - ✓ Non-penetrating filtration surgery (deep sclerectomy and viscoanulostomy)
- **Clear lens extraction by phacoemulsification with IOL implantation**

Prophylactic treatment in the normal fellow eye: Laser or surgical peripheral iridectomy.

- **Medical therapy** (topical beta blockers are the drugs of choice.) Timolol, betaxolol, cartelol.
- **Carbonic anhydrase inhibitors (Acetazolomide, Dorzolamide)**
- **Acetazolomide is used orally not topically.** All 2006
- **Prostaglandin analogues (latanoprost)**
- **Pilocarpine and adrenergic agents. (Epinephrine and Dipivefrine)**
- Atropine is contraindicated.
- **Timolol is a beta blocker.** PGI 2002
- **Argon or diode laser trabeculoplasty and trabuculectomy are surgical options**

Dorzolamide is a carbonic anhydrase inhibitor AI 2006

- It is an anti-glaucoma agent and topically applied in the form of eye drops.
- **Side effects:** ocular burning, stinging, or discomfort immediately following ocular administration. Superficial punctate keratitis, signs and symptoms of ocular allergic reaction, conjunctivitis and lid reactions blurred vision, eye redness, tearing, dryness, and photophobia. Other ocular events and systemic events were reported infrequently, including headache, nausea, asthenia/fatigue; and, rarely, skin rashes, urolithiasis, and iridocyclitis.
- **It is a sulfonamide** and, although administered topically, is absorbed systemically. Therefore, the same types of adverse reactions that are attributable to sulfonamides may occur with topical administration.
- Fatalities have occurred, although rarely, due to severe reactions to sulfonamides including Stevens-Johnson syndrome, toxic epidermal necrolysis, fulminant hepatic necrosis, agranulocytosis, aplastic anemia, and other blood dyscrasias.
- Sensitization may recur when a sulfonamide is readministered irrespective of the route of administration. If signs of serious reactions or hypersensitivity occur, discontinue the use of this preparation. Dorzolamide hydrochloride is an **inhibitor of human carbonic anhydrase II.**

⇨ Brinzolamide (Ophthalmic Suspension)

1%, the most frequently used.

Reported adverse events associated with were

- Blurred vision and bitter,
- Sour or unusual taste.
- Blepharitis, dermatitis, dry eye, foreign body sensation,
- Headache, hyperemia, ocular discharge, ocular discomfort, ocular keratitis, ocular pain, ocular pruritus and rhinitis were reported.

Carbonic anhydrase (CA) is an enzyme found in many tissues of the body including the eye. It catalyzes the reversible reaction involving the hydration of carbon dioxide and the dehydration of carbonic acid. **Brinzolamide**

is a highly specific competitive and reversible inhibitor of CA II	**AIIMS 2011**
In humans, carbonic anhydrase exists as a number of isoenzymes, the most active being carbonic anhydrase II (CA-II), found primarily in red blood cells (RBCs), but also in other tissues.	
Inhibition of carbonic anhydrase in the ciliary processes of the eye decreases aqueous humor secretion, presumably by slowing the formation of bicarbonate ions with subsequent reduction in sodium and fluid transport. The result is a reduction in intraocular pressure (IOP).	

➲ Lens associated Glaucoma

- ✓ **Phacomorphic glaucoma:** Lens swells and obliterates the angle ☛☛
- ✓ **Phacolytic glaucoma:** Lens dissolution escapes into aqueous☛☛
- ✓ **Phactopic glaucoma:** Iris becomes firmly contracted over posterior surface of lens. ☛☛

⇨ Eponym Glaucoma's

- **Hundred day glaucoma:** Neovascular glaucoma
- **Hypersecretory glaucoma:** Epidemic Dropsy
- **Ghost cell glaucoma:** Vitreous Hemorrhage
- **Angle recession glaucoma:** Blunt trauma
- **Glaucoma Fleckens:** After Acute congestive glaucoma
- **Malignant glaucoma:** Ciliary block glaucoma

⇨ Choroidoretinitis is seen in

- Syphilis
- Cytomegalovirus
- Toxoplasmosis
- Sarcoidosis (**Candle wax spot**) **PGI 1987**
- Tuberculosis

➲ Cornea

- ▶ **Dendritic ulcers** are pathogonomic **of herpes simplex virus.**
- ▶ **Acanthameoba** causes **pseudo dendritic corneal ulcers.**
- ▶ **Decreased corneal sensation** is a feature.

⇨ Band Shaped Keratopathy

Band shaped keratopathy in cornea is due to deposition of calcerous salts after hyaline infiltration. **AIIMS 2006**

Seen in:

- ✓ **Chronic uveitis**
- ✓ **Hyperparathyroidism**
- ✓ **Vitamin D toxicity**
- ✓ **Sarcoidosis**

⇨ Keratoconus

▶ Keratoconus is protrusion of central part of cornea with thinning.	UPSC 2002
▶ Corneal nerves visible	PGI 1989
Seen in association with	
✓ Downs	
✓ Turners	
✓ Ehler danhlos	
✓ Marfans	
✓ Osteogenesis imperfecta	
✓ Mitral valve prolapsed	
Features:	
▶ Munsons sign	PGI 2002
▶ Fleischer ring	COMED 2007
▶ Vogt lines	
▶ Oil droplet reflex are seen.	

⇨ Vitamin A Deficiency Affects Cornea

Causes:

- Night blindness,
- Bitots spots,
- Conjuctival xerosis,
- Corneal ulceration/Keratomalacia,
- Corneal scar,
- Xerophthalmic fundus.

Amidarone therapy causes whorl like opacities in cornea called cornea verticsallis COMED 2008

⇨ Kindly Know that

▶ Satellite lesions, dry corneal ulcer	▶ Fungal corneal ulcer	PGI 2006
▶ Dalen Fuchs nodules	▶ Sympathetic ophthalmitis	
▶ Dendritic ulcer	▶ Herpes simplex	
▶ Snow ball opacities in vitreous	▶ Pars planitis, sarcoid, Amyloidosis, candidiasis, lyme disease	
▶ Flesher ring, Munsons sign, Vogt line	▶ Keratoconus	
▶ Habbs straie	▶ Bupthalmos	

⇨ Epiretinal Membrane

Epiretinal Membrane

- This is a fibrocellular tissue that grows across the **inner surface of the retina, causing metamorphopsia and reduced visual acuity from distortion of the macula.**
- With the ophthalmoscope one can see a **crinkled, cellophane-like membrane** on the retina. Epiretinal membrane is most common in patients over 50 years of age and is usually unilateral.
- Most cases are **idiopathic, but some occur as a result of hypertensive retinopathy, diabetes, retinal detachment, or trauma.**
- When visual acuity is reduced to the level of about 6/24 (20/80), vitrectomy and surgical peeling of the membrane to relieve macular puckering are recommended. Contraction of an epiretinal membrane sometimes gives rise to a macular hole.
- Vitrectomy may improve visual acuity in some patients with macular hole. Fortunately, fewer than 10% of patients with a macular hole develop a hole in their other eye.

➲ Lens:

⇨ Important Indices

— Power of lens: + 16 D	
— Power of cornea: + 44 D cornea is the **most important refractive surface of eye.**	
— Power of eye: + 60D	
— Refractive index of air: 1	
— Refractive index of aqueous humor: 1.33	
— Refractive index of vitreous humor: 1.33	
— Refractive index of cornea: 1.37	
— Refractive index of lens: 1.39	
— Respiratory coefficient of lens: 1	AIIMS 1983
— **Equatorial diameter of lens: 9 mm**	JK BOPEE 2001
— Maximum refractive power is in **center** of lens	AIIMS 2009

⇨ Lens

❒ Lens is **avascular**	
❒ Lens has **no nerve supply**	
❒ Lens derives nutrition from **aqueous humor, perilimbal capillaries and oxygen in air.**	AI 88
❒ Lens **thicker anteriorly than posteriorly.**	AIIMS 1987
❒ Oldest cells are present in **centre** and youngest cells in periphery.	
❒ **Crystallins** and **Major intrinsic protein MIP 26** enhance lens transparency.	
❒ Glutathione, Peroxidase, catalase, ascorbic acid, α tocopherol and βcarotene are protective against free radicals.	

⇨ Cataracts

Majority are age related and due to UV light

Systemic Causes:

- DM, Hypoglycemia, Hypocalcemia, Galactosemia, Hypothyroidism, Hypoparathyroidism, Alports, Downs Syndrome, Dysytrophia myotonica, Lowes syndrome, Wilsons Disease
- Steroids, Chloroquin, Amidarone, Busulfan, Chlorambucil, Copper, Gold, Iron.
- Infection (Congenital rubella, CMV, Toxoplasmosis)
- Smoking, HTN, Diabetes mellitus — AI 2007

Ocular Causes:

- Trauma
- Radiation
- High myopia
- Atopic dermatitis, Icthyosis, Rothmunds Syndrome, Weners syndrome (Dermatological causes)
- Cataract is **the most common cause of blindness** in India.

⇨ Typical Features of Various Cataracts are

Diabetis	Snow flake cataract	**AI 1988**
Galactosemia	Oil drop cataract	**KERALA 1990**
Wilsons disease	Sunflower cataract	**AIIMS 1986**
Infra red	Glass workers cataract	
Atopic Diseases	Syndermatotic cataract	
Myotonic Dystrophy	Christmas tree pattern	
Trauma	Rossette Cataract	
Shield cataract	Atopic dermatitis	

MC congenital cataract	**Punctate/Blue Dot cataract**	
MC cataract in adults	**Cortical cataract**	**PGI 1984**
MC visually significant congenital cataract	**Zonular/ Lamellar cataract**	
Nuclear cataract	**Associated with Rubella infection**	
Coronary cataract	**Develops at puberty**	

⇨ Complicated Cataract

- ✓ Complicated Cataract: refers to opacification of the lens **secondary to other intraocular disease.**
- ✓ The opacity in complicated cataract is **irregular in outline** and variable in density.
- ✓ A slit lamp examination shows **"Bread Crumb appearance"**.
- ✓ A characteristic sign is the appearance of iridescent colored particles so called **"Polychromatic lusture"** of reds, greens and blues. **DELHI 1992**
- ✓ Posterior subcapsular cataract is visually handicapping and presents as marked diminution of vision.
- ✓ Here patient sees better in dark.

Posterior Hyperplastic Primary Vitreous Cataract:

- It is due to **embryological persistence** of Vitreous and Hyaloid.
- Almost always **unilateral.** AIIMS 2006
- Associated with **glaucoma, cataract, microphthalmus.**
- Does not calcify.
- It is a feature of **Pataus syndrome.**
- It is associated with a **poor visual prognosis.** AIIMS 2006

Lamellar cataract is also called as **zonular or perinuclear cataract.**

- Bilateral lamellar cataracts account for **50% of visually significant cataracts.**
- They are associated **with Malnutrition and hypoparathyroidism.** MAHE 2007
- **Linear opacities IN ZONULES (Like spokes of wheel) called riders are a feature.** AIPGME 2012

⇨ Cataract Surgeries

- **ICCE: (Intracapsular cataract extraction): Whole lens removed with intact capsule**
- **ECCE: (Extracapsular cataract extraction): Lens removed, capsule left behind**
- **Phecoemulsification: Whole lens removed with intact capsule.**

Phecoemulsification: Emulsifies lens nucleus and cortex by ultrasonic vibration.

After cataract is opacity persisting or developing after ECCE.

- ❒ **Sommering s Ring** is a feature.
- ❒ **Elschings Pearls** are a feature.
- ❒ **Nd-Yag LASER capsulotomy** is done AIIMS 2005

Lens Dislocation:

- ❒ **Inferior:** Homocystinuria
- ❒ **Superior:** Marfans **(Supereo temporal)** COMED 2007
- ❒ **Forward:** Marchesani Weil Syndrome, Trauma, Hypermature cataract, Ehler Danhlos syndrome also cause lens Dislocation

- ❒ **Anterior lenticonus:** Anterior conical projection of centre of lens. **(Alports Syndrome)**
- ❒ **Posterior lenticonus:** Posterior conical projection of centre of lens. **(Lowe Syndrome)**
- ❒ **Microspherophakia:** Instead of normal biconvex shape, lens is spherical **(Marfans Syndrome)**
- ❒ **Ectopia Lens:** Subluxation of Lens, **(Marfans, Familial, Ehler Danhlos Syndrome, Trauma)**

- **Hard lens** is made of **PMMA (Poly methyl methacrylate)**
- **Soft lens** is made of **HEMA (Hydroxy methyl methacrylate)**
- **Modern IOL** are made of silicon, acrylic acid. PGI 2003

⇨ Contact Lens

- ❒ **MC infection is pseudomonas infection.** ☚☚
- ❒ Most common predisposing factor for **acanthameoba** is **use of contact lens**. KCET 2012
- ❒ Other complications related to use of contact lens:
  - ✓ **Over wear syndrome**
  - ✓ **Giant papillary conjunctivitis** ☚☚
  - ✓ **Allergic conjunctivitis**

⇨ Papilledema

Causes: Raised ICT:

- ❒ ICSOLS (Intracranial space occupying lesions), Post, Cranial Fossa Tumors,
- ❒ Intracranial infections (Cavernous sinus Thrombosis, cerebral abscess) COMED 2008
- ❒ Malignant Hypertension, Toxemia of pregnancy ☚☚
- ❒ Pseudo tumor cerebri (**Tetracycline, Nalidixic acid, OCP, Vitamin A.)**
- ❒ **Foster Kennedy Syndrome** (Optic atrophy on same side and papilledema on other side)

Clinical Features:

- ❒ Color sense affected early JIPMER 1995
  - ✓ Headache, nausea, Projectile vomiting ☚☚
  - ✓ **Painless, Progressive loss of vision**
  - ✓ **Amourosis fugax**
  - ✓ **Enlargement of blind spot** Kerala 2004
  - ✓ Progressive contraction of visual field KAR 2004
  - ✓ Visual acuity and puppilary reaction remain normal until optic atrophy occurs.
  - ✓ Leads to postneuritic ophthalmopathy

- ► Axonal swelling AI 2007
- ► Stasis of axoplasmic flow
- ► Extracellular edema are a feature

- ❒ **Blurring of margins of optic disk.** ☚☚ AI 1989
- ❒ **Hyperemia of disk** ☚☚ AIIMS 1992
- ❒ **↓Physiological cup** ☚☚
- ❒ **Venous pulsations absent. Flame shaped and punctuate hemorrhages** ☚☚
- ❒ **Elevated disc (Mushroom/dome shaped)** AIIMS 1985
- ❒ **Cotton wool spots**
- ❒ **Macular fan**

4

OPHTHALMOLOGY

⇨ Pappilitis/Optic Neuritis

Causes: Idiopathic Plus:

- Multiple sclerosis, Devics disease, Leucodystrophies, Post viral infections, Vitamin B complex deficiency,
- Diabetes
- Syphilis
- Drugs: **Quinine, Chloroquine, Ethambutol, digitalis, INH, NSAIDS, Tobbaco, alcohol, arsenic**
- **Pseudopappilitis is seen in hypermetropia.** Orissa R

Features

- **(Monocular) unilateral decrease in visual acuity** over hours or days
- **Poor discrimination of colors, "Red Desaturation"** ☛☛
- **Inflammation of optic nerve**☛☛
- **Pain worse on eye movement** ☛☛
- **Relative afferent pupillary defect /Marcus Gun pupil**☛☛ **(EARLY)** **SGPGI 2005**
- **FULL afferent puppilary defect is seen in optic nerve lesion.** **AI 2010**

Defects:

- ❒ **Defective** contrast sensitivity
- ❒ **Decreased** color vision
- ❒ **Defective** depth perception of moving objects **(Pulfrich phenomenon)**☛☛
- ❒ Worsening of symptoms with exercise **(Uthoff Phenomenon)**☛☛
- ❒ Visual evoked potentials show **latency and delay in amplitude.**

⇨ Toxic Optic Neuropathy

This can result in acute visual loss with bilateral optic disk swelling and central or cecocentral scotomas. Such cases have been reported to result from exposure to **ethambutol,** **AI 1989**

Methyl alcohol (moonshine), ethylene glycol (antifreeze), or carbon monoxide.

Many agents have been implicated as a cause of toxic optic neuropathy, but the evidence supporting the association for many is weak. The following is a partial list of potential offending drugs or toxins:

- ✓ **Disulfiram, ethchlorvynol,**
- ✓ **Chloramphenicol,**
- ✓ **Amiodarone,**
- ✓ **Monoclonal anti-CD3 antibody,**
- ✓ **Ciprofloxacin,**
- ✓ **Digitalis,**
- ✓ **Streptomycin,**
- ✓ **Lead, arsenic, thallium,**

- ✓ D-penicillamine,
- ✓ Isoniazid, emetine, and
- ✓ Sulfonamides.

Deficiency states, induced either by **starvation, malabsorption, or alcoholism**, can lead to insidious visual loss.

⇨ **Remember: All the Conditions have been asked in Different PG Examinations**

- ► Optic neuritis is inflammation of optic nerve.
- ► Pappilitis is inflammation affecting optic nerve head.
- ► Neororetinitis is pappilitis+ inflammation of retinal nerve fiber layer.
- ► Optic atrophy is degeneration of optic nerve fibers.
- ► Primary optic atrophy is characterized by chalky white disc with sharp clearly defined margins and deep cup.
- ► Secondary optic atrophy is characterized by dirty / grey disk with blurred margins and obliterated cup.
- ► Wolfram syndrome is Hereditary optic atrophy.
- ► DIDMOAD Syndrome is diabetes mellitus, diabetes Insipidus, optic atrophy and deafness.
- ► Foster Kennedy syndrome is optic atrophy on side of lesion and Papilledema on opposite side.
- ► Pseudo Foster Kennedy syndrome is unilateral Papilledema associated with ↑ICT.
- ► Lebers heridetary optic neuropathy (LHON) is bilateral optic neuritis transmitted as mitochondriopathy.
- ► Morning glory syndrome is mal formation of optic disc, absence of lamina cribrosa — AI 2007

But lamina cribrosa is normally seen in:

- ✓ Coloboma iris — PGI 2011
- ✓ Coloboma retina
- ✓ Nanophthalmia — PGI 2011
- ✓ Optic nerve agenesis

- ► De Morseir syndrome is optic nerve hypoplasia +absence of corpus callosum +absence of septum pellucidium.

➲ Macular Degeneration

- ► This is a major cause of **gradual, painless, bilateral central visual loss in the elderly.**
- ► It occurs in a **nonexudative (dry)** form and an **exudative (wet)** form.
- ► **The nonexudative process** begins with the accumulation of extracellular deposits, called **drusen**, underneath the retinal pigment epithelium.

- **Exudative macular degeneration**, which develops in only a minority of patients, occurs when neovascular vessels from the choroid grow through defects in Bruch's membrane into the potential space beneath the retinal pigment epithelium.
- **Leakage from these vessels produces elevation of the retina and pigment epithelium, with distortion (metamorphopsia) and blurring of vision.**

<u>Verteporfin</u>

Verteporfin is indicated for **treatment of age-related macular degeneration in patients with predominantly classic subfoveal choroidal neovascularization**

Verteporfin is a **photosensitizing agent** composed of two isomers.

It **accumulates preferentially in neovasculature, including choroidal neovasculature.**

Activation of verteporfin by **nonthermal light** (689 nanometers wavelength) in the presence of oxygen generates highly reactive, short-lived singlet oxygen and reactive oxygen radicals.

The activated particles cause local damage to neovascular endothelium and subsequent vessel occlusion.

Damaged endothelium releases procoagulant and vasoactive factors causing platelet aggregation, fibrin clot formation, and vasoconstriction.

These factors contribute to the temporary occlusion of choroidal neovascularization.

Distribution: Verteporfin is transported in the plasma primarily by lipoproteins.

⇨ Cherry Red Spot (SEEN IN)

- CRAO
- Berlins edema
- Metachromatic dystrophy
- Niemann Pick Disease **AI 2010**
- Taysachs disease **AI 2010**
- Sand hoffs disease
- Quinidine Toxicity
- Sarcoidosis

Remember:

- **Fleischers ring:** Keratoconus
- **Pterygium:** Stockers line
- **Ferrys line:** Filtering Bleb
- **Kayser Fleischer Ring:** Wilsons Disease
- **Krukenbergs Spindle:** Pigment dispersion syndrome

⇨ Lish Nodules

- ❐ Are **melanocytic hamartomas of Iris.**
- ❐ They are **not** seen on naked eye examination.
- ❐ They are seen on **slit lamp examination.**
- ❐ They are seen in Neurofibromatosis (Von Reckling Hausens Disease).

⇨ Fundoscopy Appearances to be remembered:

Fundoscopy:
► **Chloroquine toxicity: Bulls Eye Maculopathy**
► **CMV Retinitis: Pizza fundus, Tomato Ketch up Retinopathy**
► **CRAO: Cattle trucking appearance**
► **CRVO: Blood and Thunder fundus**
► **Morning glory appearance: Optic disk coloboma**
► **Bony spicule pigmentation: Retinitis Pigmentosa**
► **Salt and pepper fundus: Congenital syphilis, Rubella**
► **Tesselated fundus: Myopia, Retinitis pigmentosa**
► **Mulberry apprearance: Tuberous sclerosis**

➲ Uveal Tract:

⇨ Episcleritis

Episcleritis

- ► Is an **inflammation of the episclera**, a thin layer of connective tissue between the conjunctiva and sclera.
- ► Episcleritis resembles conjunctivitis but is a more localized process and discharge is absent.
- ► Most cases of episcleritis are idiopathic, but some occur in the setting of an autoimmune disease.

⇨ Scleritis

Scleritis

Refers to <u>**a deeper, more severe inflammatory process**</u>, frequently associated with a connective tissue disease such as

Rheumatoid arthritis, (MC) AIIMS 2005

Lupus erythematosus, polyarteritis nodosa, Wegener's granulomatosis, or relapsing polychondritis.

The inflammation and thickening of the sclera can be diffuse or nodular.

In anterior forms of scleritis, the globe assumes a violet hue and the patient complains of severe ocular tenderness and pain.

With posterior scleritis the pain and redness may be less marked, but there is often proptosis, choroidal effusion, reduced motility, and visual loss.

Episcleritis and scleritis should be treated with **NSAIDs.**

If these agents fail, **topical or even systemic glucocorticoid therapy** may be necessary, especially if an underlying autoimmune process is active.

- **Uveitis Involving the anterior structures of the eye, this is called iritis or iridocyclitis.**

The diagnosis requires slit-lamp examination to identify inflammatory cells floating in the aqueous humor or deposited upon the corneal endothelium (keratic precipitates).

- **Circum ciliary congestion**
- **Cells and flare in aqueos are a feature.** **PGI 2007**

⇨ Acute Anterior Uveitis

Presents with

- ✓ Deep anterior chamber with
- ✓ Miotic, **AIIMS 1993**
- ✓ Sluggishly reacting pupil and
- ✓ Hazy cornea due to keratitic precipitates.
- ✓ **Occlusio pupillae** due to organization of exudates across pupillary area, ectropion and **festooned pupil.**

Anterior uveitis develops in

- **Sarcoidosis,**
- **Ankylosing spondylitis,** **PGI 1988**
- **Juvenile rheumatoid arthritis,** **PGI 1988**
- **Inflammatory bowel disease,**
- **Psoriasis,**
- **Reiter's syndrome, and**
- **Behcet's disease.**

It is also associated with **herpes infections, syphilis, Lyme disease, onchocerciasis, tuberculosis, and leprosy.**

- Treatment is aimed at reducing inflammation and scarring by judicious use of **topical glucocorticoids.** Dilation of the pupil by atropine reduces pain and prevents the formation of synechiae. **AIIMS 2000**
- **"Secondary glaucoma"** is the **most common complication of recurrent anterior uvetis.**
- **"Pilocarpine"** and other cholinergics are **contraindicated.**
- **"Steroids" are the drug of choice** followed by mydriatics. **JK BOPEE 2011**

➲ Posterior Uveitis

This is diagnosed by **observing inflammation of the vitreous, retina, or choroid on fundus examination.** It is more likely than anterior uveitis to be associated with an **identifiable systemic disease.**

Posterior uveitis is a manifestation of autoimmune diseases such as

- **Sarcoidosis,** PGI 2004
- **Behcet's disease,** CMC 2005
- **Vogt-Koyanagi-Harada syndrome, and** PGI 2004
- **Inflammatory bowel disease**

It also accompanies diseases such **as toxoplasmosis, onchocerciasis, cysticercosis, coccidioidomycosis, toxocariasis, and histoplasmosis**; infections caused by organisms such as Candida, Pneumocystis carinii, Cryptococcus, Aspergillus, herpes, and cytomegalovirus; and other diseases such as syphilis, Lyme disease, tuberculosis, cat-scratch disease, Whipple's disease, and brucellosis.

In multiple sclerosis, chronic inflammatory changes can develop in the extreme periphery of the retina (pars planitis or intermediate uveitis).

Voclosporin, a novel immunomodulatory drug inhibiting the calcineurin enzyme, was developed to prevent organ graft rejection and to treat autoimmune diseases. The chemical structure of voclosporin is similar to that of cyclosporine A, with a difference in one amino acid, leading to superior calcineurin inhibition and less variability in plasma concentration. Compared with placebo, voclosporin may significantly reduce inflammation and prevent recurrences of inflammation in patients with noninfectious uveitis.

⇨ "Hypopyon Associated with Uveitis" is seen in

- Ankylosing spondylitis
- Behcets syndrome
- Reiter syndrome
- Inflammatory Bowel diseases
- Sarcoidosis
- Trauma
- Herpes simplex virus

Features of Pauci articular JRA:

- It is the **most common type** and accounts for 60% cases.
- **Involves < 4 joints.**
- Rheumatoid factor **is negative.**
- Risk of developing **chronic uveitis is highest**. Especially with ANA positivity, early onset and HLA DR 5 positivity.

In **poly articular** JRA Uveitis occurs in only 5% cases.

In **systemic** JRA, Uveitis is rare.

⇨ Vogt Koyangi Harada Syndrome

A disease of melanocyte containing tissue. (soon) AIIMS 1998

- **Skin Changes:** Vitiligo, Alopecia, Poliosis
- **Occular changes:** Uveitis, Retinal detatchment, Depigmented fundus, Dalen fuchs nodules
- **Otological changes:** Deafness, vertigo, Tinitus
- **Neurological changes:** Meningitis, Encephalitis

➲ Sympathetic Ophthalmitis

- **Bilateral granulomatous panuveitis.**
- **Ciliary body is injured** PGI 1997
- After **penetrating trauma** in **ciliary region. (Dangerous zone)** AIIMS 2007
- **Keratatic precipitates** or **retrolental flare** are ist signs. AI 1997
- Traumatized eye is **"Exciting eye".**
- Fellow eye is **"Sympathizing eye".**
- **Keratitic precipitates are seen early.** PGI 1998
- **"Dalen Fuchs nodule"** are characteristic
- **Early excision of injured eye** is the best prophylactic measure.
- **Steroids** (Systemic) followed by topical steroids and cycloplegics are used for treatment.
- **Example: Difficulity in reading in one eye after sustaining an injury in other eye after 3-4 weeks. AI 2003**

➲ EYE Tumors

- ❒ MC intraocular malignancy in children: Retinoblastoma AP 1988
- ❒ MC tumor of orbit/periorbit in children: Capillary hemangioma
- ❒ MC primary orbital malignancy in children: Rhabdomyosarcoma
- ❒ MC cause of orbital metastasis in children: Neuroblastoma
- ❒ MC benign orbital tumor in adults: Cavernous hemangioma
- ❒ MC eyelid tumor is: BCC
- ❒ MC tumor of lacrimal glands: Benign mixed tumor KAR 90

➲ Retinoblastoma: Important for 2011/2012

- Retinoblastoma develops from **"Neuroectoderm"** from **"Photoreceptor cells"** of Retina. **(Primitive Neuroectodermal Tumor)**
- **There is mutatation of Rb gene which is a tumor suppressor gene.**
- Retinoblastoma metastasizes to brain via **optic nerve.**

- Retinoblastoma is **bilateral in 30-40 % of cases.** UPSC 1986
- Majority of cases of Retinoblastoma are **sporadic** (85-95 %)
- Only a minor are familial.
- Familial ones are usually bilateral. PGI 2002
- The gene for Retinoblastoma is located on **chromosome 13**
- **Knudsons Hypothesis applies to Retinoblastoma.** UP 2004
- Pathological features of Retinoblastoma are:
  - ✓ **Flexner Wintersteiner Rossettes** AI 2008
  - ✓ **Homer Wright Rossettes**
  - ✓ **Pseudo Rossettes** PGI 1998
  - ✓ **Flurettes**

- The most common manifestation of Retinoblastoma is **Amauratic cats eye reflex** or **"Leukokoria" (Don't confuse with Leucorrhea).** PGI 2006
- Metastasis in the form of Orbital invasion, Invasion of regional Lymph nodes, Invasion of Brain, Meninges, bone marrow, is common.
- Treatment of Retinoblastoma depends **on size**
- Diffuse Retinoblastoma is treated with **Ennucleation.** PGI 2002
- **Ennucleation** Removal of **eye ball with portion of Optic Nerve** from Orbit. PGI 1997
- **Small tumors are removed by Brachytherapy.** UP 2007
- Enlargement of Orbit and Orbital canal is a feature
- Treatment of metastatic disease is chemotherapy UPSC 2003
- Treatment of bilateral disease is chemotherapy JIPMER 2002
- **Malignancies associated with Retinoblastoma are:**
  - ✓ **Pinealoblastoma (MC)** AI 2010
  - ✓ **Osteosarcoma**
  - ✓ **Malignant Melanoma**
  - ✓ **Soft tissue tumors**
  - ✓ **Brain Tumors**

⇨ Differential Diagnosis of Leukokoria

- ❒ **Congenital cataract giving rise to leukocoria.**
- ❒ **Persistent anterior fetal vasculature is an important cause of congenital leukocoria.**
- ❒ **Coats disease is unilateral, more common in boys and tends to present later than retinoblastoma.**
- ❒ **Retinopathy of prematurity, if advanced, may cause retinal detachment and leukocoria.**
- ❒ **Toxocariasis. Chronic toxocara endophthalmitis**

- Uveitis
- Retinal dysplasia
- Incontinentia pigmenti
- Retinoma.

⇨ Malignant Melanoma

- Is commonest intraocular primary malignant tumor in adults.
- It involves vortex veins.

⇨ Orbital Pseudotumor

- This is an **idiopathic, inflammatory orbital syndrome**
- Symptoms are **pain, limited eye movements, proptosis, and congestion.**
- Imaging often shows **swollen eye muscles (orbital myositis) with enlarged tendons**
- The **Tolosa-Hunt syndrome** may be regarded as an extension of orbital pseudotumor through the superior orbital fissure into the cavernous sinus.
- Biopsy of the orbit frequently yields **nonspecific evidence of fat infiltration by lymphocytes, plasma cells, and eosinophils.**
- A dramatic response to a therapeutic trial of **systemic glucocorticoids** indirectly provides the best confirmation of the diagnosis.

Paraneoplastic Eye Syndromes Include:

- Opsoclonus-myoclonus (OM)
- Cancer-associated retinopathy (CAR)

Opsoclonus-Myoclonus:

- **The symptoms of OM** include diplopia, blurred vision, and oscillopsia, with physical finding of opsoclonus, myoclonus of the head, trunk and limbs, hyperreflexia, dysmetria, ataxia, and equivocal Babinski signs. The syndrome is associated with **antineuronal antibodies (anti-Ri)** .OM can be seen with **breast cancer and gynecologic malignancies.**
- **Cancer-associated retinopathy** presents with visual symptoms and rapidly progresses to bilateral, unexplained vision loss. Optic atrophy can be seen on the funduscopic examination. CAR has been associated with an **autoantibody reactive to a retinal antigen ("recoverin").**

Retinal Detachment

Is separation of neurosensory retina from retinary pigment epithelium.

RD is of three types:

- **Rhegmatogeneous:** Formation of hole in retina/Tear in retina. **JK BOPEE 2011**
- **Exudative:** Retina pushed from bed by fluid accumulation.
- **Tractional:** Mechanical detachment

Causes:

- Myopia, **PGI 2007**
- Trauma, cataract surgery, **PGI 2007**
- Hypertension, **KERALA 1994**
- Malignant neoplasms of eye,
- Penetrating trauma,
- Diabetes,
- Eales disease, **PGI 2007**
- Toxemia of pregnancy predispose to RD.
- Photopsia, floaters **(muscae volitantes)** are present **JIPMER 2003**
- Vitreous shows **Tobacco dusting** which is also called as **"Shafers Sign"**.
- **Indirect optholmoscopy is the investigation of choice.** **PGI 2003**
- **Primary aim of RD surgery is closure of break.** **MP 1998**

Exudative Detatchment Is Seen In

- TOXEMIA OF PREGNANCY
- HYPERTENSION
- PAN
- MALIGNANT MELANOMA OF CHOROID **PGI 2011**
- RETINOBLASTOMA
- GLOBE PERFORATION
- SYMATHETIC OPHTHALMITIS
- ORBITAL CELLULITIS
- POSTERIOR SCLERITIS **PGI 2011**
- HARADAS DISEASE

4

OPHTHALMOLOGY

⇨ 'Eales' Disease

- Idiopathic, bilateral, occlusive periphlebitis and neovascularization causing recurrent vitreous hemorrhage in young males.
- Age group commonly involved : 20-50 years
- Etiology : Idiopathic; strongly associated with tuberberculoprotein allergy

Stages:

- ❐ **Stage 1: Periphlebitis (mainly in superotemporal quadrant)**
- ❐ **Stage 2: Occlusive vasculitis**
- ❐ **Stage 3: Neovascularization and vitreous hemorrhages**
- ❐ **Stage 4: Retinal detachment**

Treatment:

- ❐ Stage 1 and 2: Systemic steroids
- ❐ Stage 3: Photocoagulation
- ❐ Stage 4: Vitreoretinal surgery

⇨ Retinitis Pigmentosa

This is a general term for a disparate group of rod and cone dystrophies characterized by progressive night blindness (**nyctalopia**).

- ❐ **Visual field constriction with a ring scotoma,** ☛☛
- ❐ **Loss of acuity, and** **AIIMS 1999**
- ❐ **An abnormal electroretinogram (ERG).** ☛☛
- ❐ It occurs sporadically or in an **autosomal recessive, dominant, or X-linked pattern.** ☛☛
- ❐ **Irregular black deposits of clumped pigment in the peripheral retina, called bone spicules** ☛ **AIIMS 1999**
- ❐ Most cases are due to a mutation in the gene for rhodopsin, the rod photopigment, or in the gene for peripherin, a glycoprotein located in photoreceptor outer segments.
- ❐ There is no effective treatment for retinitis pigmentosa. Vitamin A (15,000 IU/day) slightly retards the deterioration of the ERG but has no beneficial effect upon visual acuity or visual fields.

✓ Some forms of retinitis pigmentosa occur in association with rare, hereditary systemic diseases (**olivopontocerebellar degeneration**)

✓ **Bassen-Kornzweig disease,**

✓ **Kearns-Sayre syndrome,**

✓ **Refsum's disease.**

➲ Central Serous Retinochoriodopathy

- It is a disease which may have **short course** and **recover spontaneously**.
- It is spontaneous detachment of **neurosensory retina** in macular region with or without retinal pigment epithelium detachment.
- Typically effects younger **20-40 years age** group with **type A personality.**
- Presents with **sudden painless loss of vision, scotomas, micropsia and metamorphosia**

Ophthalmoscopy Reveals:

Mild elevation of macular area

Absent or distorted foveal reflex

Flourscein Angiography Shows:

- **Ink blot or enlarging dot pattern**
- **Smoke stack pattern**
- **Mushroom or umbrella configuration**

Treatment is **reassurance** for spontaneous recovery or **Argon Laser photocoagulation**

⇨ Parinaud's Syndrome

Is a distinct **supranuclear** vertical gaze disorder from damage to the posterior commissure.

It is a classic sign of hydrocephalus from aqueductal stenosis.

Pineal region tumors (germinoma, pineoblastoma), cysticercosis, and stroke also cause Parinaud's syndrome.

Features include:

- **Loss of upgaze (and sometimes downgaze),**
- **Convergence-retraction nystagmus on attempted upgaze,**
- **Downwards ocular deviation ("setting sun" sign),**
- **Lid retraction (Collier's sign),**
- **Skew deviation,**
- **Pseudoabducens palsy, and**
- **Light-near dissociation of the pupils.**

Disorders of vertical gaze, especially downwards saccades, are an early feature of progressive supranuclear palsy, Parkinson's disease, Huntington's chorea, and olivopontocerebellar degeneration.

⇨ Herpes Zoster (Ophthalmicus)

- Herpes zoster from reactivation of latent varicella **(chickenpox)** virus causes a **dermatomal pattern of painful vesicular dermatitis.**
- Ocular symptoms can occur after zoster eruption in any branch of the trigeminal nerve but are particularly common when vesicles form on the nose, reflecting **nasociliary (V1) nerve involvement (Hutchinson's sign).**
- **Herpes zoster ophthalmicus** produces corneal dendrites, which can be difficult to distinguish from those seen in herpes simplex.

- Stromal keratitis, anterior uveitis, raised intraocular pressure, ocular motor nerve palsies, acute retinal necrosis, and postherpetic scarring and neuralgia are other common sequelae.
- Herpes zoster ophthalmicus is treated with antiviral agents and cycloplegics. In severe cases, glucocorticoids may be added to prevent permanent visual loss from corneal scarring.

Herpetic Keratitis.

- Herpes simplex keratitis is usually caused by **HSV-1** and is accompanied by conjunctivitis in many cases. It is considered the most common infectious cause of blindness in the United States. The characteristic lesions of HSV keratoconjunctivitis are **dendritic ulcers best detected by fluorescein staining.** **AIIMS 2011**
- Deep stromal involvement also has been reported and may result in visual impairment. Widespread, often **bilateral, necrotizing retinitis** caused by herpes simplex (HSV) can occur. The corneal involvement may be recognized by the **characteristic dendrite, a branching epithelial ulcer**. Topical antiviral agents promote healing, but recurrence is frequent, with increasing risk of corneal stromal involvement and scarring. Topical steroids activate epithelial herpes infections and should not be used without ophthalmologic consultation in any patient with a red eye.

Tunnel Vision

Tunnel vision is the **concentric diminution of the visual fields**

Causes

- Papilledema
- Glaucoma
- Retinitis pigmentosa
- Choroidoretinitis
- Optic atrophy secondary to tabes dorsalis
- Hysteria

Factitious (Functional, Nonorganic) Visual Loss

Factitious (Functional, Nonorganic) Visual Loss

- Claimed by **hysterics or malingerers.**
- Malingerers comprise the vast majority, seeking sympathy, special treatment, or financial gain by feigning loss of sight.
- The diagnosis is suspected when the
  - ✓ **History is atypical,**
  - ✓ **Physical findings are lacking or contradictory,**
  - ✓ **Inconsistencies emerge on testing, and a**
  - ✓ **Secondary motive can be identified.**

⇨ Optic Disk Drusen

- These are **refractile deposits** within the **substance of the optic nerve head.**
- They are unrelated to drusen of the retina, which occur in age-related macular degeneration. Their diagnosis is obvious when they are visible as glittering particles upon the surface of the optic disk.
- However, in many patients they are hidden beneath the surface, producing **an elevated optic disc with blurred margins that is easily mistaken for papilledema.**
- **Ultrasound or CT scanning** are sensitive for detection of buried optic disk drusen because they contain calcium.
- In most patients, optic disk drusen are an **incidental, innocuous finding,** but they can produce visual obscurations.
- On perimetry they give rise to **enlarged blind spots and arcuate scotomas** from damage to the optic disk.
- With increasing age, drusen tend to become more exposed on the disc surface as optic atrophy develops. **Hemorrhage, choroidal neovascular membrane, and AION are more likely to occur in patients with optic disk drusen.**

➲ Anterior Ischemic Optic Neuropathy

- **AION** is segmental infarction of **anterior part of optic nerve.** (Fragment the word AION).
- It results from infarction of **short posterior ciliary arteries**
- It may occur as a result of atherosclerosis, in association with giant cell arteritis, anemia, collagen vascular disorders, migrane, malignant Hypertension.
- There is sudden visual loss.
- Visual fields show **altitudnal hemianopia** usually inferior or superior.
- Treatment is by high dose corticosteroids.

⇨ Diabetic Retinopathy

- Diabetic retinopathy is the **most common cause of blindness** in adults aged 35-65 years-old. **Hyperglycemia** is thought to cause increased retinal blood flow and abnormal metabolism in the retinal vessel walls. This precipitates damage to endothelial cells and pericytes.
- Endothelial dysfunction leads to increased vascular permeability which causes the characteristic exudates seen on fundoscopy.
- **Pericyte dysfunction** predisposes to the formation of microaneurysms.
- Neovasculization is thought to be caused by the production of growth factors in response to retinal ischemia
- Person with NIDDM should have ophthalmic examination as early as possible. **AI 2006**
- Person with IDDM should have fundus examination five years after diagnosis definetly. **PGI 2006**
- **INCIDENCE increases with disease duration.** **AIIMS 1992**

4

OPHTHALMOLOGY

Background Retinopathy
➡ Microaneurysms (dots)
➡ Blot hemorrhages (<=3)
➡ Hard exudates
Pre-proliferative Retinopathy
➡ Cotton wool spots (soft exudates; ischaemic nerve fibers)
➡ Blot hemorrhages
➡ Venous beading/looping
➡ Deep/dark cluster hemorrhages
➡ More common in Type I DM, treat with laser photocoagulation
Proliferative Retinopathy
➡ Retinal neovascularization - may lead to vitrous hemorrhage
➡ Fibrous tissue forming anterior to retinal disk
➡ More common in Type I DM, 50% blind in 5 years
Maculopathy
➡ Based on location rather than severity, anything is potentially serious
➡ Hard exudates and other 'background' changes on macula
➡ More common in Type II DM

➲ Ophthalmologic Disease in HIV infections

- ❒ Ophthalmologic problems occur in **approximately half of patients** with advanced **HIV** infection.
- ❒ The most common abnormal findings on funduscopic examination are **cotton-wool spots.** (Hard white spots that appear on the surface of the retina and often have an irregular edge.) PGI 2001
- ❒ They represent **areas of retinal ischemia secondary to microvascular disease.**
- ❒ One of the most devastating consequences of **HIV** infection is **CMV retinitis.** MP 2K
- ❒ The majority of cases of CMV retinitis occur in patients with a **CD4+ T cell count <50/uL.**
- ❒ Therapy for CMV retinitis consists of **intravenous ganciclovir or foscarnet, with cidofovir as an alternative.**
- ❒ Both HSV and varicella zoster virus can cause a rapidly progressing, bilateral necrotizing retinitis referred to as the **"Acute Retinal Necrosis Syndrome".**

➲ EYE in Thyroid Diseases

Hyperthyroidism is blessed with lots of Eye signs. Important ones are:

- ❒ **Lid retraction: Dalrymple sign**
- ❒ **Lid lag: Von Grafes sign** PGI 2004
- ❒ **Infrequent blinking: Stellwag sign**
- ❒ **Poor convergence: Mobius sign** PGI 1987

- Tremor of closed lids: Rosenbach sign
- Extraoccular muscle palsy: Ballets sign
- Audible bruit over closed eye: Riesmans sign
- Unequal puppilary dilatation: Knie sign
- Increased lid pigmentation: Jellienek sign

Other Features:

- External ophthalmoplegia PGI 2004
- Proptosis
- Exophthalmus
- Large extraoccular muscles PGI 2004
- Myopathy
- Inferior rectus is the muscle mc involved. AP 1996

Guanetidine is used in treatment of thyroid ophthalmopathy.

Pupil in Various Conditions:

Acute Conjuctivitis: Normal

Acute Iridocyclitis: Miotic (small) and sluggishly reacting.

Acute Glaucoma: Dilated and Fixed.

Sjogrens Syndrome

Dry eye or **Keratitis Sicca** or **Aqueous deficiency dry eye** occurs in **"Sjogrens syndrome".** Mucosal involvement is widespread and clinical manifestations include:

- Dry mouth
- Dry nose
- Dry eyes
- Dry skin
- Dry throat
- Dry sex (vaginal involvement)
- Both dry eye and dry mouth are a feature of Sjogrens syndrome.

- This occurs as a result of **decreased function of Lacrimal glands.**
- Cornea will be thickened and there will decreased visual acuity.
- Most common cause includes Sjogrens syndrome and sometimes Rheumatoid arthritis and SLE Produce similar conditions.

Other important causes of **"aqueous deficiency dry eye"** are:

- Aplasia ,Injury of Lacrimal glands, ☛☛
- Aplasia of Trigeminal Nerve☛☛
- **Medications:** ANTIHISTAMINICS, ANTICHOLINERGICS, BETA BLOCKERS. ☛☛
- Sjogrens syndrome,Riley Day syndrome, ☛☛
- **Mucin Deficiency:** Steven Johnsons Syndrome, Trachoma, Burns, Pemphigoid, Vitamin A deficiency. **AIIMS 2006**

Remember:

- **Tears are produced in new born after 4 weeks.** **KERALA 1988**
- **Tear film has 3 layers.** **KERALA 2003**

Test used for detection of Dry eye syndrome is <u>**Schrimers test.**</u>

⇨ Hypertensive Retinopathy

Characteristic changes seen with hypertensive retinopathy include:

- Narrowing of the aterioles due to smooth muscle contraction, hyperplasia, or fibrosis
- Abnormalities (apparent "nicking") where the arterioles and venules cross; called "A-V nicking"
- Increased tortuosity of blood vessels as they spread out over the retina.

The Keith-Wagner and Barker (KWB) classification system evaluates the retinal changes seen with hypertension.

- **Group 1 Changes**: increased light reflex from the arterioles; moderate arteriolar narrowing; focal narrowing.
- **Group 2 Changes**: to the above changes, add A-V crossing changes; arterioles are reduced to about half size.
- **Group 3 Changes**: to the above changes, add cotton wood spots; hemorrhages.
- **Group 4 Changes**: to the above changes, add papilledema.

⇨ Important Signs

- ✓ **Gunns sign:** Crossing of artery over vein with compression of underlying vein☛☛
- ✓ **Gvists sign:** Increased tortuosity of small venules surrounding maculae☛☛
- ✓ **Siegrest sign:** Hyperpigmented flecks and choridal vessels arranged in radial fashion in Hypertension and Temporal arteritis☛☛
- ✓ **Salus Sign:** Venous deflection☛☛
- ✓ **Bonnets sign** : is right angled deflection of vein under artery☛☛

⇨ Leber's Hereditary Optic Neuropathy (LHON) ☛☛

- ✓ LHON typically presents with **painless, subacute, bilateral visual loss with central scotomas and dyschromatopsia.**
- ✓ **Mitochondrial** disease.
- ✓ **Males** are affected three to four times more commonly than females.

River blindness is due to: ☛☛

- ✓ Oncerchiasis volvolus. AIIMS 1997
- ✓ Transmitted by black fly
- ✓ Mazotti test is helpful in diagnosis
- ✓ Ivermectin is drug of choice

➲ Blindness/Low Vision

- ❒ Blindness according to **WHO**: One whose VA in better eye with best possible correction is **<3/60** on snellens chart.
- ❒ Blindness in **India** is: VA<6/60 in better eye with best possible correction.
- ▶ MC cause of **ocular morbidity** in India: Refractive error AIIMS 2002
- ▶ MC cause of **blindness in children** in India: Vitamin A deficiency PGI 1997
- ▶ MC cause of **blindness in adults** in India: Cataract AI 1998
- ▶ MC cause of low vision in India: Refractive error

Evisceration

Is removal of contents of eyeball leaving behind the sclera. ☛☛☛☛

Indications are:

- ➨ **Panophthalmitis** AIIMS 03
- ➨ **"Frills excision" is done for pan ophthalmitis.** JK 2001
- ➨ Bleeding anterior staphyloma
- ➨ Expulsive Choroidal hemerrhage.

Enucleation:

Is removal of eye ball with a part of optic nerve from the orbit. ☛☛☛☛

- ❒ Indications are:
- ❒ Retinoblastoma in children PGI 2002
- ❒ Malignant melanoma in adults PGI 2002
- ❒ Sympathetic ophthalmitis
- ❒ Endophthalmitis (DOES NOT INVOLVE SCLERA) AI 2010
- ❒ Pthisis bulbi PGI 2002
- ❒ Blind and disfigured eye
- ❒ Blind eye
- ❒ **Contraindicated in pan ophthalmitis.**

➲ Trauma to Orbit

- ➨ **Blow out #:** Isolated comminuted # of orbital floor and medial wall. **"Hanging drop" or "Tear drop" sign on Waters view.**
- ➨ Orbital hematoma, caroticocavernous fistula
- ➨ Iridodialysis
- ➨ Subluxation/dislocation of lens
- ➨ **Rosette cataract**

4

OPHTHALMOLOGY

➠ **Vossius ring (Lens concussion)**	**COMED 2007**
➠ Macular edema/hole	
➠ **Commotio retinae (Berlins edema)** milky white cloudiness involving posterior pole with cherry red spot in foveal region. **(Concussion Injury)**	**AIIMS 1989**
➠ **Optic nerve evulsion**	
➠ Globe rupture	
➠ Bilateral black eye **(Panda eye/ Raccoon eye)**	
➠ Unilateral Black eye	
➠ **Berlins edema**	**AIIMS 1996**
➠ **D shaped pupil is seen in IRIDODIALYSIS**	**JIPMER 1993**

Blow Out Fracture of Orbit

The **medial wall** of the orbit is extremely thin except posteriorly.

- **The lacrimal groove** lies anteriorly: it opens below into the inferior meatus of the lateral wall of the nasal cavity via the nasolacrimal canal.
- **Anterior lacrimal,** **PGI 2011**
- **Frontal process of the maxilla,**
- **Orbital plate of the ethmoid labyrinth.** **PGI 2011**

Floor of the Orbit

The floor is mostly formed by the

- **Maxilla**
- **Zygomatic bone**
- **Palatine bone**

The floor is thin and largely roofs the maxillary sinus. Infraorbital groove, canal and foramen contain the infraorbital nerve and vessels.

The Orbit is Invariably Involved in

- **Depressed fractures of the zygomatic bone**
- **Le Fort II #**
- **Le Fort III #**
- **Fractures of the frontal bone**
- **Extensive nasal complex injuries.**
- A fracture of the **orbital floor without associated rim involvement is known as a 'blow-out' fracture.** **PGI 2011**
- Fortunately the **optic foramen which is situated within the lesser wing of the sphenoid bone is surrounded by dense bone and is only rarely involved** in fractures. Direct injury to the optic nerve is **therefore unusual.**

Macular Edema

Involvement of fovea by edema (Diabetic Maculopathy) is the most common cause of visual impairment in diabetic patients.

Clinically significant macular edema (CSMO) is defined as:

- Retinal edema within 500 µm of the fovea.
- Hard exudates within 500 µm of the fovea.
- Retinal edema that is one disc area (1500) or larger, any part of which is within one disc diameter of the centre of fovea.
- **Diabetic retinopathy is due to microangiopathy affecting the retinal capillaries, arterioles venules.**
- **Severity of retinopathy is not related to levels of blood sugar.**
- **Pregnancy and hypertension may accelerate changes of diabetic retinopathy.**
- **Microaneurysms in macular area are the earliest detectable lesion.** **High Yield for 2011/2012**

Chloroquine and Eye Ocular Manifestations

- ✓ **Keratopathy,**
- ✓ **Retinal toxicity,**
- ✓ **Blurred vision,**
- ✓ **Corneal deposits,**
- ✓ **Central serous retinopathy ,**
- ✓ **Pigmentary bulls eye retinopathy,** **PGI 2007, PGI 1999**
- ✓ **Optic atrophy**

In patients with kidney function.

Occurs after duration of treatment of 5 years. **AIIMS 2011**

Cumulative dose is greater than 460gm. **AIIMS 2011**

Important Questions asked in Previous Examinations (Repeated Multiple Times)

- ❐ **Retinopathy of Prematurity** ☛☛ Oxygen
- ❐ **Bulls Eye Maculopathy** ☛☛ Chloroquine **PGI 1999**
- ❐ **Nystagmus** ☛☛ Phenytoin
- ❐ **Optic Neuritis** ☛☛ Ethambutol
- ❐ **Posterior Subcapsular Catracts** ☛☛ Steroids
- ❐ **Corneal deposits** ☛☛ Amiadarone
- ❐ **Blue Vision (Cyanopsia)** Sidanefil
- ❐ **Yellow Vision (Xanthopsia)** Digitalis
- ❐ **Whorled keratopathy** ☛☛ Amidarone **JIPMER 2K**

⇨ Optic Neuritis

Followed by optic glioma followed by optic nerve meningioma are the most common cause of optic nerve enlargement.other causes are:

- **Intracranial hypertension**
- **Sarcoidosis**
- **Hemorrhage**
- **Hemangioblastoma**
- **Advanced graves disease**

⇨ Mydriatics

▶ **Tropicamide:** Quickest and shortest	
▶ **Phenylephrine**: No cycloplegia	**AIIMS 2001**
▶ **Atropine:** Used as an ointment in children	**AI 1999**
▶ **Commonest complication of topical steroids: Glaucoma**	**AI 1995**
▶ Drug used for **blepharospasm: Botulinium toxin**	**NIMHANS 1996**

⇨ Associations Asked

— **Candle wax spots**: Sarcoidosis	**PGI 1987**
— **Fleisher ring**: Keratoconus	**COMED 2007**
— **Arlts line**: Trachoma	**PGI 2002**
— **Sago grains**: Trachoma	**PGI 1981**
— **Roths spots**: Bacterial endocarditis	**PGI 1988**
— **Epibulbar dermoids**: Goldenhars syndrome	**AIIMS 1986**
— **Dalen Fuchs nodules**: Sympathetic ophthalmitis	**AI 1991**
— **Scintillating scotoma**: Migrane	**AMU 1995**
— **Ring scotoma**: Retinitis pigmentosa	**AI 1991**
— **Angiod streaks**: Pseudoxanthoma elasticum	**AIIMS 2005**
— **KF ring** : Wilsons disease	
— **Schwalbes ring**: Descements membrane	**BHU 1986**
— **Arcus senilis**: Old Age	**PGI 1985**

➲ Latest Topics (For 2011 Onwards)

NARP Syndrome: High Yield for 2011-2012 AIPGME

- NEUROPATHY, ATAXIA, AND RETINITIS PIGMENTOSA
- Gene locus is unknown
- Is a rare <u>mitochondrial</u> inheritance

Clinical Symptoms:

- Apnea
- Ataxia
- Blindness, visual loss, visual impairment
- Dementia
- Early death
- Encephalopathy
- Mental retardation
- Muscle weakness
- Peripheral neuropathy
- Retinitis pigmentosa
- Seizures

Abnormal Findings in plasma: Deranged Citrulline levels

⇨ Diseases Associated with RP: Retinitis Pigmentosa — AIIMS 2010

- RP + neuropathy + ataxia = **NARP Syndrome**
- RP + Diabetes + ataxia + dysarthia = **Friedreichs ataxia**
- RP + acanthosis + abetalipoproteinemia = **BassenKornweigz syndrome**
- RP + Cardiomyopathy + icthiosis = **Refsums disease**
- RP + Congenital deafness = **Ushers syndrome**
- RP + Ptosis + external opthalmoplegia + diabetes = **Kearns Sayre Syndrome**
- RP + Dental anomalies + polydactyly + hypogonadism = **Bardet Biedl syndrome**

⇨ Ocular Feature of Multiple Sclerosis

- optic neuritis
- Papillitis
- Retinal sheathing of vessels
- Pale optic disk
- Internuclear ophthalmoplegia

Incomitant Strabismus Syndromes High Yield for 2011-2012 AIPGME

Duane's Syndrome

- In Duane's syndrome VI cranial nerve innervation of the lateral rectus muscle is variably defective, and an anomalous branch of the III cranial nerve supplies the lateral rectus muscle.
- On attempted adduction of the eye the medial rectus and lateral rectus muscle both contract and the eye retracts into the orbit, with narrowing of the palpebral aperture.
- On attempted abduction there is variable lateral rectus weakness, which may be mistaken for VI cranial nerve palsy caused by aquired neurological disease.
- Surgical treatment is reserved for those children who develop a significant compensatory head turn (towards the side of the affected eye), or strabismus in primary position.

4

OPHTHALMOLOGY

Moebius Syndrome

- Moebius syndrome consists of congenital absence of cranial nerve nuclei, including the VI and VII nerve nuclei.
- Abduction is absent in each eye, and there is bilateral facial palsy.

Brown's Syndrome

- In Brown's syndrome there is a congenital anomaly of superior oblique tendon and trochlea function.
- When the affected eye is adducted it shoots downwards.
- The condition is usually treated conservatively as some spontaneous recovery may occur. In severe cases superior oblique tenotomy surgery is performed.

➲ Foster Kennedy Syndrome: High Yield for 2011-2012 AIPGME

This syndrome is due to optic nerve compression, olfactory nerve compression, and increased intracranial pressure (ICP) secondary to a mass (such as meningioma or plasmacytoma, usually an olfactory groove meningioma). Features:

- Optic atrophy
- Papilledema **in the opposite eye**
- Central scotoma (loss of vision in the middle of the visual fields) in the same eye
- Anosmia (loss of smell) on the same side

Pseudo-Foster Kennedy syndrome is defined as one-sided optic atrophy with papilledema in the other eye but with the absence of a mass. Pseudo-Foster Kennedy Syndrome is described as unilateral optic disk swelling with contralateral optic atrophy in the absence of an intracranial mass causing compression of the optic nerve. This occurs typically due to bilateral sequential optic neuritis or ischaemic optic neuropathy.

➲ Aniridia High Yield for 2011/2012

- Aniridia is an autosomal dominant condition caused by mutations in the **PAX 6 homeobox gene.**
- Sporadic cases have a high incidence of associated abnormalities, including **Wilm's tumor, genitourinary abnormalities and mental retardation.**
- Aniridia represents a **defect of neural crest cell development.**
- Progressive loss of vision over decades is usual in aniridia patients.

⇨ Stargardt's Disease

- **Stargardt's disease** is an autosomal recessive disease with onset in late childhood.
- Symptoms are limited to reduced visual acuity
- Typically there are **creamy fishtail shaped flecks in the retina (fundus flavimaculatus)** with additional retinal pigment epithelium atrophy at the macula.
- Fundus fluorescein angiography may be helpful in the diagnosis of early cases.
- There is a characteristic **'dark choroid' appearance** due to reduced transparency of the retinal pigment epithelium.
- Phenotype variation is related to different mutations in the ABCR gene. **High Yield for 2011/2012**

⇨ Common Occular Side Effects of Important Drugs

❒ **Corticosteroids**	Posterior subcapsular cataract Glaucoma Pseudotumor cerebri Myopia	
❒ **Chloroquine**	Bulls eye maculopathy Retinal pigmentary changes Decreased color sensation	**AP 1997**
❒ **Quinine**	Cherry red spot	
❒ **Chlorpromazine**	Anterior subcapsular cataract	
❒ **Digitalis**	Yellow vision Central scotoma	
❒ **Rifampicin**	Orange colored tears	
❒ **OCP**	Thrombosis of retinal vessels Papilledema	
❒ **Gentamycin**	Macular toxicity	**AI 2006**

⇨ Clinical Opjthalmology

❒ A **14 year old boy** complains of **pain during reading.** On examination, his **both eyes are normal and vision with Snellen's reading is 6/5.** He still complains of pain on occluding one eye. The diagnosis is: **AIIMS**

Pseudomyopia

❒ A **16 year old boy** complains of pain in the right eye. After refractometry, **he was prescribed a +3.5 D sphere lens.** The cover test is normal. There is **no heterophoria.**The diagnosisis: **AIIMS**

Anisometric amblyopia

❒ A patient complains of **pain both eyes with congestion. Blurring of vision, photophobia and mucopurulent discharge** since one day. **Many cases** have been reported from the same community. The causative agent is most probably:

Enterovirus 70

❒ A male patient with a history of **hypermature cataract** presents with a 2 day history **of ciliary congestion, photophobia, blurring of vision** and on examination has a deep anterior chamber in the right eye. The left eye is normal. The diagnosis is:

Phakoanaphylactic uveitis

A **60 year old male** patient operated for **cataract 6 months** back now **complains of floaters and sudden loss of vision.** The diagnosis is:

Retinal detachment

❒ A 12 year old boy presents with **recurrent attacks of conjunctivitis** for the last 2 years with intense **itching and ropy discharge**. The diagnosis is

Vernal conjunctivitis

❒ A **25 year old lady** presents with **severe sudden onset of pain, corneal congestion, photophobia and deep anterior chamber** in the right eye. The left eye is normal. **X-ray pelvis shows sacroiliitis**. The diagnosis is: **PGI**

Anterior uveitis

❒ A neonate, 30 days old, presented with **excessive lacrimation and photophobia. He has a large and hazy cornea**. His both lacrimal duct systems are normal. The diagnosis is :

Congenital glaucoma

❒ A patient has **normal anterior chamber and hazy cornea in one eye and shallow anterior chamber** and **miotic pupil in fellow eye**. the diagnosis is: **AIIMS**

Acute anterior uveitis

❒ A **young man** with **blurring of vision in right eye, followed by left eye after 3 months, showing disk hyperemia, edema, circumpapillary telangiectasia** with **normal pupillary response with centrocecal scotoma on perimetry**, the cause is:

Leber's hereditary optic neuropathy

❒ **A 20 yrs old female presents with proptosis and Abducens nerve palsy**. On MRI scan, **hyperintense lesions** were seen on T2 weighted images which showed intense homogenous contrast enhancement. Most probable diagnosis is: **AIIMS**

Schwannoma

❒ An **orbital tumor** has the following characteristics: **Retrobulbar location within the muscle cone, well defined capsule, presents with slowly progressive proptosis, easily resectable, occurs most commonly in the 2nd to 4th decade**. The diagnosis is:

Cavernous hemangioma

❒ A patient presented with **unilateral proptosis which was compressible and increases on bending forward. No thrill or bruit** was present. **MRI shows a retroorbital mass with enhancement**. The likely diagnosis is: **AIIMS**

Orbital varix

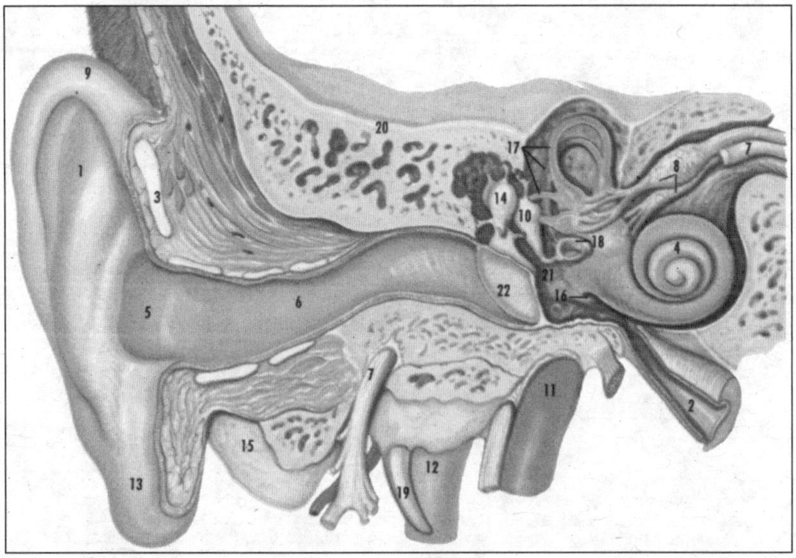

ENT

Clinical Anatomy of the Ear

External Ear

The Auricle: HIGH Yield for 2011-2012

- Forms from **six tubercles of His**
- Malformations include **microtia, a misshapen auricle, or anotia, the absence of the auricle.** Both may be associated with accessory auricles, which are small residual tubercles that may lie sometimes over the cheek without function.
- Either of these congenital abnormalities of the auricle may be associated with meatal atresia, the absence of the bony meatus.
- They are commonly associated together in a variety of congenital conditions and syndromes.
- They may present as a unilateral problem, e.g. **First arch syndrome**, or as a bilateral problem, e.g. **Craniofacial dysostosis or Treacher Collins syndrome.**

External Ear

External Ear

The External auditory canal makes a slightly **S-shaped curve. 24 mm in length**

Nerve Supply is auriculo temporal nerve and vagus. **PGI 1986**

The outer **third has a cartilaginous skeleton**, and the inner **two thirds has a bony skeleton.**

Cartilaginous part is smaller than bony part. **KAR 1989**

Fissures of santorini are present here

Bony Part:

- **No** Hair
- **No** Sebacous glands **COMED 2008**
- **No** Cereminous glands
- **Anterior recess and Foramen of Huschke are present in the bony part.**

The plane of the tympanic membrane makes an **angle of 40-45 degrees** with the long axis of the external auditory canal.

The Tympanic Membrane

The tympanic membrane is divided into the **pars tensa and the pars flaccida.**

The pars tensa is composed of three layers: **the outer stratified squamous epithelium, which is continuous with the skin of the canal; the fibrous layer; and the inner mucous membrane**, which is continuous with the rest of the mucous membrane of the middle ear. The fibrous layer thickens toward the periphery of the tympanic membrane to form the annulus tympanicus, which rests in the sulcus tympanicus, a groove in the most medial aspect of the canal. The fibrous layer ends at the anterior and posterior malleolar folds.

Pars flaccid is also called as Sharpnells membrane. **DELHI 2008**

The **Tympanic membrane is derived from** 3 layers **(ecto, endo and mesoderm)**

The **Tympanic membrane is** pearly grey/white **in color**

The Tympanic membrane has point of maximum convexity which lies at tip of handle of malleus called Umbo	AIIMS 96
Cone of light is formed by handle of Malleus	
Cone of light is anteroinferior	Delhi 2008
Nerve supply of TM is auriculotemporal nerve and auricular branch of vagus.	AI 1995
Myringotomy incision is made in Postero inferior quadrant	
The footplate of the stapes articulates with the "oval window"	
Secondary tympanic membrane closes "round window"	
Normal color of TM is pearly white.	CUPGEE 1996
Surface area of TM is 55 m^2	MANIPAL 2006

Tympanic Membrane: High Yield for 2011-2012

- Directed downwards, forwards and laterally.
- Point of maximum convexity is **umbo.**
- Greater part is tense: **Pars tensa.**
- Part between two malleolar folds is **Pars flacida.**
- Composed of 3 layers. (cuticular,fibrous, mucus)
- Derived from all **3 germ layers** (endo, meso, ectoderm)
- Nerve related to tympanic membrane is **chorda tympani**
- Cone of light is seen in which part of tympanic membrane **Anteroinferior** TN 2005

In Tympanic Membrane

- Cone of light is antero-inferior
- Sharpnell's membrane is also known as pars flaccida Delhi 2008
- Anterior malleal fold is longer than posterior

Middle Ear

Roof

Is formed by A thin plate of compact bone, the tegmen tympani, separates the cranial and tympanic cavities In youth, the unossified petrosquamosal suture may allow the spread of infection from the tympanic cavity to the meninges.

Floor

The floor of the tympanic cavity is a narrow, thin, convex plate of bone which separates the cavity from the superior bulb of the internal jugular vein.

A small aperture for the tympanic branch of the glossopharyngeal nerve lies near the medial wall.

Lateral Wall

The lateral wall consists mainly of

- The tympanic membrane,
- Openings of the anterior and posterior canaliculi for the chorda tympani
- Petrotympanic fissure

Medial Wall

The medial wall of the tympanic cavity is also the lateral boundary of the internal ear. Its features are the

- Promontory, (The promontory is a rounded prominence furrowed by small grooves which lodge the nerves of the tympanic plexus. It lies over the lateral projection of the basal turn of the cochlea)
- Fenestra vestibuli (oval window), AIIMS 2010
- Fenestra cochleae (round window) and the AIPGE 2009
- Facial prominence
- Sinus tympani

Anterior Wall

- Canal for tensor tympani PGI 2011
- Bony canal of auditory tube
- Processus cochleaformis

Posterior Wall

Its main features are the

- Aditus to the mastoid antrum,
- The pyramid, and the
- Fossa incudis.

The aditus to the mastoid antrum is a large irregular aperture which leads back from the epitympanic recess into the upper part of the mastoid antrum

⇨ Communications

Anteriorly with nasopharynx through auditory tube.

Posteriorly with mastoid antrum through aditus (path) to mastoid antrum

➲ Infections Related to 4 Sides of Middle Ear Cavity

- **Superiorly:** Meningitis through tegmen tympani
- **Inferiorly:** Internal Jugular vein thrombosis
- **Posteriorly:** Mastoid Abscess
- **Laterally :** Tympanic membrane rupture with pus discharge

5

ENT

➲ Development of the Ear: High Yield for 2011-2012

- The **otic vesicle** develops from the surface ectoderm during the **fourth week.** The vesicle develops into the **membranous labyrinth** of the internal ear.
- The otic vesicle divides into a dorsal utricular part, which gives rise to the **utricle**, **semicircular ducts**, and **endolymphatic duct**, and a ventral saccular part, which gives rise to the **saccule** and **cochlear duct**. The cochlear duct gives rise to the **spiral organ**.
- The **bony labyrinth** develops from the mesenchyme adjacent to the membranous labyrinth. The epithelium lining the tympanic cavity, mastoid antrum, and pharyngotympanic tube is derived from the endoderm of the **tubotympanic recess**, which develops from the first pharyngeal pouch. The **auditory ossicles** develop from the dorsal ends of the cartilages in the first two pharyngeal arches. The epithelium of the **external acoustic meatus** develops from the ectoderm of the first pharyngeal groove.
- The **tympanic membrane** is derived from three sources: endoderm of the first pharyngeal pouch, ectoderm of the first pharyngeal groove, and mesenchyme between the above layers.
- The **auricle** develops from the fusion of six **auricular hillocks**, which form from mesenchymal prominences around the margins of the first pharyngeal groove.

➲ Meatal Stenosis

- Meatal stenosis may occur either as a congenital abnormality or as a result of chronic otitis externa.
- Down syndrome children have very narrow external auditory meati and they often have middle ear problems. This sometimes makes the fitting of grommet tubes impossible and hence careful monitoring of their hearing is important.

⇨ The Middle Ear

The **Middle ear space** is irregular and compressed laterally. ☛☛

- The part superior to the level of the tympanic membrane is the **Epitympanum**, or attic. ☛ **Prussacks space** lies in epitympanum. **MAH 2002**
- The **Mesotympanum** lies directly medial to the tympanic membrane. (Narrowest part) ☛ **PGI 97**
- The **Hypotympanum** is inferior to the level of the tympanic membrane. ☛
- The basal turn of the cochlea makes an impression on the medial wall of the middle ear, termed the **"Promontory."** ☛☛
- The **"Tegmen", or roof, of the tympanum** is opposite the middle cranial fossa. **KAR 2006**
- The tegmen tympani extends posteriorly to become the tegmen of the antrum and mastoid process. The **middle ear communicates with the mastoid process through the antrum.** ☛
- **Malleus, incus and stapes** are the ossicles of middle ear.

- All mastoid air cells communicate one through another with the antrum. Pneumatic cells also extend into the petrous pyramid from the antrum, attic, and hypotympanum. **The floor of the middle ear is the roof of the jugular fossa.**
- **Stapedius** is a muscle which **prevents hyperacusis.** AIIMS 2006
- It gets damaged in **injury to facial nerve**

The Seventh (Facial) Nerve: High Yield for 2011-2012

The seventh nerve consists of:

- **Motor fibers** to the muscles of facial expression including the **orbicularis oculi** which closes the eye, but not the levator palpebrae superioris.

The nerve supplies also motor fibers to the digastric (posterior belly), platysma and stapedius muscles.

- **Chorda tympani (carrying taste-fibre from the anterior two thirds of the tongue) joins the nerve the facial canal of the temporal bone.**
- **Efferent autonomic fibers to the sublingual and submandibular salivary glands, and** lacrimal gland.

- **The stapedius muscle is innervated by the facial nerve.**
- **This muscle is located in the middle ear and attaches to the neck of the stapes.**
- **Contraction of the stapedius reduces the amplitude of oscillation of the stapes and thus reduces the perceived loudness of a sound.**
- **Paralysis of this muscle may result in hyperacusis.**

Examination

1. **INSPECTION**

- The face appears asymmetrical:
- The nasolabial fold is characteristically diminished or absent.
- The angle of the mouth may be deviated towards the normal side. It may sag with the saliva dribbling away.
- The lower eyelid may droop with tears flowing over it.

2. **MOTOR FUNCTIONS**

The patient is asked to perform a series of the following movements, from above downwards:

- To look upwards or wrinkle his forehead, comparing the wrinkles on both side and elevation of the eyebrows.
- To close the eyes tightly, while the examiner attempts to open the eyelids.
- To show the teeth with a broad smile (mouth closed). Asymmetrical retraction of the corners of the mouth can readily be observed.
- To blow the cheeks without letting the air escape from the mouth, while the examiner tries to empty them.
- To whistle (to test pursing of lips).

5

ENT

3. TASTE

The patient is asked to protrude the tongue and the examiner holds it with a piece of guaze. This is to prevent the patient from withdrawing his tongue and allowing the saliva to carry the test substance to other parts of the tongue.

The test substance is applied to the tongue. 4 substances are used: sweet (sugar) sour (acid) salt and bitter.

➲ Types of Facial Weakness

Weakness in the facial muscles may result from:

❒ **Upper Motor Neuron Lesion:**

- Here only the muscles of the lower part of face are affected. The eye closure is normal.
- This is because the muscles of the lower part (unlike those of the lower part) are activated through the upper motor neuron fibers of both sides.
- Spontaneous emotional expression is unaffected.

❒ **Lower Motor Neuron Lesion:**

- All the muscles of the face (upper and lower) are affected on the same side.

⇨ Canalis Nervi Facialis

Canalis nervi facialis, Facial canal, Aqueductus fallopii, Fallopian aqueduct. **High Yield for 2011-2012**

It is a bony canal in the temporal **bone through which the facial nerve passes Starts at internal acoustic meatus.** Ends at stylomastoid foramen. It is the longest bony canal for a nerve in our body. As the presence of a rigid bony canal does not provide for any space for expansion, **inflammatory swelling of facial nerve can cause ischemia of nerve**

When the bony canal is dehiscent, infections of the middle ear can affect the facial nerve. **AIPGMEE 2010**

➲ Inner Ear

INNER EAR is present in **petrous part of temporal bone.** **PGI 1997**

Facial nerve gets injure here in <u>transverse fractures</u> of temporal bone. **AI 2007**

The bony labrynth is a cancellous bone. **PGMEE 2006**

The **cochlea makes two and three-quarter turns** in the human. ☛

A cross section through the modiolus, or central bony framework, demonstrates in each turn the **scala vestibuli, the scala media, and the scala tympani.** ☛☛

The scala vestibuli is separated from the scala media by **Reissner's membrane.** ☛☛

The scala media is separated from the scala tympani by the **Basilar membrane.**

The organ of Corti, with its hair cells and their supporting cells, **rests on the basilar membrane.** **AP 1990**

The hairs of the hair cells are in contact with the tectorial membrane. Dendrites of the first-order neurons, of which the cell bodies are in the spiral canal of Rosenthal in the modiolus, arborize around the base of the hair cells. ☛☛

The axons terminate in the **dorsal and ventral cochlear nuclei** in the medulla.

The pathway to the auditory cortex consists of at least four orders of neurons and includes the **superior olivary complexes**, the **lateral lemnisci**, the **inferior colliculi**, and the **medial geniculate bodies.** Crossing of the midline occurs at the level of the brain stem nuclei and the inferior colliculi. In humans the auditory cortex lies in the posterior portion of the superior temporal gyrus in the sylvian fissure, which is termed **Heschl's gyrus.**

Eustachian Tube:	
Opposite of External auditory canal.	
Outer1/3 Bony, Inner 2/3 cartilaginous	
Develops from **1 st pharyngeal Pouch**	PGI 97
Runs **downwards, forwards and medially in adults**	
▶ **Shorter, wider and more horizontal in infants**	
▶ **Opens during swallowing**	PGI 2002
▶ **Muscle opening eustachian tube is Tensor Palati.**	PGI 2001

⇨ Patency of Eustachian Tube is Tested by:

- ✓ Valsalva maneuver
- ✓ Frenzel maneuver
- ✓ Toynbees maneuver
- ✓ Politerization
- ✓ Eustachian tube catheterization

⇨ Mastoid Cells

In acute otitis media, the infection almost invariably extends through the mastoid antrum into the mastoid cells. There is destruction of the bony partitions between the mastoid air cells. Progression of the acute infectious stages in the mastoid process is so regularly aborted by antibiotic therapy that clinically apparent acute mastoiditis has become a rare condition.

➲ The Eight (Vestibulo-Cochlear) Nerve

The eighth nerve consists of 2 parts which have different functions Cochlear and vestibular nerves. **The Cochlear part is concerned with hearing**. An affection results is tinnitus and deafness. **The vestibular part is concerned with equilibrium**. Its affection may result in vertigo.

➲ "The Cochlear Pathway"

⇨ Main Relay Centers

- Inner and outer hair cells of the **organ of Corti** in the internal ear → **bipolar cells** in spiral ganglion whose axons form the **cochlear nerve** which enters the brain stem at the junction of pons and medulla.
- The cochlear nerve ends in 2 nuclei: **The Ventral Cochlear Nucleus and the Dorsal Cochlear Nucleus**

5

ENT

—	**Trapezoid body** which crosses to the outer side and forms the **Lateral lemniscus** of the opposite side mainly; but notice that :
—	**Medial geniculate body. (M.G.B.)** is the **thalamic centre (nucleus) of hearing.**
—	The axons of the medial geniculate body form the **"Auditory radiation"** which passes in the internal capsule to reach the **"Auditory area" in Heschl's gyrus or "area 41"** on the **superior temporal gyrus**

The saccule is spherical and is connected with the scala media through the **canalis reuniens of Hensen.** ☛☛

The **saccular duct joins the utricular duct** to form the **endolymphatic duct**. The utricle is larger than the saccule and is ovoid. ☛☛

The utricle has **five openings** for the **three ampullated ends of the semicircular canals** ☛☛

The membranous labyrinth contains endolymph. ☛☛

The space between the bony labyrinth and the membranous labyrinth is filled with **perilymph.** The perilymphatic space communicates with the subarachnoid space through the cochlear aqueduct, which enters the scala tympani. ☛☛

- **The endolymph** is chemically similar to intracellular fluid, with a **high K+ concentration** and a **low Na+ concentration,**
- The **perilymph resembles extracellular fluid, with a low K+ and a high Na+** **UP 2007**

- ✓ **Angular acceleration** is sensed by: Semi circular canals☛ **COMED 2007**
- ✓ **Horizontal Linear acceleration** is sensed by: Utricle☛
- ✓ **Vertical Linear acceleration** is sensed by: saccule☛
- ✓ **Gravity and position of head in space** is sensed by: utricle and saccule. ☛

⇨ Congenital Disorders of Ear

- **Bat ear/ Lop ear:** Abnormally long protruding ear
- **Microtia**: small pinna
- **Macrotia**: abnormally large pinna
- **Anotia**: absent pinna
- **Preauricular sinus**: incomplete fusion of tubercles
- **Preauricular appendages**: skin covered tags containing cartilage.

➲ First Arch Syndrome: High Yield for 2011/2012

Abnormal development of the **components of the first pharyngeal arch** results in various congenital anomalies of the eyes, ears, mandible, and palate that together constitute the first arch syndrome

This syndrome is believed to result from insufficient **migration of neural crest cells into the first arch during the fourth week.** There are two main manifestations of the first arch syndrome:

- **In Treacher Collins syndrome (mandibulofacial dysostosis),** caused by an autosomaldominant gene, there is malar hypoplasia (underdevelopment of the zygomatic bonesof the face) with down-slanting palpebral fissures, defects of the lower eyelids, deformed external ears, and sometimes abnormalities of the middle and internal ears.

- **In Pierre Robin syndrome,** an autosomal recessive disorder, is associated with hypoplasia of the mandible, cleft palate, and defects of the eye and ear are present. Many cases of this syndrome are sporadic. In the Robin morphogenetic complex, the initiating defect is a small mandible (micrognathia), which results in posterior displacement of the tongue and obstruction to full closure of the palatal processes, resulting in a bilateral cleft palate

PINNA

- Blunt trauma to the pinna causes a **subperichondrial hematoma.**
- When bleeding occurs between the cartilage and the perichondrium, the pinna becomes a **reddish purple** shapeless mass.
- Because the perichondrium carries the blood supply to the cartilage the cartilage undergoes **avascular necrosis** if the hematoma is present on both sides of the cartilage, and with time the pinna becomes shriveled. ☛

- Hematoma may become organized and calcify which produces the **cauliflower ear characteristic of wrestlers and boxers**☛☛ PGI 2011
- **Cauliflower ear is Perichondritis in wrestlers** MANIPAL 2006

Infectious Diseases

External Otitis. Infection of the ear canal occurs in a

- **Diffuse form** involving the entire canal, termed **otitis externa diffusa**, and ☛
- A **localized form due to furunculosis**, termed **otitis externa circumscripta.** ☛☛

Malignant External Otitis. ☛ COMED 2007

- An unusually virulent form of external otitis due to **infection with P. aeruginosa**☛ AIPGME 2012
- Occurs in,
- **Immunosuppressed,**
- **Diabetics,** particularly elderly diabetics with poor metabolic control. AIIMS 2006
- It produces pain, **purulent otorrhea, and hearing loss.** ☛
- Facial nerve is most common cranial nerve involved. ☛ AIPGME 2011
- **Granulation tissue found.** PGI 2006

Acute Suppurative Otitis Media (ASOM)

Mc organism in **children: Strep. Pneumonia**☛

MC organism in **neonates: Group B streptococci**☛

A myringotomy is indicated when bulging of the tympanic membrane persists despite antibiotic therapy or when the pain and systemic symptoms and signs such as fever, vomiting, and diarrhea are severe. ☛

The infectious complications of acute otitis media are:

- **Acute mastoiditis,**
- **Petrositis**
- **Labyrinthitis,**
- **Facial paralysis,**

5

ENT

— Conductive and sensorineural hearing loss, — Epidural abscess, — Meningitis, — Brain abscess, — Lateral sinus thrombosis, — Subdural empyema, and — Otitic hydrocephalus.
Mastoid reservoir phenomenon seen. PGI 1999

⇨ Serous/Secretory Otitis Media/Glue Ear

Manifested as **effusions in the middle ear**.
↓ Mobility of Tympanic membrane
▶ **Air bubbles** behind TM.
▶ **Marginal perforation seen** MAHE 2005
— **Straw/amber** colored TM.
— **Blue tympanic membrane.**
— **B shaped tympanogram.** MAHE 2005
— **Medical treatment not effective much here.** UP 2007
— **Myringotomy with ventilation tube insertion is used as treatment.** AIIMS 2007, MAH 2012

Chronic Otitis Media. Chronic otitis media means **a permanent perforation of the tympanic membrane.** AIIMS 85

Safe CSOM	Unsafe CSOM
▶ Copious **odorless** discharge	▶ **Purulent** discharge
▶ **Tubo Typmanic Type**	▶ **Atticoantral** Type
▶ **Central** Perforation	▶ **Marginal** Perforation COMED 2006
▶ Cholesteatoma **absent**	▶ Cholesteatoma **present**
▶ Complications **rare**	▶ Complications **common**

➲ Cholesteatoma/Epidermosis/Keratoma: High Yield for 2011-2012

- A **cholesteatoma** occurs when the middle ear is lined with **stratified squamous epithelium.(white, amorphous debris in the middle ear)**
- The stratified squamous epithelium **desquamates** in this closed space.
- **Basically a bone erosion.** PGI 2006
- The desquamated epithelial debris cannot be cleared and accumulates in ever enlarging concentric layers. This debris serves as a culture medium for microorganisms.

➡ Cholesteatomas have the ability to destroy bone, including the tympanic ossicles, probably because of the elaboration of collagenase.	
▶ **Usually found in apex of petrous temporal bone.**	PGI 2006
▶ **Attic/posterior superior marginal region is usually involved.**	PGI 1988
➡ Pars flaccida and marginal perforations are frequently associated with cholesteatomas.	
➡ **Lateral semi circular canal** is the commonest to perforate.	PGI 2000
➡ The presence of a cholesteatoma greatly **increases the probability of the development of a serious complication** such as purulent labyrinthitis, facial paralysis, or intracranial suppurations. Intracranial infections include meningitis, brain abscess, lateral sinus thrombosis, subdural empyema, and epidural abscess.	
➡ **Modified Radical Mastoidectomy is used for treatment.**	PGI 1986

⇨ Complications of CSOM

▶ Commonest complication is **Mastoiditis**	COMED 2008
▶ **Commonest cause of brain abscess is CSOM.**	PGI 2000
— **Lucs abscess (Root of Zygomatic Process)**	
— **Bezolds abscess (Sternomastoid)**	AIIMS 92
— **Citellis abscess (Digastric triangle)**	
— **Labrynthitis**	
— **Petrositis**	
— **Gradiengos syndrome (Photophobia, Lacrimation, V and VI Cranial Nerve Involvement)**	KCET 2012
— **Osteomylelitis**	
— **Septicemia**	
— **Lateral sinus Thrombosis**	

➲ Gradenigo's Syndrome High Yield for 2011-2012

Is petrous apicitis	
Is a complication of otitis media **and** mastoiditis involving the **apex of the petrous** temporal bone. Symptoms of the syndrome include:	
— Retro orbital pain due to pain in the area supplied by the ophthalmic branch of the trigeminal nerve (fifth cranial nerve),	
— Ipsilateral paralysis **of the** abducens nerve (sixth cranial nerve),	KCET 2012
— **Otitis media.**	
Other Symptoms can Include	
❒ Photophobia,	
❒ Excessive lacrimation,	
❒ Fever, and	
❒ Reduced corneal sensitivity.	
❒ The syndrome is usually caused by the spread of an infection into the petrous apex of the temporal bone	

5

ENT

➲ Lateral Sinus Thrombosis: High Yield for 2011-2012

Lateral sinus thrombosis. (LST)
(Grisinger's sign) Tenderness and oedema over mastoid are pathgnomonic of lateral sinus thrombosis.(LST) **JK BOPEE 09, TN 03**
Classic symptoms of LST include a **"picket fence" fever** pattern; chills; progressive anemia (especially with beta-hemolytic strep); and, symptoms of septic emboli, headache and papilledema may indicate extension to involve the cavernous sinus.
The Toby-Ayer test is measured by monitoring the CSF pressure during a lumbar puncture. No increase in CSF pressure during external compression of the internal jugular vein on the affected side, and an exaggerated response on the patent side, is suggestive of LST. **Manipal 01, JIPMER 81, AIIMS 84**

Radical mastoidectomy, Here the **middle ear, including the attic and the antrum, and the mastoid air cell area are converted into one cavity** that communicates with the exterior through the ear canal.
Modified radical mastoidectomy if the cholesteatoma lies superficial to the remnants ofthe tympanic membrane and ossicles, a **modified radical mastoidectomy** can be performed. The modified radical mastoidectomy spares the tympanic membrane remnants and ossicles and preserves the remaining hearing.
It is the commonest operation done for CSOM **PGI 97**

— **Schwartz operation** is simple or cortical mastoidectomy.	**PGI 1998**
— **Radical mastoidectomy** is done for: **Attico antral cholesteatoma.**	**UPSC 1988**

➲ Ramsay Hunt Syndrome: High Yield for 2011-2012

❐ **VZV infection** of the head and neck that **involves the facial nerve often** (CN VII). **Kerala 2007**
❐ Other cranial nerves (CN) might be also involved, including **CN VIII, IX, V, and VI** (in order of frequency).
❐ This infection gives rise to **vesiculation and ulceration** of the external ear and ipsilateral anterior two-thirds of the tongue and soft palate, as well as ipsilateral facial neuropathy (in CN VII), radiculoneuropathy, or geniculate ganglionopathy.
❐ Acute peripheral facial neuropathy associated with erythematous vesicular rash of the skin of the ear canal, auricle (also **termed herpes zoster oticus**). **JKBOPEE 2012**

⇨ Most Common Organisms

▶ **Otomycosis**	Aspergillus niger>candida	**Delhi 96**
▶ **Furuncle**	Staph aureus	
▶ **Ramsay Hunt Syndrome**	Herpes Zoster virus	**JKBOPEE 2012**
▶ **Malignant Otitis externa**	Pseudomonas aureginosa	**Comed 07**
▶ **Bullous myringitis**	Viral (Influenza virus)	**AIIMS 87**
▶ **Haemorrhagic otitis externa**	Influenza	**PGI 98**
▶ **Perichondritis**	Pseudomonas aeruginosa	**NIMHANS 2006**

- H. Inflluenza **used to be** the most common cause of bacterial meningitis under 5 years.
- Since the introduction of vaccine its occurrence has **greatly decreased.**
- Risk factors for H. Influenza include **Otitis media**, Sinusitis, Pharyngitis and other URTI.
- As such its occurrence also is **associated with significant Sensorineural hearing loss in up to 20 percent of cases.**
- It is recommended to give Steroids immediately along with antibacterials to **decrease hearing loss**

Aspergellosis in Ear: High Yield for 2011-2012

- Aspergillus is **mold with septate hyphae.**
- **Asexual conidia** are arranged in chain, carried on elongated cells called sterigmata born on expanded ends of conidiophores.
- **Aspergillus fumigatus** is MC cause of aspergillosis.
- Commonest human disease caused by aspergillosis is **otomycosis.**
- Aspergillus infection is characterized by **hyphae invasion of blood vessel, thrombosis, necrosis, and hemorrhagic infarction.**

Otosclerosis: High Yield for 2011-2012

▶ **Autosomal dominant** ☛☛☛	
▶ **Begins in "fossula antefenestrum."**	**PGMEE 2006**
▶ **Common in females.**	
▶ **Family history positive.**	**PGI 2006**
The most common cause of a progressive conductive hearing loss usually bilateral in an adult with a normal ear drum. ☛☛	
Reversible conductive deafness seen.	**PGI 2006**
Otosclerosis is a disease of the bone of the otic capsule, with a predilection for the anterior part of the oval window. ☛☛	
Flammingo pink tympanic membrane seen.	**AI 1988**
But in majority TM is normal (Kindly remember)	
Paracusis wilsii (ability to hear better in noisy environment) ☛ ☛	**KAR 95**
(Positive Schwartz test)	
Carharts notch at 2000 Hz present ☛☛	**AI 03, PGI 98**
Gelles test is done for otosclerosis.	**JIPMER 1998**
Stapedectomy is surgery of choice ☛☛	**UPSC 85, AIIMS 87**
Sodium flouride is of benefit.	
Used in pinkish tympanic membrane.	**AI 2010**
Other operations done are: Fenetration and stapedotomy.	**PGI 2003**

➡ Commonest site of Otosclerosis: ☛☛ Oval window	COMED 07
➡ Commonest bone affected in otosclerosis: ☛☛ Stapes	UPSC 88

5

ENT

⇨ Meniere's Disease/Endolymphatic Hydrops/Ear Glaucoma

Meniere's disease is characterized by **triad of**

- ► Hearing loss,
- ► Tinnitus, and
- ► Recurrent prostrating vertigo. ☛ ☛ ☛ **AMC 91, JIPMER 89**

Tinnitus is non pulsatile. **AIIMS 2006**

Low frequency sensorineural hearing loss is seen. **KAR 2001**

The pathologic change in the inner ear is **generalized dilation of the membranous labyrinth,** or **endolymphatic hydrops.** ☛☛ **PGI 2003**

Only one ear is involved in **85%** of patients with Meniere's disease.☛☛

- ► **Females** are more commonly effected☛☛
- ► **Diplacussis** (Same sound perceived as two different pitch in two ears)☛
- ► **Henneberts sign**: Vertigo and Nystagmus induced by pressure to stapedial foot plate☛☛ **DNB 2011**
- ► **Tulios phenomenon**: Vertigo and Nystagmus induced by loud noise☛☛

⇨ Benign Paroxysmal Positional Vertigo and Nystagmus ☛

Vertigo that occurs with **changes in position** may follow lesions in the inner ear, eighth nerve, brain stem, or cerebellum. ☛☛

Positional vertigo and nystagmus arising from **the inner ear** is termed benign paroxysmal positional vertigo and nystagmus. ☛☛

The patient experiences vertigo **when lying on or rolling over onto the affected ear or when tilting the head back to look up.** There is a **latency of a few seconds** after assuming the provocative position before the vertigo and nystagmus begin. ☛☛

The vertigo is characterized by an intense sensation of spinning, and the **nystagmus is rotary and counterclockwise when the affected right ear is placed under and clockwise when the affected left ear is placed under.** ☛☛

The **quick component of the nystagmus is always toward the affected** ear. ☛☛

The finding of basophilic calcium-containing concretions in the ampulla of the posterior semicircular canal has led some to refer to this condition as **cupulolithiasis.** ☛

⇨ Bell's Palsy

Bell's palsy is a **unilateral facial paralysis** that develops suddenly and is accompanied by pain in the postauricular area. **(LMNL)** UPSC 2001

It is thought to be of **viral etiology.**

All divisions of the nerve are paralyzed; this distinguishes the disease from a supranuclear lesion. The lesion is in the internal auditory meatus or the intratemporal course of the nerve. The initial pathologic changes are **hyperemia and edema.**

- **Acute onset** DELHI 2008
- **Spontaneous remission**
- **Increased predisposition in Diabetes Mellitus** DELHI 2008

The **edema compresses the blood supply to the nerve** because of the bony confines of the fallopian canal. A conduction block develops without death or degeneration of the axons. Release of the pressure on the nerve produces rapid recovery of function. This type of paralysis is termed **neurapraxia.**

Corticosteroid therapy is initiated as soon as possible after the onset of the paralysis and is continued for 10 days to minimize the inflammatory reaction.

Is an indication for decompression of the facial nerve by removing the bone of the fallopian canal. **Approximately 85% of all patients with idiopathic facial nerve paralysis recover spontaneously.**

⇨ Temporal Bone Trauma can Lead to

- ✓ **Facial nerve palsy**
- ✓ **Hearing loss**
- ✓ **Hemotympanum**
- ✓ **TM perforation**
- ✓ **CSF rhinorrhea**
- ✓ **CSF otorrhea**
- ✓ **Nystagmus**
- ✓ **Battle sign**
- ✓ **Raccoon sign**

HIGH Yield for 2011-2012

➲ Perilymph Fistula: High Yield for 2011-2012

- In this condition perilymph leaks into the middle ear through the oval or round window.It can follow:
- As a complication of stapedectomy , or ear surgery when stapes is accidentally displaced. It can also occur as well as a result of sudden pressure changes in middle ear e.g. **barotraumas,**
  - ✓ **Diving,**
  - ✓ **Forceful valsalva, or**
  - ✓ **Raised ICT**

➲ Crocodile Tears: High Yield for 2011-2012

Injury to facial nerve may be associated with aberrant nerve regeneration. Fibers that normally innervate salivary glands may regenerate to innervate lacrimal gland. This leads to crying when patient is eating. (GUSTATORY TEARING)

⇨ Chemodectomas

These nonchromaffin paragangliomas are termed **glomus jugulare or glomus tympanicus** tumors, depending on their site of origin. PGMEE 2007

The glomus <u>tympanicus</u> tumor arises from the **area of Jacobson's nerve in the tympanic plexus on the promontory of the middle ear.**

The glomus <u>jugulare</u> tumor arises from the glomus jugulare body in the jugular bulb. Both tumors consist of rich networks of vascular spaces surrounded by epithelioid cells.

Usually the neoplasms grow slowly, and symptoms may not be evident until the neoplasm is quite large.

- **Pulsatile tinnitus,**
- **Facial nerve paralysis,**
- **Otorrhea,**
- **Hemorrhage,**
- **Vertigo, and**
- **Paralysis of cranial nerves IX, X, XI, and XII are often the presenting symptoms and signs.**

Characteristically, a **"red mass"** that **pulsates and blanches with compression with a pneumatic otoscope** can be seen in the ear canal or middle ear. **(Brown sign)**

The pulsation can also be demonstrated with tympanometry. There may be evidence of bone erosion in the mastoid process, middle ear, or petrous pyramid on CT. The extent of the lesion is best demonstrated with MRI with enhancement with gadolinium. Angiography is a necessary part of the preoperative evaluation.

⇨ Glomus Tumor: (Continued)

- One of the **most common benign tumor** of middle ear.
- **Squamous cell carcinoma is the commonest.** UP 2007
- Arises from **glomus bodies** in the jugular bulb of internal jugular vein PGI 2004
  - ✓ **Red reflex,**
  - ✓ **Rising sun appearance,**
  - ✓ **Bluish reflex through tympanic membrane** is a feature.
- **Earliest symptom** is **deafness and tinnitus.**
- Deafness is of <u>conductive</u> type
- **Vertigo** and **cranial nerves <u>IX and XII</u>** may get involved.
- **Multi centric with lymphatic metastasis.** PGI 2004
- **Modified radical mastoidectomy and excision of petrous temporal bone are standard Procedures.** MAHE 2007

➲ Acoustic Neurinomas/Vestibular Schwannoma: High Yield for 2011-2012

They arise more often from the **vestibular division** of the eighth nerve.	PGI 88
Superior Vestibular nerve is most commonly involved	JK BOPEE 05, AI 2010
These neoplasms are derived from **Schwann cells.**	
Compromise Most of **CP angle tumors**	
▶ **Cranial nerve V is involved first**	AI 07
▶ **(Loss of corneal reflex)**	Kerala 04
▶ **Deafness** is the earliest symptom	AI 84
▶ **Deafness is Retrocochlear type.**	PGI 99
The **NF2 gene** (Schwannomerlin, Schwannomin, MERL_HUMAN, merlin Moesin-Ezrin-Radixin-Like Protein) is located on the long (q) arm of chromosome **22.**	
Upon microscopic examination, the acoustic neurinoma presents two distinctive architectural patterns, designated **Antoni A and Antoni B.** Both are created by spindle cells with elongated nuclei and fibrillated cytoplasm, predominantly those of Schwann cells. The two tissue patterns differ in cellular weave and density.	
▶ **Antoni A** tissue is compact, with a prominence of interwoven fascicles.	
▶ **Antoni B** tissue is porous and less structured.	
In **Neurofibromatosis type II**, bilateral acoustic neuromas are the hallmark	
There is public concern that **use of mobile phones** could increase the risk of brain Tumors. If such an effect exists, acoustic neuroma would be of particular concern because of the proximity of the acoustic nerve to the handset	
HITSELBERGER'S SIGN - In Acoustic neuroma- loss of sensation in the ear canal supplied by Arnold's nerve (branch of Vagus nerve to ear)	
The most useful (i.e., sensitive and specific) test to identify acoustic neuromas is an **Gadolinium enhanced MRI of the head.**	Kerala 97
Surgical removal is the treatment of choice.	
However stereotactic radiotherapy by using gamma knife or X knife may be used.	

⇨ Tunning Fork Tests are

— **Schwaback test**	
— **Rinne's test**	
— **Weber's tes**	
— **Gelles test**	DNB 2002

➲ Memorize

❐ AC>BC	Normal
➠ AC <BC (**Negative Rinne**) ☛☛ ➠ Sound lateralized to deaf ear(**Weber**) ➠ Absolute Bone conduction (ABC)normal☛☛	Conductive deafness
➠ AC>BC☛ ➠ Sound lateralized to better ear☛☛ ➠ Absolute Bone conduction (ABC)Shortened☛☛	Sensorineural deafness

⇨ For Feigned Hearing Loss: Stengers Test is done

Types of Tympanograms

Type A: Normal☛	
Type As: Ossicular Fixation: Otosclerosis	**JK BOPEE 09**
Type Ad: Ossicular Discontuinity☛	
Type B: Middle Ear Effusion or thick Tympanic membrane☛	
Type C: Retracted Tympanic Membrane☛	

➲ Ototoxic Drugs: High Yield for 2011-2012

❐ Salicylates,	
❐ Quinine and its synthetic analogues,	
❐ Aminoglycoside antibiotics, (Gentamicin, neomycin, kanamycin)	**AP 1984**
❐ Loop diuretics such as furosemide and ethacrynic acid, and	**UPSC 1988**
❐ Cancer chemotherapeutic agents such as cisplatin	
❐ Interferons	
❐ Deferoxamine	

⇨ Hereditary Prenatal Causes of Deafness:☛☛

There are large numbers of syndromes in which deafness is a recognized factor

❐ **Leopard syndrome:**

- ✓ **Lentigenes,**
- ✓ **ECG abnormalties,**
- ✓ **Occular Hypertelorism,**
- ✓ **Pulmonary stenosis,**
- ✓ **Abnormal genitalia,**
- ✓ **Growth retardation,**
- ✓ **Sensorineural deafness.** ☛

- ❒ **Pendred syndrome: Deafness +goiter** ☛ PGI 2002
- ❒ **Ushers Syndrome**: Deafness+mental retardation+seizures +retinitis pigmentosa+cataracts ☛ SRMC 2002
- ❒ **Warden burgs Syndrome: White ForeLock**+Hyperpigmented Patches+deafness +displacement of inner canthi ☛
- ❒ **Klippel-Feil syndrome**. A **short neck** limits head movements, the **hairline is low** at the back, there may be paralysis of the external rectus muscle in one or both eyes and there is sensorineural hearing loss which may be severe. ☛
- ❒ **Alport's syndrome** is **X-linked dominant** and affects boys more severely than girls. There is severe progressive glomerulonephritis and a progressive sensorineural loss which does not show itself until the boy is about 10 years old. ☛ SRMC 2002
- ❒ **Refsum's syndrome** consists of **ichthyosis, ataxia, retinitis pigmentosa, night blindness, mental retardation and a sensorineural deafness.**
- ❒ **Jervell and Lange-Neilsen syndrome** is autosomal recessive with a cardiac arrhythmia and a profound sensorineural deafness. These children may present with syncopal attacks and if untreated, these attacks can be fatal. ☛

➲ Other Syndromes

- Crouzons
- Aperts
- Klippel Feil
- Downs
- Goldenhars
- Peirre robinson
- Vander Hoves
- Sticklers
- Wilder vanch Syndrome

⇨ Presbycusis

- ❒ **Presbycusis** (age-associated hearing loss) is the **most common cause of sensorineural hearing loss in adults.** UPSC 2006
- ❒ In the early stages, it is characterized by **symmetric, gentle to sharply sloping high-frequency hearing loss.**
- ❒ With progression, the hearing loss involves all frequencies.
- ❒ More importantly, the hearing impairment is associated with **significant loss in clarity.**
- ❒ There is a **loss of discrimination for phonemes, recruitment (abnormal growth of loudness), and particular difficulty in understanding speech in noisy environments.**
- ❒ Hearing aids may provide limited rehabilitation once the word recognition score deteriorates below 50
- ❒ Significant advancements and improvements in cochlear implants have made them the treatment of choice.

5

ENT

⇨ Important Questions Asked:❋

Ramsey Hunt's syndrome is caused by **herpes zoster virus.**

- It is characterized by a **facial palsy** and is often associated with facial pain and the appearance of vesicles on the ear drum, ear canal and pinna.
- Vertigo and sensorineural hearing loss (**VIIIth nerve**) accompany it **PGI 1986**
- Treatment with aciclovir is effective if given early☛☛

➲ Laboratory Assessment of Hearing:☛☛☛High Yield for 2011-2012

Pure tone audiometry assesses hearing acuity for pure tones. ☛

PTA establishes the

- **Presence and severity of hearing impairment, unilateral vs. bilateral involvement, and the type of hearing loss.** ☛
- **Often, the conductive hearing loss involves all frequencies, suggesting involvement of both stiffness and mass.** ☛☛
- **In general, sensorineural hearing losses such as presbycusis affect higher frequencies more than lower frequencies.** ☛

An exception is Meniere's disease, which is characteristically associated with low-frequency sensorineural hearing loss. Noise-induced hearing loss has an unusual pattern of hearing impairment in which the loss at 4000 Hz is greater than at higher frequencies. ☛☛ **KAR 2001**

Vestibular schwannomas characteristically affect the higher frequencies, but any pattern of hearing loss can be observed. ☛☛

Speech audiometry tests the clarity with which one hears.

- **The speech reception threshold (SRT)** is defined as the intensity at which speech is recognized as a meaningful symbol and is obtained by presenting two-syllable words with an equal accent on each syllable. **The intensity at which the patient can repeat 50% of the words correctly is the SRT. An individual with normal hearing or conductive hearing loss can repeat 88 to 100% of the phonetically balanced words correctly.** Patients with a sensorineural hearing loss have variable loss of discrimination depending on the severity of hearing loss and the site of lesion.
- **Deterioration in discrimination ability at higher intensities above the SRT also suggests a lesion in the eighth nerve or central auditory pathways.** ☛☛☛

Tympanometry

- Measures the impedance of the middle ear to sound and is particularly useful in the identification and diagnosis of **middle-ear effusions.**
- **It provides information about the status of the tympanic membrane and the ossicular chain.** Normally, the middle ear is most compliant at atmospheric pressure, and the compliance decreases as the pressure is increased or decreased; this pattern is seen with normal hearing or in the presence of sensorineural hearing loss.
- **Compliance that does not change with change in pressure suggests middle-ear effusion.** ☛☛

During tympanometry, an intense tone (80 dB above the hearing threshold) elicits **contraction of the stapedius muscle.** The change in compliance of the middle ear with contraction of the stapedius muscle can be detected. The presence or absence of this **acoustic reflex** is important in the anatomic localization of facial nerve paralysis as well as hearing loss.

Otoacoustic emissions (OAE) can be measured with sensitive microphones inserted into the external auditory canal. The emissions may be spontaneous or evoked with sound stimulation.

The presence of OAEs indicates that the **outer hair cells of the organ of Corti are intact** and can be used to assess auditory thresholds and to **distinguish sensory from neural hearing losses.** AI 2010

Evoked Responses Electrocochleography measures the **earliest evoked potentials generated in the cochlea and the auditory nerve.** Receptor potentials recorded include the cochlear microphonic, generated by the outer hair cells of the organ of Corti, and the summating potential, generated by the inner hair cells in response to sound☛☛

Brainstem auditory evoked responses (BAERs) are useful in differentiating the **site of sensorineural hearing loss.** PGI 1997

Imaging Studies CT is ideal for the **detection of bone erosion** often seen in the presence of chronic otitis media and cholesteatoma. ☛

MRI is superior to CT for imaging of retrocochlear pathology such as vestibular schwannoma, meningioma, other lesions of the cerebellopontine angle, demyelinating lesions of the brainstem, and brain tumors☛☛

➲ Otoacoustic Emissions Testing: High Yield for 2011-2012

- Is used for **infant screening.**
- Its popularity for screening is based on the fact that it is a **noninvasive measure of cochlear (outer hair cell) function** and thus is **representative of peripheral hearing.**
- Otoacoustic emissions tests are **independent of neural and central auditory system** effects, can be relatively low cost to administer, and can be performed over a relatively broad, frequency-specific range (1,000 to 6,000 Hz).
- Unlike the ABR, OAE amplitudes are more robust at birth than in adulthood. Transient evoked otoacoustic emissions (TEOAEs) are used in the most common OAE screening test of infants (15), although distortion product otoacoustic emissions (DPOAEs) tests continue to increase in popularity.
- Transient evoked oto-acoustic emissions are reported to have excellent sensitivity
- Otoacoustic emissions are low-intensity sounds produced by the cochlea in response to an acoustic stimulus.
- A moderate-intensity click or an appropriate combination of two tones can evoke outer hair cell movement, or motility.
- Outer hair cell motility affects basilar membrane biomechanics; the result is a form of intracochlear energy amplification and cochlear tuning for precise frequency resolution. Outer hair cell motility generates mechanical energy within the cochlea that is propagated outward through the middle ear system and the tympanic membrane to the ear canal. Vibration of the tympanic membrane produces an acoustic signal (the OAE), which can be measured with a sensitive microphone.

5

ENT

➲ Auditory Brainstem Response: High Yield for 2011-2012

- The ABR is a surface-recorded averaged response representing the activity of the distal portion of the auditory pathway.
- As a rule, five to seven peaks occurring within a time frame of less than 10 ms make up the ABR. For neurodiagnostic purposes, the first five positive polarity peaks (waves I through V) are typically considered.
- The ABR may be recorded with standard or disposable surface electrodes placed high on the forehead below the hairline or at the vertex (noninverting electrode); on the medial surface of the ipsilateral earlobe; or on the medial surface of the contralateral earlobe (ipsilateral and contralateral inverting electrodes) and on the center of the forehead (ground electrode).
- These electrodes may be used for a typical two-channel montage with the ipsilaterally referenced channel emphasizing wave I (synonymous to the N1 of the electrocochleogram) and the contralaterally referenced channel emphasizing the separation between waves IV and V.
- **Waves I and II of the ABR reflect the activation of the distal and proximal segments of the cochlear nerve**, respectively.
- **Waves III and IV reflect the activation of the cochlear nucleus complex and the superior olivary complex.**
- **Wave V is associated primarily with the activation of the lateral lemniscus** and not the inferior colliculus as was previously considered.

➲ The Phonic Ear: HIGH Yield for 2011-2012

- Teaching the deaf has been revolutionized by the advent of the phonic ear.
- This is a radio-aid type of hearing device where the mother or the teacher wears a microphone and a transmitter and the child wears the radio receiver.
- This means the child can sit anywhere in the class and be in direct radio contact with the teacher and hence the degree of amplification can be greatly enhanced.
- Many children with quite severe hearing handicap can therefore now be educated in their own local school rather than having to go to specific schools for the hearing impaired.

⇨ Cochlear Implants

- This is the latest and most powerful form of hearing aid in which a small fenestration is made surgically in the basal turn of the cochlea and electrodes on a very delicate wire are inserted into the cochlea itself.
- These devices are extremely expensive and require considerable expertise and a huge amount of time for each individual electrode to be specifically tuned to the child's needs.
- Used for persons with severe to profound sensorineural hearing loss and those who cannot benefit from hearing aids
- It works by producing meaningful electric stimulation of auditory nerrve where degeneration of hair cells in cochlea has progressed to a level such that amplification provided by hearing aids is no longer effective. Cochlear dysplasia is not a contraindication to cochlear aids. **AIIMS 2010**

⇨ Remember the Tests

"Tober Ayer test" is positive in: **Lateral sinus thrombosis**	DNB 2001
"Hallpike test" is done for: **Vestibular function**	DNB 2002
"Recruitment test" is positive in: Meniere's disease	Kolkata 2002
"Stenger's test" is used to detect malingering	TN2007
Caloric test detects damage to chochlea	**MH PGM CET 2005 Jan, MH 2000**
Cottle's test is Improvement in nasal patency by retracting the lateral part of the cheek and thus testing the vestibular component of nose.	MH 2008

⇨ Lateral Sinus Thrombosis is Associated with Signs AP 2008

- Greisinger sign
- Lily-Crowe sign
- Tobey Ayer test

⇨ Ear Signs☛☛

- **BROWN SIGN**—blanching of redness on increasing pressure more than systemic pressure see in **Glomus jugulare**☛
- **HITSELBERGER'S SIGN** - In **Acoustic neuroma**- loss of sensation in the ear canal suppllied by Arnold's nerve (branch of Vagus nerve to ear) ☛
- **LIGHT HOUSE SIGN**--- seeping out of secretions in **Acute Otitis media** ☛
- **LYRE'S SIGN** - splaying of carotid vessels in **Carotid body tumor**☛
- **MILIAN'S EAR SIGN- Erysipelas** can spread to pinna (cuticular affection), where as cellulitis cannot. ☛☛
- **TRAGUS SIGN- External Otitis** , Pain on pressing Tragus☛☛
- **WAQUINO'S SIGN** is the blanching of the tympanic mass with gentle pressure on the carotid artery. Seen in **Glomus tumors.** ☛☛
- **BEZOLD'S SIGN** Inflammatory edema at the tip of the mastoid process in **Mastoiditis** ☛☛

⇨ Anatomy of the Nose and Paranasal Sinuses

- The skeleton of the nose consists of the **nasal bones, the ascending processes of the maxilla, the upper lateral cartilages, the lower lateral cartilages, and the septal cartilage**. The nasal septum is the medial wall of each nasal cavity.
- **The lateral wall** of each nasal cavity provides the attachment for the **three turbinates.** ☛
- **Nasal mucosa is largely supplied by branches of external carotid artery.** AI 1992
- **Pale, edematous nasal mucosa indicates nasal allergy.** PGI 1990
- **Warming, moistening and filtration are functions of nasal cavity.** KAR 1989
- **Deviated dorsum and septum is crooked nose.** PAL 1993
- **Depressed nasal bridge is seen in trauma, abscess and syphilis.** JIPMER 1981

- The **nasolacrimal duct** opens into the **inferior meatus**. The middle meatus lies between the middle turbinate and the inferior turbinate. PGI 1998
- The **ostia of the maxillary and anterior ethmoid cells** and the **nasofrontal duct** are in the **middle meatus**. The superior meatus lies between the superior turbinate and the middle turbinate. PGI 1998
- The **ostia of the Posterior ethmoid cells** are in the **superior meatus.**
- The **ostium of the sphenoid sinus** is in the posterior part of the superior meatus, the **sphenoethmoid** recess. KERALA 1998

Terms Relating to Disorders of Smell Include

- **Anosmia**, an absence of the ability to smell;
- **Hyposmia**, a decreased ability to smell; hyperosmia (an increased sensitivity to an odorant); dysosmia (Distortion in the perception of an odor); phantosmia, perception of an odorant where none is present; and
- **Agnosia**, inability to classify, contrast, or identify odor sensations verbally, even though the ability to distinguish between odorants or to recognize them may be normal.
- **Parosomia perception of bad smell.** MAHE 2001

Choanal Atresia: High Yield for 2011-2012

CHARGE Association:

- Coloboma [of eyes],
- Hearing deficit,
- Choanal atresia,
- Retardation of growth,
- Genital defects [males only],
- Endocardial cushion defect

Other anomalies associated with choanal atresia include polydactyly, nasal-auricular and palatal deformities, Crouzon's syndrome, craniosynostosis, microencephaly, meningocele, meningoencephalocele, facial asymmetry, hypoplasia of the orbit and midface, cleft palate, and hypertelorism.

Onodi Cells

- Are the **posterior most cells of the ethmoid sinus.** It is located **superolateral to the sphenoid sinus** and is in close relation to the optic nerve. Clinical importance:
- Attempt to remove the onodi cells during sinus surgery **may cause injury to the optic nerve** The onodi cells are a **potential cause for incomplete sphenoidectomy**
- **The anatomical landmarks of the sphenoid sinus correlate with that of onodi cells.**
- A surgeon may mistakenly believe that the <u>sphenoid sinus</u> has been reached

Structures Forming Nasal Septum

- Vomer
- Perpendicular plate of ethmoid
- Nasal spine of frontal
- Rostrum of sphenoid
- Nasal
- Palatine and maxilla
- Septal cartilage
- Inferior nasal cartilage
- Lower end formed by skin

CSF Rhinorrhea

- Refers to the **drainage of** cerebrospinal fluid **through the** nose.
- It is characterized by nasal discharge, which will test positive for **glucose and, uniquely, beta-2 transferrin**
- It is a **sign of** basal skull fracture.
- Management includes watchful waiting - leaks often stop spontaneously; if this does not occur then neurosurgical closure is necessary.

Olfactory Pathway

The unmyelinated axons of the receptor cells form the fila of the olfactory nerve, pass through the **cribriform plate**, and terminate within spherical masses of neuropil, termed **glomeruli**, in the olfactory bulb. The glomeruli are the focus of a high degree of convergence of information, since many more fibers enter than leave them. The main second-order neurons are the **mitral cells.** The primary dendrite of each mitral cell extends into a single glomerulus. Axons of the mitral cells project along with the axons of adjacent tufted cells to the limbic system, including the **anterior olfactory nucleus, the prepiriform cortex, the periamygdaloid cortex, the olfactory tubercle, the nucleus of the lateral olfactory tract, and the corticomedial nucleus of the amygdala.**

A secondary potential site of olfactory chemosensation is located in the **epithelium of the vomeronasal organ, a tubular structure that opens on the ventral aspect of the nasal septum.** Sensory neurons located in the vomeronasal organ **detect pheromones**, nonvolatile chemical signals that in lower mammals trigger innate and stereotyped reproductive and social behaviors, as well as neuroendocrine changes.

Ozena, or Atrophic Rhinitis,

- Is characterized by **atrophied mucosa overlaid by foul-smelling dry crusts** (Greek ozein, "stench").
- **Klebsiella ozaenae** is often isolated from nasal cultures.
- **Youngs operation done in atrophic rhinitis.** **DNB 1990**

Rhinoscleroma :Klebsiella rhinoscleromatis

- It is a **chronic granulomatous disease** of the upper respiratory tract mucosa
- **Mikulicz cells (foamy histiocytes)** are seen in the submucosa of biopsy specimens. **JIPMER 2002**

5

ENT

- **Russel bodies are also a feature.** ☛ **MAH 2012**
- Rhinoscleroma can be treated with streptomycin, trimethoprim-sulfamethoxazole, a quinolone, or tetracycline for 2 months. ☛☛

Glanders: Pseudomonas mallei ☛

- A respiratory disease of horses. Infection is rare in humans; nasal inoculation may produce a purulent nasal discharge followed by granulomatous intranasal lesions that ulcerate. ☛
- Treatment is with sulfadiazine. ☛☛

Neonatal congenital syphilis

- May present as **rhinitis (snuffles)**, and the generalized osteochondritis that follows may result in a **"saddle-nose" deformity.** ☛☛

Rhinosporidiosis : ☛☛☛

- **Rhinosporidium seeberi** is a fungus-like organism, not yet cultured, that causes **Rhinosporidiosis.** "☛☛
- **Pedunculated nasal masses"** that grow over months or years cause obstruction and a foul odor and must be surgically excised. ☛☛

Blastomyces dermatitidis, ☛☛

- A fungus prevalent in the Mississippi and Ohio River valleys, usually causes **pulmonary disease** but may cause **chronic ulcerative lesions of the skin and nasal mucosa.** ☛☛

Mucormycosis, ☛

- A life-threatening fungal illness that occurs **primarily in diabetic patients**, may present as **black eschars** in the nasal cavity ☛☛ **AI 1997**

➲ Important Points Related to Nose

Oblique # of nasal septum: **Jarjavey #**	**PGI 1997**
Horizontal # of nasal septum: **Chaevellet #**	
Rhinophyma: Sebaceous gland hypertrophy.	
CSF Rhinorrhea:	
✓ # Cribrifiorm plate of ethmoid, Naso ethmoid#	**PGI 2003**
✓ Beta 2 transferrin levels high.	**AI 2007**
✓ Contains glucose	**PGI 2002**
✓ Less proteins	
Apple jelly nodules on nasal septum. Lupus vulgaris	**PGI 1996**

➲ Mucormycosis: High Yield for 2011-2012

- ❒ Rhizopus and Rhizomucor species are ubiquitous, appearing on decaying vegetation, dung, and foods of high sugar content.
- ❒ **Mucormycosis** is uncommon and is largely confined to patients with serious preexisting diseases.
- ❒ **Mucormycosis** originating in the paranasal sinuses and nose predominantly affects **patients with poorly controlled diabetes mellitus,organ transplantation, who have a hematologic malignancy, or who are receiving long-term deferoxamine therapy** **AI 1997**

- ❒ **Vascular invasion by hyphae** is a prominent feature.
- ❒ Ischemic or hemorrhagic necrosis is the foremost histologic finding.
- ❒ **Mucormycosis** originating in the nose and paranasal sinuses produces a characteristic clinical picture. **Low-grade fever, dull sinus pain, and sometimes nasal congestion or a thin, bloody nasal discharge are followed in a few days by double vision, increasing fever, and obtundation.**
- ❒ Examination reveals a unilateral generalized reduction of ocular motion, chemosis, and proptosis. The nasal turbinates on the involved side may be dusky red or necrotic.
- ❒ A sharply delineated **area of necrosis**, strictly respecting the midline, may appear in the hard palate. The skin of the cheek may become inflamed. Fungal invasion of the globe or ophthalmic artery leads to blindness.
- ❒ Opacification of one or more sinuses is detected by computed tomography (CT) or by magnetic resonance imaging (MRI).
- ❒ Carotid arteriography may show invasion or obstruction of the carotid siphon. Coma is due to direct invasion of the frontal lobe.

➲ Granulomatous diseases of the Nose: High Yield for 2011-2012

The nose can be affected by many disease processes causing a granulomatous response. The insults can be infectious, immunogenic, fungal and idiopathic in nature some examples are:

- Rhinoscleroma
- Lupus vulgaris
- Rhinosporidiosis
- Wegener's granulomatosis

➲ Trauma and Foreign Bodies☛☛

Nasal Fracture. The nose is a vulnerable leading part. **Fractures of the nasal bones are the most common fractures of the facial bones.** Fractures of the nose may involve the ascending processes of the maxillae and the nasal processes of the frontal bones as well as the nasal bones. A fracture of the nose is **usually an open fracture.** ☛

The **most common deformity** is a **deviation of the nasal bones to the right,** with depression of the nasal bones on the left, characteristically occurring with a right hook. Fractures of the nose may be associated with **septal fractures and hematomas.** ☛

Trauma to the facial bones is often associated with a cerebrospinal fluid rhinorrhea.

Septal hematomas lie between the quadrangular cartilage and the perichondrium. When the perichondrium has been elevated from both sides of the septal cartilage, the cartilage undergoes avascular necrosis. Septal hematomas **frequently become infected, and abscess formation produces avascular and septic necrosis of the septal cartilage**, which causes a **saddle deformity of the nose.** Septal hematomas are **incised and drained as soon as the diagnosis is made.** ☛☛

Septal abscesses are located between the cartilage and the perichondrium. They may involve both sides of the cartilage. Septal abscesses are incised and drained under general anesthesia as soon as the diagnosis is established. Incisions are made bilaterally if there is pus on both sides of the septum. ☛☛

➲ Acute Bacterial Sinusitis❋

⇨ Pains of Sinusitis:

Symptoms of acute sinusitis include purulent nasal or postnasal drainage, nasal congestion, and sinus pain or pressure whose location depends on the sinus involved.
✓ **Maxillary sinus pain** is often perceived as being located in the cheek or upper teeth;
✓ **Ethmoid sinus pain**, between the eyes or retroorbital;
✓ **Frontal sinus pain**, above the eyebrow;
✓ **Sphenoid sinus pain**, in the upper half of the face or retroorbital with radiation to the occiput. Sinus pain is frequently worse when the patient bends over or is supine

➲ Important Points about Sinusitis

- **Maxillary Sinus is the commonest sinus involved followed by frontal, ethmoid and sphenoid.** UPSC 2007
- **Muco pus in middle meatus is a feature of maxillary sinusitis.** UP 2007
- **Periodicity is seen in frontal sinusitis.** COMED 2006
- **Frontal sinusitis doesn't occur at birth.** JIPMER 1986
- **Definitive diagnosis of sinusitis is done by Sinoscopy.** Manipal 2001

In children and adults, **Streptococcus pneumoniae** and Haemophilus influenzae (not type b), the most common pathogens respectively

Chronic sinusitis is characterized by symptoms of **sinus inflammation lasting 3 months.**

Orbital complications of sinusitis, such as **orbital cellulitis and orbital abscess**, usually arise from ethmoid sinusitis, since the ethmoid is separated from the orbit by only a very thin bone (the lamina papyracea). Patients present with fever, unilateral periorbital edema and erythema, conjunctival injection and chemosis, and proptosis.

Another extracranial complication of sinusitis is **frontal subperiosteal abscess (Pott's puffy tumor) from frontal sinusitis.**

Intracranial complications such as

- **Epidural abscess,**
- **Subdural empyema,**
- **Meningitis,**
- **Cerebral abscess, and**
- **Dural-Vein thrombophlebitis may result from sinusitis**, particularly from frontal or sphenoid infections. Because the sphenoid sinus sits between the two cavernous sinuses, **sphenoid sinusitis is a major cause of cavernous sinus thrombophlebitis.**

FESS (Functional Endoscopic Sinus Surgery): High Yield for 2011-2012

Indicated in:	
▶ Nasal polyps	PGI 2003
▶ Non responsive chronic sinusitis	
▶ Recurrent sinusitis	
▶ Sinus biopsy	
▶ Sinus cyst	
▶ Antrochonal polyp	
▶ Mucocele	PGI 2003
▶ Pyocele	
▶ Control of epistaxis	
▶ Foreign body removal	
▶ Endoscopic septoplasty	

Important Points to Remember in a Case of Nasal Polyps

- If a polypus is **red and fleshy, friable and has granular surface, especially in older patients,** think of **malignancy.**
- Simple nasal polyp may masquerade a malignancy underneath. Hence **all polypi should be subjected to histology.**
- A simple polyp in a child may be **glioma, an encephalocele or a meningoenccephalocele.** It should always be **aspirated and fluid examined for CSF.**
- **Multiple nasal polypi** in children may be associated with **mucovisidosis.**
- **Epistaxis and orbital symptoms** associated with a polyp should always arouse the **suspicion of malignancy.**

Various Diseases Associated with Polyp Formation

- **Chronic rhinosinusitis**
- **Asthma**
- **Aspirin intolerance**
- **Cystic fibrosis**
- **Kartagener's syndrome**
- **Young's syndrome**
- **Churg-strauss syndrome**
- **Nasal mastocytosis**

5

ENT

➲ Differential Diagnosis Between Mucous and Antrocoanal Polypi:

High Yield for 2011-2012

S.NO	FEATURES	MUCOUS POLYP	ANTROCOANAL POLYP
1.	Basis	➨ Usually allergic	➨ Usually infective
2.	Origin	➨ Ethmoid sinuses and middle meatus	➨ Maxillary sinus
3.	Age	➨ Usually adult	➨ Usually young.
4.	Side	➨ Usually bilateral	➨ Usually unilateral **JKBOPEE 2012**
5.	Number	➨ Usually multiple	➨ Usually single
6.	Surface epithelium	➨ Ciliated columnar	➨ Stratified squamous
7.	Examination	➨ Easily seen on anterior rhinoscopy	➨ Easily seen on posterior rhinoscopy

⇨ Epistaxis: ☛☛☛

Ninety percent of the time, epistaxis occurs from a plexus of vessels **(Keisselbachs plexus)** in the **anteroinferior** Part of the septum. (Littles area) **Kerala 1988**

Which is an area of anastomosis between ICA and ECA ☛☛

Arteries contributing to Littles area: **UPSC 2005**

- ▶ Sphenopalatine, **JK BOPEE 2011**
- ▶ Anterior ethmoidal,
- ▶ Superior labial,
- ▶ Greater palatine artey

Recurrent epistaxis is seen in: **AI 1996**

- ✓ DNS
- ✓ Atrophic rhinitis
- ✓ Maxillary carcinoma

- ➨ In the other 10% of cases, nasal bleeding occurs from the **posterior part of the nose,** particularly from far posterior in the inferior meatus at the junction of the inferior meatus and the nasopharynx. ☛
- ➨ **Wood ruffs area (under the posterior end of inferior turbinate where sphenopalatine artery anastomoses with posterior pharyngeal artery may be source of posterior epistaxis. MAH 2012**
- ➨ It is from this area that individuals with **arteriosclerosis and hypertension** are likely to bleed. ☛
- ➨ This type of bleeding may be difficult to control

Silver nitrate is preferred as the cauterizing agent, since it produces satisfactory intravascular coagulation without a severe burn of the mucous membrane. ☛

Nose pricking is the **commonest cause of epistaxis in children.** ☛

Hypertension is the **commonest cause of epistaxis in adults.**
Mc cause of epistaxis in pubescent male: Angiofibroma SGPGI 2005
Mc cause of epistaxis in pubescent female: Bleeding disorder
MC cause of epistaxis in children: trauma. UP 2007
A particularly debilitating form of epistaxis occurs in **hereditary hemorrhagic telangiectasia (Rendu-Osler-Weber disease).** Patients with this disease have frequent bleeding from the nose and gastrointestinal tract.

⇨ Posterior Epistaxis

- Posterior epistaxis if from terminal branches of **sphenopalatine artery** and internal maxillary artery
- It is more serious and is frequently associated with **hypertension, diabetes mellitus or major systemic vascular disease.**
- Sphenopalatine artery enters the lateral wall of the middle turbinate, gives a branch to posterior choana called **artery of Zuckerkandl** which is a source of posterior bleed in hypertensives.

Congenital Malformations

➲ Choanal Atresia: High Yield for 2011-2012

Choanal Atresia. Choanal atresia is a malformation in which the **opening of the nasal cavity into the nasopharynx is obstructed by a partition of mucous membrane and bone.**
The malformation may occur unilaterally or bilaterally.
If it occurs bilaterally, it produces respiratory distress in the neonate.
Newborn infants are obligatory nasal breathers. If there is obstruction to the nasal airway, asphyxia occurs.
The newborn presses his tongue against the roof of his mouth during the inspiratory effort. Fortunately, crying, with its attendant mouth breathing, often allows some ventilatory exchange.
This diagnosis should be made in the **delivery room.**
Choanal atresia should be considered in an infant who makes respiratory effort but fails to accomplish ventilatory exchange.
The immediate solution to the problem is the insertion of an oral airway.

➲ Oral Cavity

⇨ Ludwigs Angina:

- **Edema of floor of mouth.**
- Involves **submandibular, sublingual spaces.** PGI 2007
- Bilateral usually
- Is a rapidly spreading, life-threatening cellulitis of the sublingual and submandibular spaces that usually starts in an infected lower molar. **Patients are febrile and may drool the secretions they cannot swallow.**
- **A brawny, board like edema in the sublingual area pushes the tongue up and back.**
- **Airway obstruction may result as the infection spreads to the supraglottic tissues**

⇨ Vincent's Angina

- Vincent's angina, also called **acute necrotizing ulcerative gingivitis or trench mouth,**
- Have **halitosis and ulcerations of the interdental papillae.**
- **Oral anaerobes are the cause,** **KCET 2012**
- Therapy with oral penicillin plus metronidazole or with clindamycin alone is effective in both this condition and gingivitis.

⇨ Ranula

- Sublingual **JIPMER 1996**
- Thin walled, **retention cyst** **MAHE 2005**
- Due to **obstruction of mucus glands**
- Lined by columnar epithelium
- Complete excision is the ideal treatment.

➲ Cancrum Oris: High Yield for 2011-2012

- **Rapidly developing gangrene in oral cavity.**
- Post measles usually.
- Does not involve jaw.
- **Noma**, or cancrum oris, is a fulminant gangrenous infection of the oral and facial tissues that occurs in severely malnourished and debilitated patients and is especially common among children. **Beginning as a necrotic ulcer in the gingiva of the mandible**, noma is caused by oral anaerobes, especially fusospirochetal organisms **(e.g., Fusobacterium nucleatum).**
- It is treated with high-dose penicillin, debridement, and correction of the underlying malnutrition.

➲ Oral Cancer:

⇨ Predispositions for Oral Cancer

MC malignant tumor of adult males. **AI 2004**

- Smoking
- Spirits (Alcohol)
- Sharp jagged tooth
- Sepsis
- Syndrome (Plummer vinson)
- Syphilis
- Betel nut

⇨ Pre Malignant Conditions: PGI 1999

Leukoplakia PGI 2011

"Leukoplakia" applies to a white plaque that does not rub off and whose appearance does not indicate another disease. Leukoplakia can occur in any area of the mouth and usually exhibits benign hyperkeratosis on biopsy. On long-term follow-up, 2 to 6% of these lesions will have undergone malignant transformation into squamous cell carcinoma. Areas of leukoplakia with a corrugated surface or mixed with areas of erythema are often found in the lower labial or buccal vestibule of those who use smokeless tobacco.

Erythroplakia PGI 2011

Solitary red macules or plaques ("Erythroplakia") are less common in the mouth than white lesions but should be viewed with concern because they may exhibit microscopic dysplasia or represent carcinoma in situ.

Chronic Candidiasis

- ✓ Pappilomas tongue/cheek
- ✓ OMSF (Oral Submucosal Fibrosis) PGI 2011
- ✓ Surgery treatment of choice PGI 2004
- ✓ Radiosensitive PGI 2004

⇨ Anatomy of the Pharynx❋

For descriptive purposes, the pharynx can be divided into the

- ▶ Nasopharynx,

  Oval shaped AI 1984

  Eustachian tube opens into it. AIIMS 1984
- ▶ Oropharynx, and
- ▶ Hypopharynx

However, from a functional point of view, the pharynx remains united by the constrictors of the pharynx. They have a common insertion in the median pharyngeal raphe and form a musculo membranous tubular passage from the base of the skull to the opening of the esophagus.

Waldeyers ring: The lymphoid structures of the pharynx include the pharyngeal tonsil or adenoid the palatine tonsils the Tubal bands and the lingual tonsils. ☛

Foreign Bodies☛☛

Foreign bodies of the pharynx are likely to be found in four locations: the palatine tonsils, the lingual tonsils, the valleculae, and the pyriform sinuses. ☛

- ➡ Foreign bodies in the palatine tonsil are removed by grasping the foreign body with a hemostat. ☛
- ➡ Foreign bodies in the nasopharynx require general anesthesia for their removal. ☛
- ➡ Foreign bodies of the hypopharynx are removed during direct laryngoscopy under local anesthesia. ☛

5

ENT

➲ Nasopharynx: ☛☛ High Yield for 2011-2012

Important Points about Anatomy of Nasopharynx:

- Also called as Epipharynx.
- The nasopharynx lies above the soft palate and behind the posterior nares, which allow free respiratory passage between the nasal cavities and the nasopharynx.
- Elevation of the soft palate and constriction of the palatopharyngeal sphincter close the isthmus during swallowing.
- The nasopharynx has a roof, a posterior wall, two lateral walls and a floor.
- A lymphoid mass, the adenoid, lies in the mucosa of the upper part of the roof and posterior wall in the midline.
- The lateral walls of the nasopharynx display a number of important surface features. On either side each receives the opening of the pharyngotympanic tube (also termed the auditory or Eustachian tube.)
- A vertical mucosal fold, the salpingopharyngeal fold, descends from the tubal elevation behind the aperture.
- Further behind the tubal elevation there is a variable depression in the lateral wall, the Pharyngeal recess (Fossa of Rosenmüller). It corresponds to Internal carotid artery.
- The floor of the nasopharynx is formed by the upper surface of the soft palate.

⇨ The Adenoids

- Nasopharyngeal tonsil.
- No crypts and no capsule
- Adenoid hypertrophy in childhood often leads to obstruction of the eustachian tubes and the choanae. Nasal obstruction, nasal discharge, sinusitis, epistaxcis and voice change.
- **Adenoid Facies:**
  - Elongated face with dull expression,
  - Open mouth,
  - Prominent crowded upper teeth,
  - Hitched up upper lip.
- This lymphoid hyperplasia may be physiologic or secondary to infectious and allergic manifestations.
- Obstruction of the eustachian tubes leads to serous or secretory otitis media, recurrent acute otitis media, and exacerbations of chronic otitis media.

Tornwaldt's Cyst:

- Cysts occasionally form in the region of the **medial recess of the nasopharynx**. These cysts become symptomatic when they become infected.
- There may be persistent purulent drainage that has a foul taste and odor.
- **Symptoms of eustachian tube obstruction and sore throat may be prominent.**
- Excision or marsupialization of the cyst with an adenotome is the treatment of choice. ☛☛

⇨ Benign Neoplasms of the Nasopharynx

Juvenile Nasopharyngeal Angiofibroma☛

Juvenile angiofibromas are Benign, vascular neoplasms ☛	**TN 1991**
They are common in **pubescent males.** ☛	
They cause **recurrent Epistaxis.** ☛	
Mc site is the posterior part of nasal cavity close to sphenopalatine foramen. ☛	**JIPMER 2004**
Biopsy is contraindicated in Nasopharyngeal angiofibroma. ☛	
They may encroach upon the paranasal sinuses, the orbit, and the intracranial cavity. Histologically, these neoplasms are composed of fibrous tissue and numerous thin-walled vessels without contractile elements. ☛	
Millers sign seen	**PGI 2006**
The extent of the neoplasm can be determined with **CT and angiography.**	
Contrast enhanced CT is DOC.	**AIIMS 1997**
The pterygomaxillary fissure is often widened on the sagittal plane of the CT of the lateral part of the nasopharynx by the extension of the neoplasm into the infratemporal fossa. These neoplasms have a characteristic vascular pattern on angiography. ☛	
Treatment with estrogens and embolization of the internal maxillary artery at angiography have been used to reduce the operative blood loss.	
These neoplasms are **responsive to radiation therapy.** ☛☛	**PGI 2003**
Surgery is the TOC.	**PGI 2003**

➲ Nasopharyngeal Carcinoma: ☛☛☛High Yield for 2011-2012

Lymphoepithelioma or squamous cell carcinoma is the most common type. ☛	
Carcinoma of the nasopharynx occurs at relatively young ages, and there is an unusually high incidence among the **Chinese.** ☛	
Bimodal age distribution seen	**AI 2010**
MC site is lateral wall of nasopharynx (Fossa of Rosen Muller) ☛☛	**JKHND 2003**
MC Cranial nerve involved is VII CN☛	
Epstein-Barr virus Is implicated☛	**AI 2010, MAHE 2005**
Cervical Lympadenopathy is the **commonest presentation.**	
Others present with **nasal or eustachian tube obstruction.**	
Obstruction of the eustachian tube may cause a middle-ear effusion. ☛☛	
Serous otitis media seen.	**PGI 2002**
The nasal obstruction may be associated with **purulent, bloody rhinorrhea and frank epistaxis.** The more dramatic symptoms caused by cranial nerve paralysis and cervical lymph node metastasis are, unfortunately, common presenting complaints. ☛	

5

ENT

The diagnosis is made by **biopsy of the primary tumor.**

Trotters Triad

- Conductive deafness, **MH 2008**
- Palatal paralysis and **MH 2008**
- Temporo parietal neuralgia is seen.

The **treatment of choice** for carcinoma of the nasopharynx is **irradiation with a supervoltage source.** The radiation should be delivered to the primary tumor-bearing area of the nasopharynx and to both sides of the neck whether or not there is clinically demonstrated metastasis. Operations have no role in the initial therapy of carcinoma of the nasopharynx. Those cervical metastases that remain clinically palpable following radiation therapy or that subsequently become apparent should be eradicated by radical neck dissection.

⇨ Fossa of Rosenmuller

The nasopharynx communicates with the nasal cavity **anteriorly** at the choanae and with the **oropharynx** inferiorly at the lower border of the soft palate. The **Eustachian tubes** enter the nasopharynx laterally and are covered superiorly and posteriorly by cartilage known as the torus tubarius. The **Fossa of Rosenmuller** (lateral nasopharyngeal recess) is located superior and posterior to the torus and is the most common location for nasopharyngeal carcinoma.

IT corresponds to Internal carotid artery. **PGI 2011**

At the base of this recess is the Retropharyngeal lymph node (The Node of Rouvier.)

⇨ Inverted Papilloma/Ringertz Tumor

- Of the nose and para-nasal sinuses are **rare TumorsThis** is **histologically benign tumor, but tends to act clinically in a malignant fashion.**
- It is associated with **squamous cell carcinoma in 10-15% of patients.**
- Pathophysiology: inverted papiloma of the nose and paranasal sinuses is recongnized as a **neoplastic growth of the epithelium on the lateral wall of the nose that inverts into the underlying stroma rather than proliferating outward from the surface.** **(that is why the name)**
- The neoplasm is characterized by its **capacity to destroy, tendency to recur after removal.**
- **Etiology:** still remains unknown. Inflammation, allergy, tobacco and occupation exposures have been discounted as significant factors.
- Viral etiology remains inconclusive and investigations using in-situ hybridization (ISH) and PCR have been used to determine its link with HPV (Types 6 and 11).

⇨ Esthesioneuroblastoma (ENB) AIPGME 2012

Also known as **olfactory neuroblastoma**, is a rare neoplasm originating from **olfactory neuroepithelium** are **undifferentiated tumors of neuroectodermal origin** derived from the olfactory epitheliumThe symptoms of esthesioneuroblastoma (ENB) can be classified into **nasal, neurologic, oral, facial, cervical, and ophthalmologic.**

Grossly, esthesioneuroblastoma (ENB) appears as a gray to red mass in the nasal vault.The hallmark of well-differentiated ENBs is arrangements of cells into **rosettes or pseudorosettes** (sheets and clusters). True rosettes **(Flexner-Wintersteiner rosettes)** refer to a ring of columnar cells circumscribing a central oval-to-round space, which appears clear on traditional pathologic sections. **Pseudorosettes (Homer-Wright rosettes)** are characterized by a looser arrangement and the presence of fibrillary material within the lumen.

Esthesioneuroblastomas stain **positive for S-100 protein and/or neuron-specific enolase**, while the stain usually is **negative for cytokeratin, desmin, vimentin, actin, glial fibrillary acidic protein, UMB 45, and the common leukocytic antigen.**

Surgery remains the primary treatment for esthesioneuroblastoma (ENB) and offers the best chance for locoregional control as well as survival. Both open and endoscopic craniofacial resection have achieved complete surgical resection with tumor-free margins.

➲ Peritonsillar Abscess/Quinsy: ☛☛☛High Yield for 2011-2012

Peritonsillar Abscess. Called Quinsy: JKBOPEE 2012

MC organism: streptococcus. **KERALA 1988**

Peritonsillar cellulitis and abscess are complications of acute tonsillitis in which the infection has spread deep to the tonsillar capsule.

Pus forms between the tonsillar capsule and the superior constrictor of the pharynx

The tonsil is displaced medially.

The **uvula** becomes tremendously edematous and is **displaced to the opposite side**

The soft palate is very red and **displaced forward**

- There is marked **trismus** due to irritation of the **pterygoid muscles**, and the head is held tilted toward the side of the abscess. It is painful for the patient to talk and to swallow.
- **Odynophagia,**
- **Hot potato voice,**
- **Referred otalgia via IX Cranial nerve are a feature.**

Swallowing is so painful that the patient drools. The breath is foul-smelling.

Peritonsillar cellulitis or abscess is rare in children under the age of 10 to 12 years and is usually caused by a group A beta-hemolytic streptococcus or anaerobe.

Tonsillectomy done usually 6 weeks after appearance. **KERALA 1988**

⇨ Parapharyngeal Abscess ☛☛☛

Parapharyngeal abscess may occur in infants and young children as well as in adults.

- The abscess is usually secondary to streptococcal pharyngitis or tonsillitis.
- Pus forms in the parapharyngeal space secondarily from the breakdown of lymphadenitis.
- The pus is **located lateral to the superior constrictor of the pharynx and adjacent to the carotid sheath.**
- The tonsil and soft palate may be displaced medially but there may be no inflammatory reaction in the pharynx.
- There is marked swelling in the anterior cervical triangle.

5

ENT

⇨ Retropharyngeal Abscess ☛☛

- Retropharyngeal abscess occurs in infants and young children and is rare after the age of 10 years.
- These infections are **located between the constrictors of the pharynx and the prevertebral fascia.**
- Dysphagia fever torticollis bulge in posterior pharyngeal wall are a feature.

⇨ So for Revision Purposes Remember:

Streptococcal Pharyngitis.

- The most common bacterial cause is **group a beta-hemolytic streptococci.**
- Rapid Strep antigen kits have a high degree of sensitivity and specificity.
- The gold standard is **throat culture**
- Penicillin is the antibiotic of choice and amoxicillin an acceptable alternative.
- Complications of streptococcal pharyngitis include **rheumatic fever, glomerulonephritis, peritonsillar abscess, and retropharyngeal abscess.**
- All but glomerulonephritis are preventable with early antibiotic treatment.

A peritonsillar Abscess

- Should be suspected when a patient with strep pharyngitis has persistent fever and an increasingly severely sore throat.
- The patient drools, and the affected **tonsil bulges medially.**
- The uvula will deviate to the noninvolved site and the patient has a **"hot potato" voice.** Intravenous antibiotics and surgical drainage are the treatment.

Retropharyngeal Abscess

- Presents as a soft tissue mass in the lateral neck of a patient with history of recent pharyngitis.
- Lateral films of the neck confirm the diagnosis.
- Intravenous antibiotics and surgical drainage are the treatment.

➲ Anatomy of the Larynx: ☛☛☛High Yield for 2011-2012

The skeleton of the larynx consists of the **thyroid cartilage, the cricoid cartilage, the arytenoid cartilages with corniculate and cuneiform cartilages, and the epiglottis.**

Larynx:

Larynx has nine cartilages. **PGI 2011**

3 paired and 3 unpaired cartilages. **PGI 2011**

Unpaired:

- ❒ Thyroi (Elastic) **PGI 2011**
- ❒ Cricoids
- ❒ Epiglottis (Elastic) **PGI 2011**

Paired:

- ❒ Arytenoids
- ❒ Corniculate
- ❒ Cuneiform

The primary function of the larynx is

Protection of lower respiratory tract. **PGI 1988**

That of a sphincter.

During deglutition, both the true vocal cord sphincter and the false vocal cord sphincter are closed, and the epiglottis is drawn posteriorly over the closed sphincter and serves as a watershed, deflecting food and fluid into the pyriform sinuses.

The larynx serves as the **sounding source for speech**. A fundamental tone is produced by the movement of the vocal cords, which is brought about by the flow of exhaled air past lightly approximated vocal cords.

Abductor of vocal cord is **posterior cricoarytenoid.** **KERALA 1995, JK BOPEE 2011**

Adductors of vocal cord: lateral crocoarytenoid, transverse arytenoid. **PGI 1986**

Vocal cords in larynx are lined by stratified squamous epithelium. **DELHI 1996**

Singer Nodule (Vocal Cord Nodule)

This is also called Teacher's nodule or Screamer's nodule. It is a small inflammatory or fibrous growth that develops on the vocal cords of people who constantly strain their voices.

- **The internal laryngeal nerve is sensory to larynx above vocal cords.**
- **The Recurrent laryngeal nerve is sensory to larynx below vocal cords.**
- **All muscles of larynx except cricothyroid are supplied by recurrent laryngeal nerve.**
- **Cricothyroid is supplied by External laryngeal nerve.** **JKBOPEE**

Muscles Acting on Vocal Cords: HIGH Yield for 2011-2012

- **Abductor:** Posterior cricoarytenoids.
- **Adductor:** Lateral cricoarytenoid, Interarytenoid (Transverse arytnoid),

Thyroarytenoid:

- **Tensors:** Cricothyroid, Vocalis (Internal Part of Thyroarytenoid.)

Nerve Supply

All the muscles of larynx are supplied by: recurrent laryngeal nerve except cricothyroid which is supplied by external laryngeal nerve.

Sensory Supply:

- **Above vocal cords by internal laryngeal nerve**
- **Below the vocal cords by recurrent laryngeal nerve**

- Paralysis of external laryngeal nerve causes **loss of timber of voice.**
- Paralysis of recurrent laryngeal nerve causes **hoarseness of voice.**

"Bilateral" Recurrent Laryngeal Nerve Palsy is seen in

- **Thyroidectomy** **Delhi 2008**
- **Carcinoma thyroid**
- **Cancer cervical oesophagus**

5

ENT

➲ Laryngeomalacia: High Yield for 2011-2012

A **5-week-old infant** is brought to the clinic for a 4-week history of **noisy breathing** that has not improved. She has otherwise been healthy except for a current upper respiratory infection for the past 4 days, which according to the parents, has worsened the noisy breathing. On examination, she has **inspiratory stridor**. The noisy breathing improves when the infant is asleep. the most likely diagnosis is: **Laryngomalacia**

⇨ Remember Causes of Stridor

- **Laryngomalacia**
- **Vocal cord palsy**
- **Laryngeal webs**
- **Vascular rings**
- **Subglottic stenosis**
- **hypocalcemia**

▶ **Mc cause of stridor in newborn.**	**PGI 2003**
▶ **Inspiratory stridor seen.**	
▶ **Omega shaped epiglottis.**	**UP 2007**
▶ **Reassurance is the treatment modality.**	**UP 2007**

Vocal Nodules. Vocal nodules are caused by **using a fundamental frequency that is unnaturally low and using the voice too loudly and too long.** ☛☛

Vocal nodules are condensations of hyaline connective tissue in the lamina propria at the **junction of the anterior one third and the posterior two thirds of the true vocal cord.** These nodules produce hoarseness and give the voice a breathy quality. In adults, these lesions are removed during direct laryngoscopy to restore the voice. However, it is necessary to begin voice therapy prior to surgical therapy, because if the underlying misuse of the voice is not corrected, the nodules recur. In children, surgical removal is not usually necessary, because the vocal nodules regress with voice therapy, which consists of voice rest, reduction in intensity and duration of voice production, and elevation of the pitch.

⇨ Vocal Cord Paralysis

Vocal cord paralysis follows traumatic, infectious, and neoplastic involvement of the vagus and recurrent laryngeal nerves and degenerative neurologic disorders.

Unilateral vocal cord paralysis produces hoarseness and aspiration. ☛

Bilateral vocal cord paralysis causes upper airway obstruction with little adverse effect on the voice. ☛☛

▶ Bilateral <u>INCOMPLETE</u> vocal cord paralysis causes Maximum stridor.	**KERALA 1991**
▶ **Most dangeous is bilateral <u>abductor</u> paralysis.**	**UPSC 2001**
▶ **Total thyroidectomy is the mc cause of vocal cord palsy.**	**UPSC 2005**
▶ **Bilateral recurrent laryngeal nerve palsy occurs in thyroid malignancy.**	**PGI 2000**

➲ The Recurrent Laryngeal Nerves: HIGH Yield for 2011-2012

- ❒ **The recurrent laryngeal nerves** are **branches of the vagus (CN X)**, and
- ❒ **Supply all intrinsic muscles of the larynx except the cricothyroid.**
- ❒ **The right** recurrent laryngeal nerve **recurs around the right subclavian artery.**
- ❒ **The left** recurrent laryngeal nerve recurs in the thorax around **the arch of the aorta** and ligamentum arteriosum.
- ❒ Both nerves ascend to the larynx **by passing between the trachea and esophagus (Tracheo esophageal groove)** in close proximity to the thyroid gland.
- ❒ The recurrent laryngeal nerves are therefore particularly vulnerable during **thyroid surgery**, and damage may cause **hoarseness.**

⇨ Thyroplasty

- ► Thyroplasty type I: Medialization of vocal cords — AI 2003
- ► Thyroplasty type II: lateralization of vocal cords
- ► Thyroplasty type III: shorten vocal cords
- ► Thyroplasty type IV: lengthen vocal cords

Heimlich maneuver (abdominal thrust) In this maneuver, the operator places his arms around the choking individual from behind, grasps the fist of one hand in the other hand, and brings both hands up in the subxiphoid area briskly to apply pressure to the diaphragm. The pressure increases the intrathoracic pressure and may expel the foreign body. Should this maneuver fail, an alternative airway must be established by the prompt performance of a tracheostomy.

⇨ Laryngeotracheobronchitis☛☛☛

Laryngeotracheobronchitis is **Croup**☛

MC Causative agent: **Para Influenza**

Haemophilus influenzae is the most frequently isolated agent in bacterial croup, but Staphylococcus and Streptococcus may also cause croup. ☛

Painful croupy cough, Hoarsness and stridor☛

Narrowing of subglottic region on x ray☛ **(Steeple Sign)**

⇨ Epiglottitis: ☛☛☛

H. influenzae Type b is the predominant microorganism in epiglottitis. ☛☛ — COMED 2009

Epiglottitis or supraglottic laryngitis is more likely to cause abrupt and complete airway obstruction. ☛

MC cause of death is also complete airway obstruction. ☛ — DELHI 1996

- ► **Child prefers sitting position (Tripod Sign)** ☛
- ► **Lateral x ray shows swollen epiglottis (Thumb Sign)** ☛
- ► **Hospitalization with IV Antibiotics, steroids, humidification and intubation are a sequence.** ☛

❒ **Hot potato voice: Quinsy**	
❒ **Median rhomboid glossitis: Candidiasis**	
❒ **Thumb sign: Epiglottitis**	
❒ **Hour glass sign: Subglotic edema**	
❒ **Seals bark cough: Croup**	
❒ **Steeple sign: Croup**	SGPGI 2005
❒ **Trench mouth: Vincents angina**	

⇨ Laryngoceles

Laryngoceles are epithelium-lined diverticula of the laryngeal ventricle and may be located internal or external to the laryngeal skeleton. ☛

An internal laryngocele may displace and enlarge the false vocal cord and may cause hoarseness and airway obstruction. ☛

External laryngoceles pass through the **thyrohyoid membrane** and present as a mass in the neck over the thyrohyoid membrane. AI 2006

The mass rises with the larynx on swallowing. Internal and external laryngoceles may coexist. ☛☛

Laryngoceles are more common in glassblowers, wind instrument musicians, and others who develop high intraluminal pressures. Initially, laryngoceles are filled with air and expand and collapse with changes in the intraluminal pressure. ☛☛

They are expanded during the Valsalva maneuver. They appear as smooth, ovoid, air-filled masses on CT scans of the neck. ☛

⇨ Quinkes Disease/Uvular Hydrops PGI 2004

- **The uvula ("little grape")** is a small **conical pedulous process hanging from the middle of lower border of the soft palate.**
- **Angioneurotic edema and Quincke's disease**, is edematous condition that may variably involve the deeper skin layers and subcutaneous tissues as well as mucosal surfaces of the upper respiratory and gastrointestinal tracts.
- **Immediate hypersnesitivity type I reactions**, seen with atopic states and specific allergen sensitivities, are the most common causes of angioedema.
- These reactions involve the interaction of an allergen with IgE antibodies bound to the surface of basophile or mastocytes.
- Physical agents, including cold, pressure, light and vibration, or processes that increase core temperature, may also cause edema through the IgE pathway.
- **Hereditary angioedema, a genetic disorder of the complement system, is characterized by either an obsence of functional deficiency of C'1 esterase inhibitor. This allows unopposed activaation of the first component of complement, with subsequent breakdown of its two substrates, the second (C'2) and fourth (C'4) components of the complement cascade. This process, in the presence of plasmin, generates a vasoactive kinin-like molecule that causes angioedema.**

⇨ Presentation

A patient complains of a foreign body sensation or fullness in the throat, possibly associated with a muffled voice and gagging. Upon examination of the throat, the uvula is swollen, pale, and somewhat translucent (uvular hydrops). If greatly enlarged, the uvula might rest on the tongue and move in and out with respiration. There might be an associated rash or a history of exposure to phsical stimuli, allergens, or a recurrent seasonal indicence.

⇨ Pappilomas of Larynx

- HPV implicated
- Common in children and infants **NIMHANS 1998**
- Multiple
- Recurrent **PGI 2K**
- Treated by removal/Surgical excision

➲ Premalignant Lesions

- Leukoplakia
- Keratosis **PGI 2001**
- Smoking
- Pappiloma **PGI 2001**
- Chronic laryngitis

⇨ Malignant Neoplasms of the Larynx ☛☛

The majority of malignant neoplasms of the larynx are **squamous cell carcinomas.** **PGI 1988**

Carcinoma may arise from the mucous membrane of any part of the larynx; however, there is a predilection for the true vocal cords, particularly the anterior portions of the true vocal cords. For purposes of clinical staging and end result reporting, carcinomas of the larynx can be divided into :

- **Supraglottic lesions** involve the epiglottis, aryepiglottic fold, and false vocal cords. ☛
- **Glottic lesions** are limited to the area of the true vocal cords. ☛
- **Subglottic lesions** include the glottic area as well as the subglottic area. ☛
- **Hypopharyngeal lesions** may be divided into lesions of the pyriform sinus, area, and posterior pharyngeal wall. ☛

Supraglottic Carcinomas ☛☛☛

Smoking is a common factor.

Pain is the mc manifestation. **PGI 2003**

Second mc laryngeal tumor.

Early lymphatic spread seen. **COMED 2005**

They may produce hoarseness by secondary involvement of the vocal cords, or they may produce pain on swallowing as the first symptom. Often the pain radiates to the ears.

Not infrequently, a patient with a supraglottic carcinoma presents with the chief complaint of a swelling in the neck that represents a metastasis

Early supraglottic carcinoma is successfully treated with radiation therapy to the primary lesion and both sides of the neck, but in advanced lesions, better survival rates are obtained with a combination of radiation therapy and surgical therapy ☛

Glottic Cancers:

Mc cancers	
Hoarsness is the mc manifestation	**AI 2005**
Hoarsness is the earliest manifestation	**AI 2005**
Best prognosis	**COMED 2006**
No Lymphadenopathy usually	**DELHI 2005**

Subglottic Lesions:

- Represent more advanced glottic carcinomas in which the neoplasm has secondarily invaded the subglottic area as well as the supraglottic area.
- Metastasis to the same side is present in 50% of patients.
- Subglottic extension of the carcinoma requires a total laryngectomy and radical neck dissection
- With thyroid lobectomy on the same side☛

Treatment Consists of:

- **Radiotherapy**
- **Surgery**
  - ✓ **Conservative laryngeal surgery,**
  - ✓ **Total laryngectomy**
- **Combined therapy**

Total laryngectomy is a radical procedure where the whole larynx including the hyoid bone, pre-epiglottic space, strap muscles and one more rings of trachea are removed. It is indicated in the following conditions:

Total laryngectomy is **contraindicated patients with distant metastasis.**

Pyriform Sinus Carcinomas

- Tend to remain asymptomatic for long periods of time.
- Often the patient presents with dysphagia and pain on swallowing that may radiate to the ear on the same side
- A combination of preoperative or postoperative radiation therapy and operation yields better survival rates than operation alone☛

Postcricoid Carcinoma: ☛

- The presenting complaint is usually pain on swallowing and dysphagia.
- Metastasis to both sides of the neck is common. **PGI 2005**
- A combination of preoperative or postoperative radiation and surgical therapy is usually employed, and the operation required is pharyngectomy, total laryngectomy, and, if there are palpable metastases, radical neck dissection on one side followed by radical neck dissection on the other side in approximately 6 weeks☛
- Verrocous carcinoma larynx is treated by endoscopic surgery. **UP 2007**

Lasers Used in ENT

– CO_2 LASER	AI 2010, JK BOPEE 2012
– Argon LASER	
– Krypton LASER	
– Nd YAG LASER	

▶ **Laryngeal TB:** Odynophagia occurs	
▶ Turban epiglottis	Delhi 2008
▶ Mammilated appearance	Delhi 2008
▶ Mouse nibbled appearance	
▶ **Laryngitis sicca:** laryngitis atrophica caused by klibessela ozoaena	PGI 2004
▶ **Quinkes disease:** Edema of uvula not vulva.	PGI 2004
▶ **Reikes edema: edema of vocal cords**	JIPMER 1998
▶ **Kiss ulcer of larynx:** vocal abuse.	KERALA 1994
▶ **Contact ulcer** of vocal cords: voice abuse	KERALA 1995

Dysphonia: High Yield for 2011-2012

- Dysphonia, or difficulty in producing sound, is usually associated with laryngeal disease (hoarseness).
- Some children have weakness or roughness of their voice in the course of an upper respiratory tract infection, this being a manifestation of laryngitis.
- Persistent hoarseness should be investigated and this can only be done by visualization of the larynx with a fiberoptic endoscope passed along the nose, into the nasopharynx.

The causes of hoarseness in children are as follows:

1. **Vocal nodules:** These occur at the junction between the anterior third and posterior two-thirds of the vocal cords. They are usually secondary to voice abuse and in loud and noisy children are known as 'screamers' node.
2. **Polyps of the larynx:** These occur spontaneously or following intubation and cause variable hoarseness. They are removed under general anesthetic.
3. **Laryngeal papillomas:** These are a rare cause of hoarseness associated with maternal genital warts (Papilloma Virus). They present as persistent hoarseness, sometimes with aphonia and occasionally airway obstruction. Treatment is by removal and multiple operations may be required. They do not become malignant but can spread into trachea and in rare cases, into bronchus.
4. **Unilateral vocal cord paralysis:** This can follow surgical or non-surgical trauma to the neck, or occur following viral infections including mononucleosis. The voice may be breathy if the cord is abducted or well maintained if the cord is medialized. The diagnosis is usually made on fiberoptic endoscopy, and treatment consists of speech therapy.

5

ENT

Aphonia

Complete loss of voice can occasionally occur with laryngeal pathology, e.g. papillomas, and in most cases the larynx should be visualized. Complete aphonia in an otherwise healthy child should be viewed with suspicion. Functional or 'hysterical' aphonia occurs after emotional or physical trauma, e.g. tonsillectomy

Remember the Terms

- **Hysterical aphonia/functional aphonia** is a disorder common in emotionally labile females (15-30 years) where patient communicates with a whisper.
- **Dysphonia plica ventricularis** is sound produced by false vocal cords instead of true vocal cords.
- Voice is rough, low pitched and unpleasant.
- **Androphonia** is vocal pitch in females due to androgenic hormones/ reduced activity of cricothyroid muscle.
- **Puberophonia** is persistence high pitched voice in adults. Normal from puberty to adult voice undergoes a change from high pitch to low pitch.

Tracheostomy

Indicated in

- Cancer larynx
- Coma
- Diphtheria
- Double tube — AI 1999
- Made of titanium silver alloy — AI 1999
- Cuffed tube used for IPPV

In **emergency traceostomy** structures which can be damaged are: AIIMS 2007

- Isthmus of thyroid
- Inferior thyroid vein
- Thyroid imma artery

Common complication is **tracheal stenosis.** PGI 1997

Mitomycin is used for tracheal stenosis AI 2010

Cancers of Head and Neck: High Yield for 2011-2012

Epithelial carcinomas of the head and neck arise from the mucosal surfaces in the head and neck area and typically are squamous cell in origin.

Etiology and Genetics

- **Alcohol**
- **Tobacco use**

Mmarijuana and

- **Occupational exposures such as nickel refining, exposure to textile fibers, and woodworking.**
- **The DNA of human papilloma virus has been detected in the tissue of oral and tonsil cancers, and** Epstein-Barr virus (EBV) infection is associated with nasopharyngeal cancer.

- **Squamous cell head and neck carcinomas** can be divided into well-differentiated, moderately well-differentiated, and poorly differentiated categories.
- Patients with poorly differentiated tumors have a worse prognosis than those with well-differentiated tumors.
- **Salivary gland tumors** can arise from the major (parotid, submandibular, sublingual) or minor salivary glands (located in the submucosa of the upper aerodigestive tract).
- Most parotid tumors are **benign**, but half of submandibular and sublingual gland tumors and most minor salivary gland tumors are malignant.
- **Malignant tumors** include **mucoepidermoid and adenoidcystic carcinomas and adenocarcinomas.**
- The mucosal surface of the entire pharynx is exposed to alcohol and tobacco-related carcinogens and is at risk for the development of a premalignant or malignant lesion, such as **erythroplakia or leukoplakia (hyperplasia, dysplasia)**, that can progress to invasive carcinoma.
- **Cancer of the nasopharynx** typically does not cause early symptoms. However, on occasion it may cause unilateral serous otitis media due to obstruction of the eustachian tube, unilateral or bilateral nasal obstruction, or epistaxis. Advanced nasopharyngeal carcinoma causes neuropathies of the cranial nerves.
- **Carcinomas of the oral cavity** present as nonhealing ulcers, changes in the fit of dentures, or painful lesions. Tumors of the tongue base or oropharynx can cause decreased tongue mobility and alterations in speech. Cancers of the oropharynx or hypopharynx rarely cause early symptoms, but they may cause sore throat and/or otalgia.
- Hoarseness may be an early symptom of **laryngeal cancer**, and persistent hoarseness requires referral to an otorhinolaryngologist for indirect laryngoscopy and/or radiographic studies
- **Advanced** head and neck cancers in any location can cause severe pain, otalgia, airway obstruction, cranial neuropathies, trismus, odynophagia, dysphagia, decreased tongue mobility, fistulas, skin involvement, and massive cervical lymphadenopathy, which may be unilateral or bilateral
- **In patients with lymph node involvement and no visible primary, the diagnosis should be made by lymph node excision. If the results indicate squamous cell carcinoma, a panendoscopy should be performed,** with biopsy of all suspicious-appearing areas and directed biopsies of common primary sites, such as the nasopharynx, tonsil, tongue base, and pyriform sinus.

Remember for Tumors:

➲ Ohngrens Line: High Yield for 2011-2012

Is an imaginary line extending from medial canthus of eye to angle of mandible. Tumors above this line have poorer prognosis than tumors below this line.

⇨ Levels of Lymph Nodes in Neck

Level I	Submental, Submandibular
Level II	Upper Jugular
Level III	Mid Jugular
Level IV	Lower Jugular
Level V	Posterior triangular group
Level VI	Pre laryngeal, Pretracheal, Paratracheal
Level VII	Upper mediastinal nodes

➲ Costen's Syndrome

(Mandibular joint neuralgia, temporomandibular arthrosis, temporomandibular dysfunction syndrome) HIGH Yield for 2011-2012

- A syndrome of ear and sinus symptoms dependent upon disturbed function of the temporomandibular joint.
- A syndrome as consisting **of partial deafness, stuffy sensation in the ears** (especially during eating), tinnitus, clicking and snapping of the temporomandibular joint, dizziness, headache, and burning pain in the ears, throat, and nose.
- Costen ascribed the symptoms to dental malocclusion.
- This syndrome consists mainly of **temporomandibular crepitation, decreased temporomandibular mobility, preauricular and auricular pain,** pain on movement, headache, tenderness of the jaws on palpation, and, sometimes, head and nasopharyngeal symptoms.

➲ ENT Manifestations of HIV

Ear:

- Otitis media
- Kaposi sarcoma of pinna
- SNHL
- Facial palsy of viral origin

Nose:

- Sinusitis

Oral Cavity

- Candida infection
- Angular chelitis
- Recurrent apthous ulcers
- Hairy leukoplakia
- Kaposi sarcoma
- NHL

Parotid

- Parotid cyst and parotitis

Esophagus

- Esophageal candidiasis

Neck

- Cervical lymphadenopathy

Important Anatomical Terms Essential for Exams

Killian's Dehiscence: High Yield for 2011-2012

- Is known as "Gateway of Tears" **Delhi 2008**
- Is a triangular area in the wall of the pharynx between the **thyropharyngeus** part of the inferior constrictor of the pharynx and the **cricopharyngeus** muscle.
- It represents a **potentially weak spot** where a pharyngoesophageal diverticulum **(Zenker's diverticulum)** is more likely to occur.

Palatopharyngeus: High Yield for 2011-2012

- Origin: Palatine aponeurosis and post margin of hard palate
- Insertion: Upper border of thyroid cartilage and blends with constrictor fibers. Upper fibers interdigitate with opposite side (Passavant's ridge) **PGI 2011**
- Action: Elevates pharynx and larynx. Passavant's muscle closes nasopharyngeal isthmus in swallowing
- Nerve: Pharyngeal br of vagus N (X) with its motor fibers from cranial

Tympanic Plexus

Formed by tympanic branch of glossopharyngeal nerve and symparthetic plexus around internal carotid artery. It lies on the promontry.

Chorda Tympani

It is a branch of facial nerve which enters the middle ear through posterior canaliculus and lies in close association to tympanic membrane. It also carries taste sensation from anterior two thirds of tongue and supplies secretomotor fibers to submaxillary and sublingual salivary glands.

Plunging Ranula

A pseudocyst caused by extravasation of mucus from obstruction to sublingual salivary glands. It is transillumination positive. Can coexist with ranula.

Sternberg's Canal **AI 2009**

- Is antero-medial to the foramen rotundum
- It is situated at the attachment of posterior root of lesser wing to the body of sphenoid.
- The parasellar bony defect is due to persistence of the lateral craniopharyngeal canal (Sternberg's canal)
- The canal lies was identified by Sternberg (1988) between the ossification centers of the 3 parts of sphenoid bone.
- Sternberg's canal is the lateral craniopharyngeal canal connecting middle cranial fossa with the nasopharynx.
- This canal is considered as the congenital origin for the intra-sphenoidal meningocele
- Sometimes a medial craniopharyngeal canal may be observed, running from the anterior part of the hypophyseal fossa to the exterior of the skull
- Infection may be carried from the nasopharynx towards the sphenoidal sinus via the canal.

➲ Sternal Clefts: HIGH Yield for 2011-2012

- Are an defects of the sternum resulting from failure of midline fusion of the two sternal bands during embryologic development.
- This failure of fusion can lead to defects ranging from simple sternal clefts to complete defects of the sternum and pericardium with herniation of the heart through the defect. This severe form of the defect, thoracic ectopia cordis, is believed to be the result of disruption of the amnion, chorion, or yolk sac during embryologic development.
- In 1958, James Cantrell at the Johns Hopkins Hospital described five cases found to have the following common characteristics: This association of defects has come to be known as **Cantrell's pentalogy**

✓ A lower sternal defect;
✓ A midline, supraumbilical abdominal wall defect (omphalocele);
✓ A diaphragmatic defect (Hernia);
✓ A pericardial defect; and
✓ A congenital intracardiac defect.

⇨ Zygomatic Fracture

"Tripod fracture" is the 2nd most common frequently fractured bone mostly caused by direct trauma.The fracture line passes through:

- ▶ Zygomaticofrontal suture
- ▶ Orbital floor
- ▶ Infraorbital margin and foramen
- ▶ Anterior wall of maxillary sinus
- ▶ Zygomaticotemporal suture

Clinical Features:

- **Flattening of malar prominence**
- **Step-deformity** of infraorbital margin
- Anaesthesia in the distribution of infraorbital nerve
- **Trismus, due to depression of zygoma** on the underlying coronoid process
- Oblique palpebral fissure, due to the displacement of lateral palpebral ligament
- Restricted ocular movements, due toentrapment of inferior rectus muscle producing diplopia**Herniation of orbital contents into the maxillary sinus**
- **Periorbital emphysema**, due to escape of air from the maxillary sinus on nose blowing.

➲ Calcifying Epithelial Odontogenic Tumor/Pindborg Tumor (CEOT) High Yield for 2011-2012

- Is an **odontogenic tumor.**
- Arises from the epithelial element of the enamel origin.
- It is a **typically benign and slow growing, but invasive neoplasm.**

- It is more common in the **posterior mandible of adults.**
- Typically seen in the 4th to 5th decades.
- There may be a painless swelling, and it is often concurrent with an impacted tooth.
- On radiographs, it **appears as a radiolucency (Dark area) and is known for sometimes having small radiopacities (white areas) within it. In those instances, it is described as having a "driven-snow" appearance.**
- Microscopically, there are **deposits of amyloid-like material.**
- Two-thirds of the lesions are **in jaws, more commonly in the molar area with a tendency to occur in the pre-molar areas.** It appears clinically to be a slowly enlarging painless mass. In the maxilla it can cause **proptosis, epistaxis and nasal air way obstruction.**

Some Important Signs: High Yield for 2011/2012

- **BOCCA'S SIGN** - Absence of post cricoid crackle(Muir's crackle) in **Carcinoma post cricoid**
- **BOYCE SIGN** - **Laryngocoele**-Gurgling sound on compression of external laryngocoele with reduction of swelling
- **DODD'S SIGN/CRESCENT SIGN** - X-ray finding-Crescent of air between the mass and posterior pharyngeal wall.
- **Positive in AC polyp** Negative in Angiofibroma
- **FURSTENBERGERS SIGN-** This is seen when nasopharyngeal cyst is communicating intracranially, there is enlargement of the cyst on crying and upon compression of jugular vein.
- **HITSELBERGER'S SIGN** - In **Acoustic neuroma**- loss of sensation in the ear canal suppllied by Arnold's nerve (branch of Vagus nerve to ear)
- **HONDOUSA SIGN**--X-ray finding in **Angiofibroma** indicating infratemporal fossa involvement characterized by widening of gap between ramus of mandible and maxillary body.
- **HENNEBERT SIGN**- False fistula sign (**cong.syphilis, Meniere's,**) **DNB 2011**
- **IRWIN MOORE'S SIGN**-------- positive sueeze test in **chronic tonsillitis**
- **RACOON SIGN**-Indicate **subgaleal hemorrhage** and not necessarly base of skull #
- **STEEPLE SIGN**- X-ray finding in **Acute Laryngo tracheo bronchitis**
- **STANKIEWICK'S SIGN** - Indicate **orbital injury during FESS.** fat protrude in to nasl cavity on compression of eye ball from ouside
- **THUMB SIGN** --X-ray finding A/c **epiglottitis**
- **TRAGUS SIGN- EXTERNAL OTITIS** , Pain on pressing Tragus
- **TEA POT SIGN** is seen in **CSF rhinorrhea.**
- **BATTLE SIGN**- Bruising behind ear at mastoid region, due to petrous temporal bone fracture (middle fossa #)
- **OODS SIGN**----- palpable jugulodigastric lymphnodes

➲ ENT Abscesses: High Yield for 2011-2012

- Bezolds abscess in sternomastoid sheath
- Peritonsillar abscess: Quinsy (between tonsillar capsule and superior constrictor muscle) JKBOPEE 2012
- Parapharyngeal abscess: Swelling of lateral pharyngeal wall which bulges medially.
- Space of Gillete abscess: Retropharyngeal abscess (between pharynx and prevertebral fascia)
- Citteles abscess: Abscess in digastric triangle
- Lucs abscess: Subperiosteal temporal abscess (Deep to temporalis muscle)
- Dubios abscess: Thymic gland abscess in congenital syphilis
- Politzeri abscess: Internal auditory meatal abscess due to labrynthitis

➲ Tracheostomy: High Yield for 2011-2012

Is making an opening in the anterior wall of trachea and converting it into a stoma on skin surface.

It is of three types:

- Emergency tracheostomy
- Elective tracheostomy
- Permanent tracheostomy
- **A vertical incision** is made in the in the midline of neck extending from cricoids cartilage to just above the sterna notch. This is the most favoured incision and be **used in emergency or elective tracheostomy.**
- **A transverse incision** 5cm long given 2 finger breadth above the notch can be used in elective procedures. It has the advantage of cosmetically **better scar.**

➲ Important Questions Repeated and Frequently Asked

➨ In Jarjaway fracture of nasal bone, the fracture line runs: **Horizontal**	MH 2010
➨ Most common cause of congenital stridor: **Laryngomalacia**	MH 2010
➨ Nerve of 6th branchial arch **Recurrent laryngeal**	
➨ Caloric test assesses the function of: **Lateral semicircular canal**	
➨ **Tensor veli palatini** causes opening of Eustachian tube.	MH 2010
▶ **Epstein-Barr virus** Is implicated in nasopharyngeal cancer	AI 2010
▶ **Mitomycin is used for tracheal stenosis**	AI 2010
▶ CSF-Rhinorrhoea is commonest in fracture to **Cribriform plate**	UP 2008
▶ Mode of trauma in petrous bone fracture **Transverse**	UP 2008
➨ A diabetic patients presents with black necrotic mass filling the nasal cavity. Most likely fungal infection is **Mucormycosis**	UP 2008
▶ Myringitis bullosa is commonly caused by **Virus**	UP 2008
▶ Earliest nerve involved in Acoustic neuroma is **V**	UP 2008

- Tober Ayer test is positive in: **Lateral sinus thrombosis** DNB 2007
- Carhart's notch is found in: **Otospongiosis** DNB 2007
- The abductor of vocal cords is: **Posterior circoarytenoid** DNB 2007
- Hallpike test is done for: **Vestibular function** DNB 2007
- In Dacryocystorhinostomy, opening is done into: **Middle meatus** DNB 2007
- Commonest complication of CSOM is **Mastoiditis** DNB 2007
- Recruitment phenomenon is seen in **Meniere's disease** DNB 2007
- Treatement for post-cricoid carcinoma (Nasopharyngeal carcinoma) is by **Total laryngectomy + Pharyngectomy + Esophagectomy** TN 2007
- Carhart's notch is located at **2000 Hz** TN 2007
- Improvement in nasal patency by retracting the lateral part of the cheek and thus testing the vestibular component of nose is **Cottle's test** MH 2008
- Stylalgia is also called as: **Eagle syndrome** MH 2008
- Paracusis Willis is feature of: Otosclerosis

- Most Common cause of croup is: **Viral infection** Delhi 2008
- Type I Thyroplasty includes: **Medialization of vocal cords** Delhi 2008
- Gateway of Tears" is **Killian's dehiscence** Delhi 2008
- "Mulberry" mucosa is seen in: **Hypertrophic rhinitis** Delhi 2008
- In auditory evoked brain stem potential, V wave is seen by signal from **Lateral lemniscus** Delhi 2008
- **The term "Otoconis" is related to Balance** KOL 2006
- **Glottic carcinoma-presents with Hoarseness** KOL 2006
- **Antrochoanal polyp originates from Mucosa of maxillary antrum** KOL 2006
- **Laryngocele arises from:Saccule of larynx** KOL 2008
- **Treatment of choice for nasopharyngeal carcinoma: Radiotherapy** KOL 2008

- A post dental extraction patients presents with swelling in posterior one third of the sternocleidomastoid pushes medially. Most likely diagnosis is **Parapharyngeal abscess** UP 2008
- A 13 years boy presented with selling in the cheek with recurrent epistaxis. Most likely diagnosis is **Angiofibroma** UP 2008
- Bilateral chemosis and proptosis is a presenting feature following infection of the nasal vestibule Most likely cause is: **Cavernous sinus thrombosis** UP 2004
- A post dental treatement, presented with pain and swelling of SCM, examination reveals medially shift of the tonsil, Diagnosis is **Parapharyngeal abscess** UP 2002
- A diabetic patients presents with black necrotic mass filling the nasal cavity. Most likely fungal infection is **Mucormycosis** UP 2008

5

ENT

NOTES

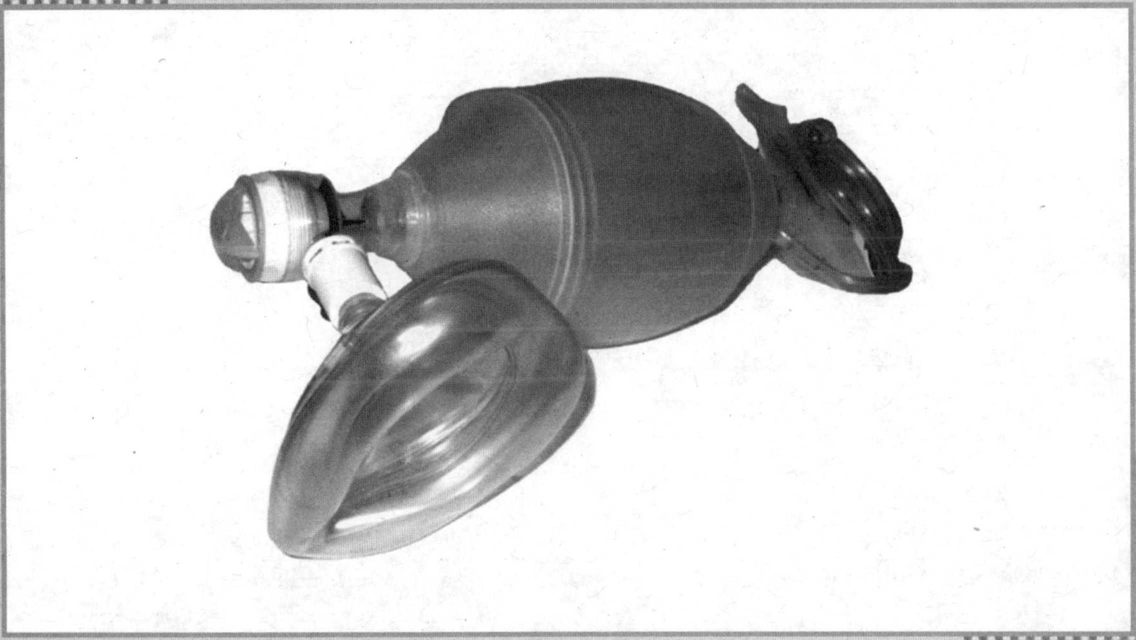

ANESTHESIOLOGY

✓ Term ANESTHESIA coined by Oliver Holmes.	TN 1995
✓ Anesthesia was first used by Morton.	
✓ Nitrous oxide was discovered by Priestley	
✓ Anesthetic properties of nitrous oxide were discovered by Humphry Davy.	MAH 2012
✓ Spinal analgesia was first described by Bier	
✓ IV anesthesia was discovered by Lundy	TN 1989
✓ IV Regional Anesthesia was discovered by Bier.	
✓ Xenon: William Ramsay	
✓ Balanced anesthesia: Evolved by Lundy	

➲ Anatomy Important in Anesthesia: High Yield for 2011-2012

❒ Extent of larynx: C3 -C6	
❒ Extent of trachea: C6-T5	
❒ Diameter of trachea: 1.2-1.6 cms	DNB 1983
❒ Angle of right main bronchus to vertical: Only 25°	AIIMS 1985
❒ Angle of left main bronchus to vertical: 45°	
❒ Carina is at level of: T4	ROHTAK 1989
❒ LP in adult is done in L3-L4 interspace.	
❒ LP in children is done in L4-L5 interspace.	

⇨ Infant Larynx

- One third of size of adult larynx.
- Suglottic area is the narrowest area in infants.
- Infant tissue is softer and more pliable.
- Epiglottis tilts more posteriorly.

Following features distinguish infant larynx from adult larynx:

✓ Epiglottis is long and leafy	Delhi 2008
✓ Subglottic region is narrowest laryngeal portion	Delhi 2008
✓ Large tongue	Delhi 2008

IDEAL GAS OBEYS PGI 1998

- ► Boyles law: Volume α 1/Pressure
- ► Charles law: Volume α temperature
- ► Avagadros law: Equal volume of gases at same temperature and pressure contain same number of molecules.

⇨ Anatomical Dead Space

AIIMS 09

- ❒ A normal individual at rest inspires approximately 12 to 16 times per minute, each breath having a tidal volume **of approximately 500 mL.**
- ❒ A portion (approximately 30%) of the fresh air inspired with each breath does not reach the alveoli but remains in the conducting airways of the lung. This component of each breath, which is not generally available for gas exchange, is called the **anatomic dead space.**

Increased by		Decreased by
✓ Old age		✓ **Intubation**
✓ Neck extension		✓ **Tracheostomy**
✓ Jaw protrusion		✓ **Hyperventilation**
✓ Bronchodilator		✓ **Neck flexion**
✓ ↑lung volume		✓ **bronchoconstriction**
✓ Atropine	**AI 1999**	
✓ Halothane	**AI 1999**	
✓ Inspiration	**AI 1999**	

➲ Lung Volumes and Capacities: High Yield for 2011-2012

	MEN	WOMEN
1. IRV	3300 ml	1900 ml
2. TV	500 ml	500 ml
3. ERV	1000 ml	700 ml
4. RV	+ 1200 ml	+ 1100 ml
5. TLC	6000ml	4200 ml

- ERV+RV=FRC
- IRV+ TV+ERV=VC
- IRV+ TV=INSPIRATORY CAPACITY

⇨ Airway is Assessed by

- Cormarck and Lehane Classification (View of Larynx at Laryngoscopy)❋
- Mallampati criterion❋
- Thyromental distance❋
- Sternomental distance❋
- Wilsons score❋

⇨ Airway Protection is by

- Head tilt, chin lift and jaw thrust maneuver
- Oropharyngeal and nasopharyngeal airways
- LMA (Laryngeal Mask Airways)
- ET (Endotracheal tube)
- Combitube

⇨ Premedication (AAAAAA)

- Anxiolysis JKBOPEE 2012
- Amnesia
- Anti emetic PGI 2002
- Antiacid
- Analgesic JKBOPEE 2012
- Anti autonomic

Allodynia:	**Perception of non painful stimulus as painful.** AIIMS 2006
Analgesia:	**Absence of perception of pain**
Anesthesia:	**Absence of all sensation**
Dysthesia:	**Unpleasant pain sensation**
Hypalgesia:	**↓response to noxious stimulus**
Hyperalgesia:	**↑response to noxious stimulus**
Hyperasthesia:	**↑response to mild stimulation**
Hyperpathia:	**Presence of hyperasthesia, allodynia, hyperalgesia**
Neuralgia:	**Pain distribution along a nerve**
Parasthesias:	**Abnormal sensation perceieved without apparent stimulus**
Radiculopathy:	**Functional abnormality of motor roots**

⇨ Minimum alveolar concentration: MAC: High Yield for 2011-2012

- **MAC is the best index of potency of anesthetics.**
- **It is unaffected by sex or duration of anesthesia.**
- **Nitrous oxide has highest MAC and Methoxyflurane the highest.**

It is alveolar vapor phase concentration of an inhaled anesthetic that prevents movement in 50% of patients in response to a standard noxious stimulus.

Factors↑ MAC:

- **Hyperthermia**
- **MAO inhibitors**
- **Hypernatremia**
- **Chronic Alcohol abuse**

Factors decreasing MAC:

- ❐ Hypoxia☛☛
- ❐ Hypothermia☛
- ❐ Metabolic acidosis☛
- ❐ Pregnancy
- ❐ Acute alcohol abuse.
- ❐ Drugs: opoids, propofol, ketamine, benzodiazepenes, lidocaine, barbiturates☛

- ► MAC measures potency of inhalational anesthetic.☛☛
- ► Oil gas partition coefficient measures anesthetic potency
- ► Blood gas partition coefficient measures solubility of general anesthetics.
- ► Gases with high blood solubility have slower rate of induction and recovery.❋❋
- ► Gases with low blood solubility have higher rate of induction and recovery.❋❋❋

⇨ Remember Colors of

Gas Color of Cylinder

- ✓ Nitrous oxide blue❋
- ✓ Cyclopropane orange❋
- ✓ Oxygen black body with white shoulder❋ JK BOPEE 2011
- ✓ Thiopentoneyellow❋
- ✓ Carbon dioxide grey❋
- ✓ Halothane purple (red)❋
- ✓ Helium brown❋
- ✓ N_2 black❋
- ✓ Air grey body with black and white shoulder

⇨ Pin Indicies

Gases	Pin Code Index
✓ Air ☛	1,5
✓ Co_2 (>7.5%)☛	1,6
✓ Co_2 (<7.5%)☛	2,6
✓ 0_2☛	2,5
✓ N_2o☛	3,5 KCET 2012

- ❐ Gas cylinders are made of steel alloy (molybdenum)
- ❐ Gase pipes are made of seam less copper tubing.

⇨ **Gases stored in Liquid Form are: ✱✱✱**

- Nitrous oxide
- Carbon dioxide
- Cyclopropane

Muscle Relaxants

Depolarizing MR

➢ Usually short acting	PGI 2000
➢ Cause Fasciculation's	
➢ No reliable antagonists.	
➢ No fade	JIPMER 1999
➢ No post tetanic facilitation	PGI 2000

Examples: Succinyl choline, Decamethonium

NON DEPOLARIZING MR

➢ Long acting	
➢ Don't cause muscle fasiculations	
➢ Neostigimine as effective antagonist	
➢ Post tetanic facilitation seen.	AIIMS 1993
➢ **Train of four used.**	AI 2008
➢ **Diaphragm is resistant to non depolarizing agents.**	JIPMER 2003

Examples: Mivacurium, Pipecuronium, Doxacurium, NGallamine

Also Remember:

Directly acting MR : Dantrolene and Quinine

Centrally acting MR is: Mephensin, Baclofen, benzodiazepine

- ✓ **Ultra short acting: succinyl choline**
- ✓ **Short acting: rapacuronium, mivacurium**
- ✓ **Intermediate acting: atracurium, cisatracurium, vecuronium, rocuronium**
- ✓ **Long acting: gallamine, pancuronium, d tubocurarine, doxacurium**

Depolarizing MR	NON Depolarizing MR
Muscle fasiculation +	Muscle fasiculation absent — PGI 2000
NOT reversed by cholinesterases (potentiate block)	**Reversed** by cholinesterases
Absent train of four fade	**Present** train of four fade — AI 2008
	Present tetanic fade — PGI 2000

➠ Absent tetanic fade☛	➠ **Present** tetanic facilitation☛
➠ **Absent** tetanic facilitation☛	➠ Effect of non depolarizing drugs causes **more** blockade
➠ Effect of non depolarizing drugs causes **less blockade**☛	➠ Diaphragm, adductors of larynx, corrugator supercilli are **resistant**☛☛

➲ Succinyl Choline: ❋❋❋❋ High Yield for 2011-2012

- Succinyl choline is a **depolarizing muscle relaxant.**☛ PGI 1997
- Action **not antagonized by** anticholinesterase agents.☛
- **Phase I block is persistent depolarization of muscle end plate and is rapid in action**
- **Phase II is slow onset, desensitization of receptor to acetyl choline.**
- **Dual block** JKHND 2006
- Order of depolarization is neck, limbs→face, jaws, eyes→trunk→respiratory
- May cause **histamine release** ☛
- Biotransformation rapidly hydrolyzed by **pseudocholinesterase.**☛☛ JK BOPEE 2001
- Onset of action: **Intravenous:** Initial effect within **0.5-1 minute Intramuscular:** Initial effect within **3 minutes**
- Elimination: **Renal;** about 10% as unchanged succinylcholine.
- **Precautions:**

Pediatric patients are especially susceptible to **succinylcholine-induced myoglobinemia, myoglobinuria, and cardiac effects.** Hyperkalemic rhabdomyolysis resulting in cardiac arrest and death has occurred in apparently healthy pediatric patients after administration of succinylcholine.

Succinylcholine is contraindicated in patients with **skeletal muscle myopathies.** Additionally, succinylcholine should not be used in patients with **major burn injury, severe trauma, extensive denervation of skeletal muscle, or upper neuron injury**. Use of succinylcholine in these patients may result in **"dangerous hyperkalemia".** ☛☛☛

Cardiac arrest has occurred when succinylcholine was used in patients with these conditions.

- Caution required in patients with cardiovascular function impairment.
- Effects may be prolonged in patients with renal function impairment, but to a lesser extent than for gallamine.
- Caution also required in Conditions that may lead to **low plasma pseudocholinesterase activity** (severe anemia, dehydration, exposure to neurotoxic insecticides or other cholinesterase inhibitors, severe hepatic disease or cirrhosis, malnutrition, pregnancy, recessive hereditary trait)
- Conditions that may be adversely affected by **increase in intraocular pressure** (open eye injury, glaucoma, ocular surgery)
- Fractures or **muscle spasm**
- **Malignant hyperthermia,**

⇨ Adverse Effects:

- Moderate risk of side effects associated with **histamine release.**☛☛
- More likely than other neuromuscular blocking agents to cause **bradycardia or cardiac arrhythmias.**☛
- Increased intraocular pressure, malignant hyperthermia, rhabdomyolysis leading to myoglobinemia and myoglobinuria, postoperative muscle pains and stiffness, and excessive salivation have been report☛☛

⇨ Important about Succinyl Choline

Succinylcholine causes Hyperkalemia❋❋	AIIMS 2003
Succinylcholine causes muscle pain❋❋	AI 1991
Succinylcholine increases Intra ocular pressure❋	
Succinylcholine increases intra gastric pressure❋	
Succinylcholine increases Intra cranial pressure❋❋	AIIMS 2002
Succinylcholine triggers Malignant Hyperthermia.❋❋	AIIMS 1993
Succinylcholine causes vagal stimulation.❋	AIIMS 2005
Succinylcholine is the shortest acting MR.❋	
Succinylcholine causes dual/biphasic block.❋	
Succinylcholine has shortest duration of action due to rapid hydrolysis by pseudocholineesterase.❋❋	

⇨ Succinylcholine is Important Factor in Triggering Hyperkalemia

Factors increasing this susceptibility are:

- ✓ **Massive trauma (Rhabdomyolysis)**❋❋ AIIMS 2000
- ✓ **Burns**❋ AIIMS 2000
- ✓ **Acidosis**❋
- ✓ **Spinal injury**❋
- ✓ **Closed head injury**❋
- ✓ **Tetanus**❋
- ✓ **Myopathies**❋
- ✓ **Prolonged immobilization**❋
- ✓ **Encephalitis/stroke**❋ PGI 2005
- ✓ **Renal dysfunction**❋
- ✓ **Necrotizing pancreatitis**❋
- ✓ This is a dangerous complication as it can lead to cardiac arrest and sudden death.
- ✓ Maximum chances of Hyperkalemia are usually in 7-14 days time following trauma and between **3 days 6 months following paraplegia.** AIIMS 1999

➲ Rocuronium: High Yield for 2011-2012

Rocuronium ✻✻

- ▶ Is indicated as an adjunct to general anesthesia to facilitate rapid-sequence or routine tracheal intubation and to induce skeletal muscle relaxation during surgery or mechanical ventilation
- ▶ Is a nondepolarizing neuromuscular blocking agent with a rapid to intermediate onset of action, depending on dose, and with an intermediate duration of action
- ▶ **Rocuronium** produces neuromuscular blockade by competing with acetylcholine for cholinergic receptors at the motor end plate
- ▶ **Mutagenicity**: No mutagenic effect was observed with the Ames test .The micronucleus test did not suggest mutagenic potential
- ▶ **Rocuronium** is recommended for intravenous administration only.
- ▶ **Produces pain on im injection.** AIPGME 2012

⇨ Atracurium and Cisatracurium

❐ Reversal not required.	
❐ Undergo spontaneous non enzymatic degradation.**(Hoffmans elimination)✻✻**	PGI 1997, JK BOPEE 2011
❐ Pharmacokinetics are independent of renal and hepatic functions and	
❐ Can be safely used in renal/liver diseases.	PGI 1997
❐ **Laudanosine** is produced as a metabolite responsible for seizure activity.✻	
❐ Atracurium **causes bradycardia.✻**	
❐ Can be **safely used in myasthenia gravis.✻**	
❐ **Can be used in patients with high serum creatinine**	AI 2010

➲ Atracurium: High Yield for 2011-2012

Is muscle relaxant with its metabolism independent of hepatic or renal metabolism.

- ✓ Available as Atracurium Besylate
- ✓ Dose - 0.5 mg/kg
- ✓ Duration - 15 -20 min.
- ✓ Metabolism: metabolized by Hoffmann's degradation (95%) in plasma and ester hydrolysis (5%)
- ✓ Metabolism produces laudanosine which crosses blood brain barrier and can produce convulsions
- ✓ Effect: Releases histamine but in significant amount at clinical doses
- ✓ Allergic reactions ranging from pruritic rash to angioneurotic edema can occur

It is relaxant of choice in:

- **Renal failure**
- **Hepatic failure**
- **Patients with atypical pseudocholinesterase**
- **Myasthenia gravis**
- **Small children**

Frequently Asked Questions

- Shortest acting non depolarizing MR: Mivacurium
- Shortest acting depolarizing MR: Succinylcholine — AI 1992
- Overall shortest acting MR: Succinylcholine
- Shortest acting local anesthetic: Chlorprocaine
- Contraindicated in renal failure: Gallamine, metocurine — AI 1991
- MR Causing ganglion block: Curare, Gallamine, Trimethapan, Pancuronium
- MR used in asthma: Atracurium, Vecuronium

D Tubocurarine

- **Causes Maximum histamine release.**
- **Causes maximum ganglion block.**
- **Causes bronchoconstriction.**
- **Does not cross placenta and used in obstretics.**

Reversal of Muscle Relaxants

PEN:

- **Pyridostigmine**
- **Edrophonium**
- **Neostigmine.** — PGI 1997

✓ Neostigimine is commonly used.

✓ Acts by **anticholineesterase activity** and prevents hydrolysis of Ach allowing it to accumulate.

✓ Antagonizes only non depolarizing MR.

✓ Usually given along with atropine/glycopyrollate.

Balanced Anesthesia

- Evolved by Lundy.
- Thiopental for induction.
- **N_2O for amnesia**
- **Mepridine for analgesia**
- **Curare for muscle relaxation**

Local Anesthetics (LA)

- LA (Local Anaesthetics) inhibit propagation of nerve impulses.
- LA in general block **Na^+ channels.** — PGI 1997
- Potency of these agents depends on lipid solubility. — PGI 2004
- Low PK means increased activity. — PGI 2004

- **Type C Fibres** followed by **Type B** Followed by **Type A** are most susceptible. **AI 1995**
- **Smaller diameter fibres** are blocked earlier than larger diameter fibres.
- **Non myelinated fibres** are also blocked earlier than myelinated fibres.
- **Absorption rates: intrapleural> intercostal> pudendal>caudal>epidural>brachial plexus>caudal AIIMS 09**

- Cocaine is a local vasoconstrictor anaesthetic.
- Addition of local vasoconstrictor such as adrenaline reduces absorption and reduces toxicity and prolongs anesthetic action.

Vasoconstrictors

"Decrease **the systemic absorption of local anaesthetics in blood, so increases the concentration thereby increasing the duration of action."**

Vasoconstrictors used are: **Adrenaline:** Duration of both sensory and motor blockade is increased by addition of epinephrine to lignocaine but only sensory block is prolonged if epinephrine is added to bupivacaine with no effect on motor blockade.

Lignocaine with adrenaline **should not be used for:**

- **Ring block of fingers, toes, penis, pinna (absolute contraindication)**
- **When an inhalational agent (halothane) which sensitizes myocardium to adrenaline is used.**
- **Myocardial ischemic patients**
- **Hyperthyroid patient**
- **Severe hypertensives**
- **Intravenous regional anesthesia (Biers block)**

Adrenaline is added for its vasoconstrictor effect along with anaesthetic in local anesthesia for the purpose o

- ✓ Reduce systemic toxicity **AP 2005**
- ✓ Delay absorption of anesthetic **AP 2005**
- ✓ Prolong the anesthetic action **AP 2005**

Amide Linked LA are:✱✱✱ AI 2007

Lidocaine	Bupvicaine	Dibucaine	Prolocaine	Mepivicaine	Ropivicaine

Ester Linked LA are:✱✱✱ AI 2003

Cocaine	Procaine	Benzocaine	Tetracaine	Chlorprocaine.

Amide LA

- ✓ Produce more intense/ longer lasting anesthesia.
- ✓ Bind to α1 acid glycoprotein.
- ✓ Not hydrolysed by esterases.
- ✓ Rarely cause hypersensitivity reactions **COMED 2006**

❒ **Shortest acting LA** is: Chlorprocaine	AI 1997
❒ **Longest acting**: Dibucaine	
❒ **LA causing Methhemoglobinemia**: Prilocaine	

➲ Lignocaine

❒ Most commonly used LA.	
❒ Amide linked.	AI 1998
❒ Also used for: VT, VES (Ventricular tachycardia, ventricular extra systoles)	
❒ 5% Concentration is used in subarachnoid space.	AIIMS 1992
❒ Maximum dose as Local anesthetic is	AIIMS 1992
❒ Maximum dose with adrenaline is 7 mg/kg	AI 1992
Causes:	
➨ **Depression,**	
➨ **Tremor,**	
➨ **Convulsions,❋❋**	PGI 2004
➨ **Bradycardia,**	
➨ **Hypotension,**	
➨ **Cardiac failure.❋**	PGI 2004
➨ **Bronchospasm,**	
➨ **Urticaria, angioedema.❋**	

➲ Bupivicaine: High Yield for 2011-2012

➨ **Bupivicaine** is LA of choice for **isobaric spinal anesthesia**☛☛	
➨ **Amide with duration greater than 2 hours**	PGI 2005
➨ Bupivicaine is **contraindicated for intravenous regional anesthesia (Biers Block).**☛☛	AIIMS 2004
➨ Bupivicaine is **highly cardiotoxic** and causes:☛☛	AIIMS 2004
✓ **AV Heart block**	
✓ **Prolong QT interval**	
✓ **Dysarythmias/VF**	
✓ **Circulatory collapse/ cardiac failure.**	
➨ Cardiotoxicity is more pronounced in pregnancy, Hypoxia and associated acidosis. There are more chances of fatal arrhythmias after iv dose. Bupivicaine binds more strongly to sodium channels and depolarizes membranes to a greater extent.	
➨ **Cardiotoxicity is not easily reversed** because of inhibition of epinephrine stimulated Camp.	PGI 2006
➨ **Amidarone is the DOC for Dysarrythmias due to Bupivicaine.**☛	
➨ **LEVO Bupivicaine is used by epidural/ intrathecal route.**	PGI 2004

➲ EMLA Cream

Is a mixture of **2.5% Lidocaine and 2.5% Prilocaine** (NOT Procaine) **PGI 2006**

It allows Anesthesia of intact skin.

It is used for:

- ❐ Making comfortable venipuncture in children
- ❐ Skin grafting
- ❐ Circumcision
- ❐ Needle phobias

- ❐ **Naturally occuring LA: Cocaine**
- ❐ **Vasoconstrictor: Cocaine** **AI 1999**
- ❐ **Safest LA: Prilocaine**
- ❐ **Maximum Methhemoglobinemia is due to: Prilocaine** **AIIMS 09**
- ❐ **Most used for Biers Block: Prilocaine**
- ❐ **Best for isobaric spinal anesthesia: Bupivicaine**
- ❐ **Contraindicated in IV regional anesthesia: Bupivicaine**
- ❐ **Not surface Anesthetics: Bupivicaine, mepivicaine, procaine**

➲ Methemoglobinemia: High Yield for 2011-2012

Methemoglobinemia results from exposure to chemicals that oxidize the ferrous (Fe^{2+}) iron in hemoglobin to the ferric (Fe^{3+}) state.

- ▶ Dapsone,
- ▶ Local anesthetics (particularly, Prilocaine benzocaine),
- ▶ Nitrites, nitrates, naphthalene, nitrobenzene and related chemicals,
- ▶ Oxides of nitrogen,
- ▶ Phenazopyridine,
- ▶ Primaquine and related antimalarials, and sulfonamides.

"Methemoglobinuria" is seen with:

- ➨ Prilocaine
- ➨ Lignocaine
- ➨ Benzocaine
- ➨ Sulfonamides
- ➨ Phenacetin
- ➨ Nitrites
- ➨ N_2O

⇨ Ketamine

- ❐ Ketamine causes almost complete anesthesia.
- ❐ Ketamine causes **dissociative** anesthesia. AIIMS 2006

➡ Is a phencyclidine.	MH 2008
➡ causes sympathetic stimulation ❋❋	
➡ **Increases salivation**❋	
➡ **Increases muscle tone**❋	
➡ **Increases cardiac output.** (Useful in hypovolumic shock)❋	
➡ Causes bronchodilatation. (Useful in asthma)❋	
➡ Causes (Hallucinations, delusions, illusions)❋	AI 1993
➡ Causes profound analgesia.	MAH 2012, PGI 2006
➡ **Increases all pressures: (BP, ICT, IOT)**❋❋❋	PGI 1997

Contraindicated in **Any condition** in which a **significant elevation of blood pressure would be hazardous**, such as:

1. Hypertension, severe or poorly controlled
2. Myocardial infarction, recent
3. Stroke,
4. history of Cerebral trauma
5. Intracerebral mass or hemorrhage AIIMS 2006

⇨ Excellent Analgesics:❋❋❋

- ❐ Ketamine☛☛
- ❐ Buprenorphine☛
- ❐ Trilene☛
- ❐ Sulfantenyl☛

Anesthetics with good analgesic properties:

- N_2O
- Ether
- Ketamine

Anesthetics with weak analgesic properties:

- Halothane
- Thiopentone
- Etomidate

⇨ Thiopentone

Ultra short acting barbiturate. Because of **rapid redistribution.**	AI 1996
Cerebroprotective	AIPGME 2012
Decreases intracranial pressure and cerebral blood flow.	
✓ Cerebral perfusion pressure is increased	
✓ Pain threshold decreased.	
Respiratory depressant. Causes laryngeal spasm.	
CVS effects:	
✓ Venous pooling	
✓ Decreased contractility	
✓ Decreased cardiac output	
✓ Negative ionotropic effect	
✓ Increases myocardial oxygen consumption.	
Musculo Excitatory:	
Lacks analgesic effect.	PGI 2005
On intra arterial im injection **first sign** is white hands and cyanosis.	AI 1997
Ist symptom is pain.	
Papaverine, prostacycline, **stellate ganglion/brachial plexus block** is used	
Can precipitate porphyria and is contraindicated in porphyria.	PGI 2004
IV injection presents as pain, rash, hypotension, spasm.	PGI 2003

Potential cerebral protective mechanisms	
➨ Decrease cerebral metabolism	
➨ Increase cerebral blood flow	
➨ Mild hypothermia	
➨ Prevent hyperthermia	
➨ Thiopentone anesthesia	AIPGME 2012
➨ Maintain normoglycemia	
➨ Inhibit release of excitatory neurotransmitters (eg, glutamate, aspartate)	
➨ Enhance release of inhibitory neurotransmitters (eg, GABA)	
➨ Block neuronal calcium influx	

⇨ Propofol

➨ Propofol is the "**agent of choice**" for day care anesthesia.	AI 2008, JK BOPEE 2011
➨ Propofol is used for **only "IV administration"** as 1% solution.	
➨ Causes pain on IV administration.	AIIMS 2006
➨ The induction dose in an adult is **1.5-2.5mg/kg.**	

- It is used **"both" for induction as well as maintenance** of anesthesia.
- Induction and recovery from propofol is **smooth**
- Incidence from nausea and vomiting is **low.**
- Propofol has **minimal effects** on hepatic and renal systems.
- Propofol supports growth of bacteria. As a result **"disodium edetate** and **sodium meta bisulfate"** are used in preparations to retard the growth of bacteria.
- Contains egg extract. **AI 2008**
- Propofol resembles barbiturates and also has **"anticonvulsant"** properties.
- Propofol is **safe** in Porphyria **SGPGI 2002**
- Propofol **does not** trigger malignant hyperthermia.

CNS Effects are:

- Decreases Cerebral blood flow
- Decreases intracranial pressure
- Decreases intraocular pressure
- Cerebroprotective **PGI 2005**

CVS Effects are:

- **Dose dependent decrease in BP** due to vasodilatation as well as myocardial depressant effect. **SGPGI 2002**

Respiratory Effects are:

- Propofol is a respiratory depressant
- Remember Propofol **has CNS, CVS and Respiratory depressant effects.**

Other features of Propofol

- ✓ **Antiemetic*** **SGPGI 2002**
- ✓ **Antipruritic***
- ✓ **Antioxidant***
- ✓ Propofol should not be used in extremely ill patients as it causes **"propofol infusion syndrome"**.

Propofol infusion syndrome:**

- ✓ Associated with long term propofol use.
- ✓ Is rare but fatal.
- ✓ Characterized by:
- ✓ **Lactic acidosis***
- ✓ **Lipaemic plasma ***
- ✓ **Cardiac failure.***

Fos propofol:

Is water soluble and hence is associated with

- ❐ ↓pain, ❋❋
- ❐ ↓ **hyperlipdemia**❋
- ❐ ↓**risk of sepsis**❋
- ❐ **It is used along with fentanyl especially for procedures like endoscopy, colonoscopy, bronchoscopy.**❋

⇨ Etomidate

- ✓ **Imidazole** derivative.
- ✓ Acts at **GABA a receptor.**☛☛
- ✓ Minimal respiratory depression.
- ✓ **Decreases intracranial pressure and cerebral blood flow**☛☛
- ✓ Does not have analgesic properties.
- ✓ Etomidate has **"Minimal effects on cardiovascular system".** **AIIMS 09**
- ✓ Mild reduction in peripheral resistance
- ✓ Myocardial contractility usually unchanged
- ✓ Cardiac output usually unchanged
- ✓ **Causes adrenocortical suppression** by inhibiting 11 β hydroxylase and 17 α hydroxylase. **PGI 2006, KCET 2012**

- ➨ Is a selective **positive allosteric modulator at GABA $_A$ receptor**
- ➨ **Sedative hypnotic** without any analgesic properties

Side Effects:

- Excitatory phenomenon causing myoclonus, hiccups and other
- Involuntary movements
- High incidence of nausea and vomiting
- Pain on injection and thrombophlebitis
- Causes adrenocortical suppression by inhibiting enzymes hydroxylases involved in cortisol and aldosterone (mineralocorticoid) production. **AIPGME 2012**
- Contraindicated in porphyria and adrenal insufficiency

- ❐ Pain on intraarterial injection: thiopental☛
- ❐ Pain on intravenous injection: etomidate (thrombophelebitis as well)☛
- ❐ Pain on intravenous injection: propofol, methohexitol, thiopental (thrombophelebitis not seen)☛

➲ Important Points

✓ Intravenous anesthetic used in shock: Ketamine☛☛	
✓ IVA safe in Porphyria: Propofol, ketamine☛☛	
✓ IVA which precipitates porphyria: Thiopentone, Methohexitone.☛	JK BOPEE 2011
✓ IVA with high incidence of venous thrombosis: Propofol☛	
✓ IVA which can cause postoperative vomiting: Ketamine☛	

➲ Stages of Anesthesia:❋❋❋

⇨ Guedels Stage of Anesthesia

Based on Ether PGI 1987

Ist Stage: stage of analgesia: onset of loss of consciousness❋❋	
2nd Stage: stage of excitation: stage of delerium❋	
3rd Stage: stage of surgical anesthesia	Eyes centrally fixed
Plane I	Beginning of intercostal muscle paralysis, corneal laryngeal reflexes lost
Plane II	Complete paralysis of intercostal muscles. Light reflex lost
Plane III	Beginning of diaphragmatic paralysis, fully dilated pupils, intercostal paralysis
Plane IV	Surgical anesthesia 3 KERALA 1998
	Lacrimation occurs in stage 3 CUPGEE 1995
4th Stage	Medullary paralysis, cardiorespiratory arrest

⇨ Ether: Morton First used Ether

Disadvantages	Advantages
► Irritant	► Good muscle relaxant
► Excessive salivation	► Wide safety margin
► Inflammable	► Cheap
► Slow induction and slow recovery	► Easy to adminiter
► Volatile liquid.	► Minimal cardiac depression
► Can be used by Endotracheal route/mask	► Hyperglycemia PGI 1988
JIPMER 1990	► Inflammable PGI 1986
	► Contraindicated in
	► Diabetes mellitus
	► Diathermy
	► Beta blocker use

6

ANESTHESIOLOGY

⇨ Chloroform

- Cardiotoxic
- Emetic
- Hepatotoxic
- Diabetogenic
- Causes malignant hyperthermia

⇨ Halothane

- ✓ **Non inflammable, colorless liquid with pleasant vapor.**
- ✓ **Decomposed by light and stabilised by thymol.**
- ✓ **Corrodes metals,**
- ✓ **Soluble in rubber, plastics.**

- **Arrythmogenic**
- **Myocardial depressant.** **KCET 2012**
- **Vagal stimulant**
- **Sensitizes heart to adrenaline.** **AI 2001**
- **↑ICT. (Less than halothane)**
- **Dissolves rubber.** **AIIMS 1993**
- May cause PPH (Relaxes uterine muscle) and **bronchodilator (used in asthma)** **KCET 2012**
- Hepatotoxic
- **Drager narko test** is used for halothane
- **Halothane and other halogenated inhalational anesthetic agents**, such as enflurane, isoflurane, sevoflurane, and desflurane, are known to cause severe **liver dysfunction.** **PGI 2001**
- When the World Health Organization (WHO) drug monitoring database was reviewed for the medications that most commonly cause fatal hepatotoxicity; **halothane was one of the 10 most common causes.** (Post operative jaundice) **PGI 1999**
- Two major types of hepatotoxicity are associated with halothane administration. The two forms appear to be unrelated and are termed.
- **Halothane and other halogenated inhalational anesthetic agents**, such as enflurane, isoflurane, sevoflurane, and desflurane, are known to cause severe **liver dysfunction.**
- When the World Health Organization (WHO) drug monitoring database was reviewed for the medications that most commonly cause fatal hepatotoxicity; **halothane was one of the 10 most common causes.**
- Two major types of hepatotoxicity are associated with halothane administration.

⇨ Type I (Mild) and Type II (Fulminant)

Type I hepatotoxicity is benign, self-limiting, and relatively common (up to 25-30% of those that receive halothane).

- ❒ This type is marked by mild transient increases in serum transaminase and glutathione S-transferase concentrations and by altered postoperative drug metabolism.
- ❒ Type I hepatotoxicity is not characterized by jaundice or clinically evident hepatocellular disease. Type I probably results from reductive (anaerobic) biotransformation of halothane rather than the normal oxidative pathway.
- ❒ It does not occur following administration of other volatile anesthetics because they are metabolized to a lesser degree and by different pathways than halothane.

Type II hepatotoxicity (also called halothane hepatitis) is associated with massive centrilobular liver necrosis that leads to fulminant liver failure; the fatality rate is 50%.

- ❒ Clinically, it is characterized clinically by fever, jaundice, and grossly elevated serum transaminase levels.
- ❒ Type II hepatotoxicity appears to be immune mediated. Halothane is oxidatively metabolized, producing trifluroacetyl metabolites to an intermediate compound. These metabolites bind liver proteins and, in genetically predisposed individuals, antibodies are formed to this metabolite-protein complex. The antibodies in turn mediate subsequent type II toxicity.
- ❒ Volatile anesthetics other than halothane also have the potential to cause type II hepatotoxicity. This risk is directly related to the relative degree of their oxidative metabolism to acetylated protein adducts.

⇨ Isoflurane

- ▶ Leads to coronary steal phenomenon (dilitazem) also causes.
- ▶ Particularly useful in neurosurgery, myasthenia gravis and renal failure.

⇨ Enflurane

Contraindicated in epilepsy.

⇨ Methoxyflurane

- ❒ **Nephrotoxic**☛☛
- ❒ **Highest fluoride content**☛
- ❒ **Causes high output renal failure.**☛☛
- ❒ **Causes oxalate stones.**☛

⇨ Desflurane

✓ **Fluorinated congener of isoflurane.**☛	**AIIMS 2004**
✓ **Low blood and tissue-gas partition coefficient.**☛	**WB 2006**
✓ **Used in OPD procedures**☛	
✓ **Minimal cardiac depression.**☛	
✓ **Less soluble**	**TN 2005**

6

ANESTHESIOLOGY

⇨ Sevoflurane

➨ Agent of choice in induction for paediatric age group and elderly.	BHR 2005
➨ Not used in closed circuits because of toxic product (olefin) production.	
➨ Non pungent	MAH 2012
➨ Inhalational agent of choice in pediatric population.	PGI 2005, MAH 2012
➨ Fast acting	JK BOPEE 2006

- ❒ Smooth induction❋❋
- ❒ Safe in children❋
- ❒ Sweet odor❋
- ❒ Speedy onset of action❋
- ❒ Safe CVS profie.❋

⇨ Adverse Effects with Sevoflurane

➨ Raised intracranial tension	
➨ Respiratory depression	Delhi 2008
➨ Nephrotoxicity	

⇨ The Physical Properties of Inhalation Anesthetics

❒ **Halothane:** Sweet smell	
❒ **Isoflurane:** Pungent ethereal odor with airway irritation	
❒ **Sevoflurane:** Non-pungent, sweet odour	MAH 2012
❒ **Desflurane:** Pungent and airway irritant	

⇨ The Triad of General Anesthesia Includes — Karnataka 2009

- ➨ Analgesia
- ➨ Amnesia
- ➨ Muscle relaxation

The advantages of **Isoflurane** for general Anesthesia in a cardiovascular patient are: AP 2005

- ➨ Decreased incidence of arrhythmias
- ➨ Vasodilatory effect
- ➨ Early recovery

⇨ Nitrous Oxide

❒ Color of cylinder of Nitrous oxide is : **blue**☛☛	PGI 2004
❒ Code: **3,5**☛☛ **(PIN index)**	PGI 2003
❒ MAC: **104**☛	
❒ Discovered by **Priestley. Also called as laughing gas**☛	TN

- ❐ Usually used in 50-65 % mixture with oxygen.
- ❐ **Lighter than air** and has high solubility in blood.☛☛
- ❐ **Entonox** is 50% N_2O and 50%O_2.☛☛ **KCET 2012**
- ❐ It is <u>not</u> used in Pneumo conditions such as pneumothorax, volvolus of gut☛
- ❐ It is a **non irritant, colorless, inorganic gas.**☛

Advantages:

- ▶ Inert gas
- ▶ Minimal CVS effects
- ▶ Rapid induction and Recovery
- ▶ Has analgesic properties
- ▶ Non inflammable anesthetic
- ▶ Safe anesthetic

Disadvantages:

Has **low Blood solubility** <u>but that is not an advantage.</u> It diffuses rapidly to alveoli from blood and dilutes alveolar air. This causes excess of N_2O in alveoli so partial pressure of O_2 in alveoli is reduced resulting in Hypoxia. **(Diffusion Hypoxia)**✱✱✱

Not used in pneumo conditions.

Side effects:

- **Diffusion Hypoxia/Second gas effect**☛☛ **COMED 2005**
- **Methemoglobinemia**☛☛
- **Bone marrow suppression**☛☛ **DNB 2001**
- **Megaloblastic anemia**☛☛ **UPSC 01**

⇨ **"Nitrous Oxide"**

Can produce signs of vitamin B12 deficiency (**megaloblastic anemia, peripheral neuropathy) following long administration.** For this reason it is not used as a chronic analgesic or a sedative in critical care settings'. Side effects of nitrous oxide:

- EXPANSION OF AIR POCKETS: Exchange with nitrogen in any air- containing cavity in the body.
- HEMATOLOGICAL EFFECTS: Nitrous oxide inactivates the cobalt in vitamin B12 and irreversibly **in activates the enzyme methionine synthetase Megaloblastic anemia has occurred with N_2O periods of 6-12hrs**
- NERVOUS SYSTEM: **increases cerebral blood flow and intracranial pressure when used alone.** When co-administered with other anesthetics, increase in cerebral blood flow is abolished. It causes **peripheral neuropathy** because of vitamin B12 defiency.

➲ Not Used In: ✱✱✱✱ AIIMS 09

- ❒ Pnemothorax
- ❒ Air embolism
- ❒ Obstructed middle ear
- ❒ Obstructed bowel
- ❒ Pulmonary bleb
- ❒ Cochlear surgeries
- ❒ Microarynqeal surgery
- ❒ Vitreoretinal surgery

► Second gas effect:

- ✓ Seen during induction of anesthesia.
- ✓ As the gas is used in high concentration, N_2O enters at high rate and any other anesthetic agent added will also be delivered at high rate. JK BOPEE 2012

► Diffusion hypoxia:

- ✓ During recovery phase N_2O having low blood solubility diffuses rapidly into alveoli and dilutes alveolar air and reduces partial pressure of oxygen causinf diffusion hypoxia PGI 1998

➲ Explosive Agents: ✱✱✱

- ✓ Ether
- ✓ Cyclopropane
- ✓ Ethylene
- ✓ Ethyl chloride

⇨ XENON Anesthesia

- Inert
- Minimal CVS effects.
- Non explosive
- Environmental friendly
- Rapid induction/recovery
- Low blood solubility
- No malignant hyperthermia

Eg: Patient with mitral stenosis had preanaesthetic checkup. Increased liver enzymes were noted. Xenon as an inhalational agent is preferred.

➲ Spinal Anesthesia: High Yield for 2011-2012

▶ **In children** spinal anesthesia is administered in L3-L4 space.	AI 1997
▶ **In adults** spinal anesthesia is administered in L4-L5 space.	
▶ Epidural, spinal, caudal is the same procedure.	
▶ **Nerve roots in cauda equina** are the sites of action.	
▶ **Autonomic pre ganglionic fibres** are earliest to be blocked (sympathetic)	AIIMS 1992
▶ Percentage of xylocaine used in spinal anesthesia is: **2%-5%.**	
▶ **Sixth cranial nerve is the commonest cranial nerve** to be effected in spinal anesthesia.	
▶ Cauda equina syndrome is possible complication.	
▶ **Touhy needle** is used during the procedure.	
▶ **High spinal anesthesia** is characterized by hypotension and bradycardia.	
▶ **Ephedrine is the agent of choice as a vasopressor.**	PGI 2004

Contraindications of spinal (centrineuraxial) anesthesia: ***	
✓ Patients refusal	AI 2003
✓ Inability of patient to maintain stiffness during needle puncture.	
✓ Raised ICP	
✓ Severe Hypovolumeia	AI 2003
✓ Severe stenotic heart disease	
✓ Marked skin sepsis and marked spinal deformity	
✓ Marked coagulopathy, blood dyscrasia.	AI 2003

⇨ Adverse Effects of Central Neuraxial Block Include — Karnataka 2009

- Hypotension
- Nausea and vomiting
- Urinary retention

In **Epidural Anesthesia**, anesthesia used is: Bihar 2004

- Buprenorphine
- Bupivacaine
- Morphine,
- Fentanyl

➲ High/Total Spinal Anesthesia

✓ If there is inadvertent intrathecal injection.	
✓ Can occur due to intrathecal injection of largr amount of drug.	
✓ Marked hypotension, apnea, dilated pupils, bradycardia are seen.	AIIMS 2001
✓ Subarachnoid lavage, iv fluids and vessopressors, head down position are used as treatment option.	

➲ Post dural Puncture Headache (PDPH)✱✱✱✱ High Yield for 2011-2012

➠ Post dural Puncture Headache (PDPH) or post LP headache is the **second most common complication** after hypotension in spinal anasthesia.	
➠ It occurs due to **low CSF pressure**./CSF leak	**AI 1995**
➠ Onset is usually in 12-72 hours.	
➠ Lasts 7-10 days.	**AI 1994**
➠ **Increased incidence** with early mobilization of patient is seen.	
➠ Use of **small gauge needles** prevents it.	
➠ Post dural Puncture headache is different as it is a **postural headache** worsened by standing or sitting and improved in supine position.	
➠ Post dural Puncture is **not** treated effectively by NSAIDS.	
➠ Post dural Puncture headache is effectively treated by **caffeine** and **Epidural Blood patch.**	
➠ PDPH occurs hours to days after puncture.	
➠ Post dural headache is caused by **decreased intracranial pressure** due to leak of CSF from puncture site.	
➠ Post dural Puncture headache depends on **needle size** and can be prevented by using thinner needles. However it is not only the needle size but also the **needle design** and **orientation** which influence the incidence of Post dural Puncture headache.	
➠ **"Sprottee needle or whitacare needle"** reduces risk of PDPH.	**PGI 2004**

⇨ Higher Incidence of Post Dural Headache is seen in

- ❒ **Pregnant patients**
- ❒ **Female sex**
- ❒ **Younger patients**
- ❒ **Larger needles**
- ❒ **Multiple punctures.**

Ephedrine is used as a vassopressor acting on α as well as β receptors. (DOC)	
Mephentramine is used if ephedrine is not available.	**AI 2006**

⇨ Doxapram

Doxapram is a **"respiratory stimulant"** and **"CNS stimulant "(analeptic)** and not a specific reversal agent.

- ✓ Doxapram is administered **intravenously**
- ✓ Doxapram causes **increase in tidal volume and respiratory rate**. (Peripheral action)
- ✓ Doxapram stimulates **chemoreceptors** in the carotids which in turn **stimulate respiratory centre** in brain stem. (Central action)
- ✓ Doxapram is a **white, odourless powder** stable in light and air with **acidic pH.**

Doxapram is used:
✓ In respiratory failure and respiratory depression.❋
✓ In treatment of COPD/COAD.❋
✓ Side effects: Pain and redness at injection site, flushing, sweating, headache, nausea diarrhea, enlarged pupils❋

⇨ Other Respiratory Stimulants are

- Almitrine☛☛
- Amiphenazole☛☛
- Demifline☛☛
- Bemegride☛☛
- Nikethemide☛
- Pentetrazol☛

⇨ BLS has three components

- **A Airway (FIRST)**
- **B Breathing**
- **C Circulation**

ATLS is advanced trauma Life Support

GCS is Glasgow Coma Scale

ABCDE is Airway, Breathing, Circulation, Disability assessment, Exposure

Adult BLS Sequence

- Ensure that the **scene is safe**
- Assess the victim's level of consciousness by asking loudly "Are you okay?" and by checking for the victim's responsiveness to pain.
- If the victim has no suspected cervical spine trauma, open the airway using the **head-tilt/chin-lift maneuver**; if the victim has suspected neck trauma, the airway should be opened with the **jaw-thrust technique.** If the jaw-thrust is ineffective at opening/maintaining the airway, a very careful head-tilt/chin-lift should be performed.
- **Assess the airway** for foreign object obstructions, and if any are visible, remove them using the **finger-sweep technique**. Blind finger-sweeps should never be performed, as they may push foreign objects deeper into the airway.
- **Look, listen, and feel** for breathing for at least 5 seconds and no more than 10 seconds.
- If the patient is breathing normally, then the patient should be placed in the recovery position and monitored and transported; do not continue the BLS sequence.
- If patient is not breathing normally, and the arrest was witnessed immediately before assessment, then immediate defibrillation is the treatment of choice.

- Attempt to administer two artificial ventilation's using the mouth-to-mouth technique, or a bag-valve-mask (BVM). The mouth-to-mouth technique is no longer recommended, unless a face shield is present. Verify that the chest rises and falls; if it does not, reposition (i.e. re-open) the airway using the appropriate technique and try again. If ventilation is still unsuccessful, and the victim is unconscious, it is possible that they have a foreign body in their airway. Begin chest compressions, stopping every 30 compressions, re-checking the airway for obstructions, removing any found, and re-attempting ventilation.
- If the ventilation's are successful, assess for the presence of a pulse at the carotid artery. If a pulse is detected, then the patient should continue to receive artificial ventilation's at an appropriate rate and transported immediately. Otherwise, begin **CPR at a ratio of 30:2** compressions to ventilation's at 100 compressions/minute for 5 cycles.
- After 5 cycles of CPR, the BLS protocol should be repeated from the beginning, assessing the patient's airway, checking for spontaneous breathing, and checking for a spontaneous pulse.

⇨ Causes of Delayed Recovery from Anesthesia — JK BOPEE

- Overdose of anaesthetic.
- Duration and type of Anesthesia.
- **Hypo** thermia
- **Hypo** calcemia
- **Hypo** kalemia
- **Hypo**/Hypernatremia
- **Hypo**xia/Hypercapnia
- **Hypo**/Hyperglycemia
- **Hypo** thyroidism
- Renal **failure**
- Hepatic **failure**
- Cardiac **failure**

⇨ Drugs Used in Postoperative Shivering are

- Clonidine
- Mepridine
- Tramadol
- Pethidine (NOT with MAO inhibitors) — AI 2010

Nitric Oxide (Old Drug but Important for PG Exams)

- ✓ Nitric oxide is **NO**
- ✓ It is also called as **EDRF (Endothelial derived relaxing factor).**
- ✓ It is produced from **arginine** by enzyme NO synthetase. — PGI 2007
- ✓ NO has a short $t_{1/2}$ **(4 seconds).**
- ✓ It acts via **c GMP** pathway. — AIPGME 05, AIIMS 93

There are 3 forms of NOS

- ❒ NOS 1: in nervous system
- ❒ NOS 2: in macrophages
- ❒ NOS 3: in endothelium

❒ It **relaxes smooth muscles** specifically	
❒ Dacreases pulmonary artery pressure	
❒ Vasodilates corpora cavernosa. Leads to penile erection	PGI 2007
❒ Inhaled NO exerts effects on pulmonary system only	
❒ It **prevents platelet aggregation**	AIIMS 04
❒ It functions as a **neurotransmitter**	
❒ It mediates **bactericidal actions of macrophages**	

⇨ Drugs Forming NO

❒ **Sodium nitroprusside.**	PGI 02
❒ **Nitroglycerine**	
❒ **Hydralazine**	

⇨ Oxygen Toxicity

- ✓ Carbon dioxide narcosis
- ✓ Bronchopulmonary dysplasia
- ✓ Alveolar edema
- ✓ Retrolental fibroplasias
- ✓ Epilepsy

❒ **Nasal cannula delivers 44% maximum oxygen concentration.**	COMED 01
❒ **Venture mask/oxygen mask delivers 60% maximum oxygen concentration**	
❒ **Ventilator delivers 100% maximum oxygen concentration**	

⇨ Oxygen is delivered by

- ✓ Oxygen tent
- ✓ Oxygen apparatus
- ✓ Poly mask
- ✓ Venturimask
- ✓ Nasal catheter
- ✓ BLB mask

➲ Hyperbaric Oxygen Therapy is given in

✓ Histotoxic anoxia	
✓ Carbon monoxide poisoning	
✓ Gas gangrene	DNB 02

6

ANESTHESIOLOGY

➲ Malignant hyperthermia (Repeated Often and High Yield for 2011-2012)

- ▶ Occurs in individuals with an inherited abnormality of **skeletal-muscle sarcoplasmic reticulum** that causes a rapid increase in intracellular calcium levels in response to halothane and other inhalational anesthetics or to succinylcholine.
- ▶ Defect in ryanodine receptors in Sarcoplasmic reticulum.
- ▶ Mitochondrial and sarcolemma damage is a feature.
- ▶ Marked rise in intracellular Ca++ occurs.
- ▶ Elevated temperature, increased muscle metabolism, rigidity, rhabdomyolysis, acidosis, and cardiovascular instability develop.
- ▶ Hyperkalemia — AIIMS 2007
- ▶ Metabolic acidosis — AIIMS 2007
- ▶ Hypertension.
- ▶ This condition is often fatal.
- ▶ Rise in end tidal CO_2*
- ▶ Tachycardia

⇨ Trigerring Agents

- ✓ Succinyl choline
- ✓ Ether,
- ✓ Cyclopropane
- ✓ Halothane
- ✓ Fluranes,
- ✓ Lidocaine and amides
- ✓ TCA,
- ✓ MAO inhibitors,
- ✓ Phenothiazines

Intravenous dantrolene is indicated to reverse the symptoms of the malignant hyperthermic crisis syndrome occurring during or following surgery or anesthesia**

Malignant hyperthermia should be treated immediately with cessation of anesthesia and intravenous administration of dantrolene sodium. Procainamide should also be administered to patients with malignant hyperthermia because of the likelihood of ventricular fibrillation in this syndrome.

⇨ Causes of Postoperative Hypertension:***

- Pre operative withdrawal of anti hypertensive's.
- Pre operative Phaeochromocytoma
- Pain
- Reaction to tracheal tube
- Excessive fluid administration.
- Hypothermia
- Hypoxemia
- Hypercarbia
- Full bladder

⇨ Neurolept Malignant Syndrome

Is a **potentially life Threatening** idiosyncratic reaction to neuroleptic drugs.

- **Fever**
- **Muscular rigidity**
- **Altered mental status**
- **Autonomic dysfunction**

- Pathological abnormality is **central D_2 receptor blockade or dopamine depletion in the hypothalamus and nigrostriatal / spinal pathways.** This leads to an elevated temperature set point, impairment of normal thermal homeostasis and extrapyramidally induced in muscle regidity.
- Is usually associated with potent neuroleptics such as haloperidol and fluphenazine, which block central D_2 receptors **but it has now been reported to occur with all drugs that affect the central dopaminergic system** (including dopamine agonists and levodopa). **In these cases neurolept malignant syndrome is precipitated by rapid withdrawl of the dopaminergic agonists.**
- **Amantadine** is a dopamine agonist and its withdrawl precipitates neurolept malignant syndrome.
- N.M.S. is also associated with other drugs that have central D_2 receptor antagonist activity **Metoclopromide**.
- It is second only to haloperidol in triggering neurolept malignant syndrome.
- Domperidone like metoclopromide is a D_2 blocker and is similar to metoclopromide in all respects except that **Domeperidone** **does not cross** **C.N.S.** and so it does not cause neurolept malignant syndrome.

➲ Granisetron: High Yield for 2011-2012

- Is a potent, selective antagonist of 5-hydroxytryptamine (serotonin) subtype 3 (5-HT $_3$) receptors.
- The most common side effect of chemotherapy administration is nausea, with or without vomiting.
- Nitrogen mustard, nitrosoureas, streptozotocin, DTIC, cisplatin, and actinomycin are **highly emetogenic** and produce vomiting in virtually all patients.
- Doxorubicin, daunorubicin, and conventional-dose cyclophosphamide are **moderately emetogenic.**
- Emesis is a reflex caused by stimulation of the **vomiting center in the medulla.** Input to the vomiting center comes from the **chemoreceptor trigger zone (CTZ)** and afferents from the peripheral gastrointestinal tract, cerebral cortex, and heart.

- In addition, a conditioned reflex may contribute to anticipatory nausea arising after repeated cycles of chemotherapy
- The serotonin receptor antagonists ondansetron and **granisetron** are the most effective drugs against highly emetogenic agent
- Granisetron is indicated for the prevention of nausea and vomiting associated with **radiation,** including total body irradiation and fractionated abdominal radiation
- Granisetron is indicated for the prevention of nausea and vomiting associated with initial and repeat courses of moderately or severely **emetogenic cancer chemotherapy.**

⇨ Latest $5HT_3$ Antagonists

- ❒ Ondansterone
- ❒ Dolasteron
- ❒ Palonosteron
- ❒ Granisetron

Stellate Ganglion Block

Stellate ganglion is so called because it is **star shaped.** It is **inferior sympathetic Cervical ganglion or cervicothoracic ganglion** when it is blocked it causes

- Ptosis-drooping of upper eyelid
- Miosis-constriction of pupil
- Anhydrosis-loss of sweating on that of face
- Enophthalmos- retraction of eyeball
- Loss of ciliospinal reflex-pinching skin on nape of does not produce dilatation of pupil; which normally takes place

⇨ Aspiration Pneumonia

- ✓ Volume of aspirate>25 ml.
- ✓ Aspirate pH<2.5
- ✓ Partially digested food.
- ✓ ↓Conscious level (anesthesia, stroke, seizures)
- ✓ At high risk for aspiration
- ✓ Children and elderly
- ✓ Diabetecs
- ✓ Pregnant
- ✓ Obese
- ✓ Leads to chemical pneumonitis, infection and bacterial pneumonitis
- ✓ Mendelsons syndrome is aspiration of gastric contents. (Prevented by Sellicks maneuver) JIPMER 1993

➲ Basic Life Support: High Yield for 2011-2012

- ❐ Known as **CPR**, is intended to maintain **organ perfusion** until definitive interventions can be instituted.
- ❐ The elements of CPR are the **maintenance of ventilation of the lungs and compression of the chest.**
- ❐ **Mouth-to-mouth respiration** may be used if no specific rescue equipment is immediately available (e.g., plastic oropharyngeal airways, esophageal obturators, masked Ambu bag).
- ❐ Conventional ventilation techniques during CPR require the **lungs to be inflated 10 to 12 times per minute**, i.e., **once every fifth chest compression when two persons are performing the resuscitation and twice in succession every 15 chest compressions when one person is carrying out both ventilation and chest wall compression.** JK BOPEE 2011
- ❐ Chest compression is based on the assumption that cardiac compression allows the heart to maintain a pump function by sequential filling and emptying of its chambers, with competent valves maintaining forward direction of flow.
- ❐ The palm of one hand is placed over the lower sternum, with the heel of the other resting on the dorsum of the lower hand.
- ❐ The sternum is depressed, with the arms remaining straight, at a rate of approximately **80 to 100 per minute.**
- ❐ Sufficient force is applied to **depress the sternum 3 to 5 cm**, and relaxation is abrupt.

⇨ During CPR

- ✓ **# Ribs, sternum, vertebrae occur**
- ✓ **Injury to lungs**
- ✓ **Rupture liver and spleen**

⇨ Advanced Life Support

Is intended to achieve adequate ventilation, control cardiac arrhythmias, stabilize blood pressure and cardiac output, and restore organ perfusion.

The activities carried out to achieve these goals include

- ✓ **Intubation with an endotracheal tube,**
- ✓ **Defibrillation/cardioversion and/or pacing, and**
- ✓ **Insertion of an intravenous line.**

- ❐ **Ventilation with O_2** (room air if O_2 is not immediately available) may promptly reverse hypoxemia and acidosis. ❋
- ❐ When possible, **immediate defibrillation** should precede intubation and insertion of an intravenous line;
- ❐ CPR should be carried out while the defibrillator is being charged.
- ❐ As soon as a diagnosis of **VT or VF is obtained, a 200-J shock** should be delivered. Additional shocks at higher energies, **up to a maximum of 360 J**, are tried if the initial shock does not successfully abolish VT or VF. ❋
- ❐ **Epinephrine, 1 mg intravenously**, is given after failed defibrillation, and attempts to defibrillate are repeated. ❋

If the patient is less than fully conscious upon reversion, or if two or three attempts fail, prompt intubation, ventilation, and arterial blood gas analysis should be carried out

After initial unsuccessful defibrillation attempts, or with persistent electrical instability, **a bolus of 1 mg/kg lidocaine** is given intravenously and the dose is repeated in 2 min in those patients who have persistent ventricular arrhythmias or remain in VF. This is followed by a continuous infusion at a rate of 1 to 4 mg/min. If lidocaine fails to provide control, other antiarrhythmic therapies should be tried.

For persistent, hemodynamically unstable ventricular arrhythmias.

- ❐ **Intravenous amiodarone** has emerged as the treatment of choice ❋
- ❐ **Intravenous procainamide** may be tried for persisting, hemodynamically stable arrhythmias; or ❋

Bretylium tosylate (may be tried as an alternative for unstable arrhythmias. ❋

➲ Retrobulbar Block

- ❐ Is **regional anesthesia for eye surgery.**☛☛
- ❐ LA is injected behind eye into **cone formed by extraoccular muscles.**☛☛
- ❐ **Lidocaine, bupivicaine and hyaluronidase** are combined.☛
- ❐ After block, onset of ptosis indicates successful needle placement
- ❐ **Optic, oculomotor, abducens, nasociliary nerve and ciliary ganglion** are affected in conal block.☛
- ❐ **Lacrimal, frontal, infraorbital and trochlear nerves** outside the cone are least affected.☛
- ❐ **Anesthesia, akinesia and abolishment of occulocephalic reflex** are determinants of successful block.
- ❐ **Superior oblique is the last muscle to get paralyzed in this block.** **AIIMS 2006**

Complications:

- ✓ Retrobulbar hemorrhage☛☛ **PGI 2004**
- ✓ Globe perforation☛☛ **PGI 2004**
- ✓ Optic nerve atrophy☛ **PGI 2004**
- ✓ Convulsions☛☛
- ✓ Occulocardiac reflex
- ✓ Pulmonary edema
- ✓ Trigeminal block
- ✓ Respiratory arrest

Brachial plexus block: needle is passed lateral to subclavian artery. (Risk of pneumothorax)

Phrenic nerve block: Neddle is passed into scalenus anterior muscle.

- ► DOC in status epilepticus: IV lorazepam
- ► DOC in anaphylactic shock: IV adrenaline

⇨ Mallampati Grading

- **Is used for assessing oral cavity before intubation.** **AI 2000**
- **Assesses size of tongue, pharyngeal pillars, uvula**
- Grading:
  - ✓ Grade I faucial pillars, soft palate, uvula seen
  - ✓ GradeII faucial pillars, soft palate
  - ✓ Grade III soft palate seen
  - ✓ Grade IV hard palate seen

⇨ Rapid Sequence Induction

- **Used to reduce risk of aspiration pneumonia.**
- **Patient is preoxygenated prior to induction.**
- **Induction by thiopentone is done.**
- **Pressure over cricoid (sellicks maneuver) to prevent regurgitation.**
- **Prior curarization with non depolarizing MR plus use of suxamethonium is done.**

⇨ Circoid Pressure

- Is one of the methods of **prevention of acid aspiration syndrome**
- It is used to prevent regurgitation by **occluding the esophagus between the cricoid cartilage and the vertebrae,** as recommended by **Sellick**
- It should be applied as the patient loose consciousness, using the tips of first two
- Fingers and thumb of an assistant to apply pressure on the cricoid cartilage.
- This method **must not be used during active vomiting** as it may lead to **esophageal rupture**

⇨ Features of Nasal Airway

- ❒ The nasal airway is **more traumatic** than oral airway. There is more mucosal damage and bleeding.
- ❒ The **incidence of infections** is also more with nasal airway as compared to oral airway. (Sinusitis, otitis media)
- ❒ The nasal airway is not usually used in anticoagulated patients due to high risk of bleeding and is better avoided.
- ❒ There is displacement of endotracheal tube in nasal airway.

However the benefits of nasal airway are:

- ✓ **It is better tolerated than oral airway.**
- ✓ **Less chances of displacement.**
- ✓ **Maintains good oral hygiene.** **AIIMS 2007**

Contraindications of nasal/oral intubation:

- ✓ Laryngeal edema☛☛
- ✓ Laryngo tracheobronchitis☛ AIIMS 1995
- ✓ Epiglottitis☛

Nasal intubation is Contraindicated in:

- Basal skull #
- CSF Rhinorrhea AIIMS 1995
- Nasal obstruction
- Adenoids
- Bleeding disorders
- Previous nasal surgery

⇨ Endotracheal Intubation

Endotracheal Tubes:

- ❒ Made of PVC.☛☛
- ❒ Resistance to air flow depends on diameter of tube.☛
- ❒ Len cuffed tubes are usually used in children. Tube size is given in millimeters.☛☛
- ❒ Tubes with high pressure low volume are associated with more ischemic damage.☛
- ❒ Tubes with low pressure high volume are associated with more chances of sore throat, aspiration, difficult insertion.☛

Also remember: Endotracheal intubation is associated with:❋❋❋

- Hypertension❋
- Tacchycardia❋
- Raised Intraoccular tension❋
- Raised Intracranial tension❋
- Arryhthmias❋

It decreases anatomical dead space.

It increases resistance to respiration. Indicated:

- ✓ To deliver PPV.☛☛
- ✓ Protection of Respiratory tract from gastric aspiration.☛☛
- ✓ Head and neck operations that preclude manual airway support.☛
- ✓ To maintain airway☛
- ✓ Tracheobronchial toilet☛
- ✓ Unconscious patients.☛

Involves: Extension of atlanto occipital joint, Flexion of lower cervical spine

⇨ **Complications of Intubation**

➠ Hypertension☛☛
➠ ↑ICT☛☛
➠ ↑IOT☛
➠ ↑Heart rate☛
➠ Arrhythmias☛
➠ Airway trauma☛☛
➠ Esophageal intubation☛
➠ Edema, stenosis☛
➠ Hoarsness☛
➠ Laryngospasm☛

Laryngeal Mask Airway

➲ Laryngeal Mask Airway: High Yield for 2011-2012

➠ LMA is a **supraglottic airway**
➠ used in **place of facemask or tracheal tube** during administration of an anaesthetic to facilitate ventilation and passage of tracheal tube in a patient with difficult airway, and to aid in ventilation during fibreoptic bronchoscopy as well as placement of bronchoscope.
➠ LMA that has an orifice through which nasogastric tube can be inserted and that **facilitates positive pressure ventilation**
➠ LMA partially protects larynx from **pharyngeal secretions** (but not gastric regurgitation) and it should remain in place until patient has regained airway reflexes.
➠ The reusable LMA which is autoclavable, is made of **silicone rubber**.
➠ It is available in many sizes- **1, 1.5, 2, 2.5, 3, 4, 5.** **PGI 2009**

⇨ **Contraindications to use of LMA:**

✓ Risk of pulmonary aspiration of gastric contents
✓ Hiatal hernia with significant gastroesophageal reflux
✓ Morbid obesity
✓ Intestinal obstruction
✓ Delayed gastric emptying
✓ Poor pulmonary compliance
✓ Increased airway resistance
✓ Glottic or subglottic airway obstruction
✓ Limited mouth opening (<1.5mm)

⇨ LMA Quick Revision Points

- Also called as Bain mask.
- Used for airway maintainence. AIIMS 2003
- Protects larynx from pharyngeal but not gastric secretions.
- Indicated in: difficult airway management during CPR. PGI 2001
- When difficult intubation is anticipated.
- Contraindicated in oropharyngeal mass/ abscess., pregnancy, hiatal hernia, full stomach
- Advantages:
  - ✓ Easy to insert.
  - ✓ Does not require MR/ Laryngoscopes
  - ✓ Specific Cervical spine positions not required.

⇨ Anesthesia Gas Delivery Systems

Mapelson A	Mapelson B	Mapelson C	Mapelson D	Mapelson E
Magill system For spontaneous breathing Flow rate=minute volume AI 2000	Not commonly used	Waters system For postoperative recovery	Bain coaxial system Assisted controlled ventilation	Ayres T tube. MAH 2012 For infants/young children Flow rate 2-3x minute volume

- ► Boyles apparatus: Continuous flow machine Low resistance circuit PGI 2006
- ► PIN index system prevents delivery of gases and prevents wrong attachment of cylinders.
- ► Gas cylinders are composed of molybdenum steel
- ► End tidal CO_2 is used as an early and reliable indicator of air embolism in anesthesia. COMED 2008
- ► Best technique to monitor babys breathing and detecting apnea is impedence pulmonometry. AI 2007

⇨ Soda Lime

- ❒ 94% $Ca(OH)_2$ + 5%NaoH + 1% KoH JIPMER 2000
- ❒ Granules size is 4-8 mesh.
- ❒ Soda lime is contraindicated with trilene due to formation of phosgene gas.

Soda lime should not be used with:

- ✓ Sevoflurane*
- ✓ Chloroform *
- ✓ Trilene*

⇨ **Bara Lime**

80 % $Ca(OH)_2$, 20% $Ba(OH)_2$
Granules size is 4-8 mesh

CO_2 absorption is increased by:

- ✓ Resistance in circuit.
- ✓ Small granule size
- ✓ Low flow rate.

CO_2 absorption is decreased by:

- ✓ High flow rate and tidal volume
- ✓ Dead space
- ✓ Channeling
- ✓ Large granule size

⇨ **Capnography: ❋❋❋** AIIMS 09

Is monitoring of partial pressure of CO_2 in expired gases.

CO_2 absorbs infra red radiation.

Flat capnograph is seen in:

- ❒ Equipment failure
- ❒ Disconnection
- ❒ Total occlusion
- ❒ Accidential extubation
- ❒ Bronchospasm

➲ Indications for Mechanical Ventilation

- Ventilation failiure
- Oxygenation failure
- Failure to Ventilate

Neurological Problems

- **Central:** Loss of ventilatory drive due to sedation, narcosis, stroke or brain injury.
- **Spinal:** Spinal cord injury, cervical-loss of diaphragmatic function, thoracic-loss of intercostals.
- **Peripheral:** Nerve injury (e.g. phrenic nerve in surgery), Guillain-Barrè syndrome (demyelination), poliomyelitis, and motor neuron disease.

Muscular Problems

- **Myopathic disorders:** Myasthenia gravis, steroid induced myopathy, protein malnutrition.

Anatomical Problems

- **Chest wall:** Rib fractures or flail chest, obesity, abdominal hypertension, restrictive dressings.
- **Pleura:** Pleural effusions, pneumothorax, hemothorax.

- **Airways:** Airway obstruction (in lumen, in wall, outside wall), laryngeal edema, inhalation of a foreign object, bronchospasm.

Gas Exchange Problems

- Ventilation perfusion mismatch, particularly **increased alveolar deadspace**
- Acute lung injury (ALI), lung contusion.

Continuous Positive Airway Pressure (CPAP): High Yield for 2011-2012

Also called **continuous distending pressure (CDP)**

Refers to the application of **continuous pressure during both inspiration and expiration** in a spontaneously breathing baby

By CPAP:

- **Alveoli are kept open**
- **Increases FRC of the lungs**
- **Better gas exchange**
- **Improve oxygenation CO_2 wash out and better blood Ph**
- **Splints** the upper airways
- **Stimulate 'J' receptors** by stretching the lung/pleura and providing positive feed back to respiratory Center by Hering-Breuer reflex
- **Improve type II pneumocyte function** and **recycling of surfactant**
- **Promote growth of premature lung Improve lung compliance**

Contraindications for CPAP:

- Progressive respiratory failure with $PaCO_2 > 60$ mm Hg/$PaO_2 < 50$ mm Hg
- Congenital malformations of the airway
- Cardiovascular instability
- Poor respiratory drive **PGI 2009**

Capnography: High Yield for 2011-2012

Determination of end tidal CO_2 ($EtCO_2$) concentration to confirm adequate ventilation is useful during all anaesthetic procedures, but particularly for GA.

It is a valuable monitor of pulmonary, cardiovascular and anaesthetic breathing systems.

Causes of Increased $EtCO_2$

- ✓ Absorption of CO_2 from peritoneal cavity
- ✓ Injection of $NaHCO_3$
- ✓ Pain, anxiety, shivering
- ✓ Increased muscle tone (as from muscle relaxant reversal)
- ✓ Convulsions
- ✓ Hyperthermia
- ✓ Increased transport of CO_2 from the lungs restoration of peripheral circulation after it has been impaired.

⇨ Causes of Decreased $EtCO_2$

- ✓ Hypothermia
- ✓ Increased depth of anesthesia
- ✓ Use of muscle relaxants
- ✓ Decreased transport of CO_2 to lungs (impaired peripheral circulation)
- ✓ Decreased transport of CO_2 through the lungs (pulmonary embolus, surgical manipulations)
- ✓ Increased patient dead space
- ✓ Hyperventilation
- ✓ Leakage in sampling line
- ✓ Blockage of sampling line

⇨ Causes of Absent $EtCO_2$

- ✓ Disconnection
- ✓ Apneic patient, stopped ventilator
- ✓ Esophageal intubation

⇨ Membrane Oxygenators

Are devices used in cardiopulmonary by pass surgeries

They improve efficiency of gas exchange and decrease trauma to blood elements.

- **Lessen RBC damage** **AIIMS**
- **Lessen Platelet trauma**
- **Lessen WBC trauma**
- **Lessen Protein denaturation.**

⇨ Gases Used to Create Pneumoperitoneum

- Carbon dioxide
- Oxygen
- Room air
- Nitrous oxide

Brain Death

- This is a state with cessation of cerebral blood flow;
- As a result, global ischemia of the brain occurs while respiration is maintained by artificial means and the heart continues to function.
- Criteria for the diagnosis of **brain death**

- They contain three essential elements:
  - ✓ Widespread cortical destruction shown by deep coma, unresponsiveness to all forms of stimulation; **JIPMER 2003**
  - ✓ Global brainstem damage demonstrated by absent pupillary light reaction and the loss of oculovestibular and corneal reflexes; and
  - ✓ Lower brainstem destruction indicated by complete apnea. The pulse rate is also invariant and unresponsive to atropine.
- The proof that apnea is due to irreversible medullary damage requires that the PCO_2 be high enough to stimulate respiration during a test of spontaneous breathing (apnea test).
- The possibility of profound drug-induced or hypothermic depression of the nervous system should be excluded, and some period of observation, usually 6 to 24 h, is desirable during which this state is shown to be sustained
- An isoelectric EEG may be used as a confirmatory test for total cerebral damage but is not absolutely necessary.
- In Nutshell:
  - ► Absent brain stem reflex **JIPMER 2005**
  - ► Absent motor activity **JIPMER 2005**
  - ► Coma
  - ► Puppilary dilatation. **PGI 2007**
  - ► Spinal cord reflexes + or –

⇨ Pain Scales

- Visual analogue scale (VAS) measures pain intensity☛☛
- Verbal and numerical rating scale☛
- Faces scale☛
- Cheops scale☛
- Mc Gill pain questionnaire☛☛

⇨ Dexmedetomine

Is a new drug which causes sedation without respiratory depression.

It Has:

- Sedative properties
- Analgesic properties
- Sympatholytic properties
- Anxiolytic properties

⇨ Intrapleural Analgesia

- Intrapleural analgesia **provides effective pain relief for many procedures, including upper abdominal and thoracic procedures.**
- Intrapleural analgesia involves placement of analgesic agents (usually a local anesthetic) in the intrapleural space, usually through a single shot or catheter.
- The action of intrapleural local anesthetic agents is believed to occur principally by diffusion through the parietal pleura to anesthetize the intercostal nerves.
- The close proximity of the thoracic sympathetic chain indicates that the sympathetic nervous system could be involved after an intrapleural blockade.
- However, little alteration of hemodynamic parameters has been noted, probably due to the unilateral nature of these blocks.

⇨ Transdermal Opioids

- **Transdermal fentanyl** has been approved for use in patients with cancer-induced pain.
- Fentanyl meets the criteria for use in a transdermal delivery system in that it is **both highly lipid soluble and potent enough for transdermal use.**
- The TTS is self-adhesive with a selectively permeable membrane, which comes in various sizes to vary the rate of delivery.
- These patches provide the predicted amount of medication in the range of 25 to 100 mg per hour.
- Because the skin is not uniform, the **rate of transfer varies with the site on which the patch is placed as well as the patient's gender, age, skin, blood flow, sweat gland activity, temperature, and pH of the skin.**
- Fever or local heating, such as the use of a heating pad, increases the release of fentanyl, which may precipitate respiratory depression.
- Respiratory depression, nausea, and vomiting all are reported side effects.

➲ Intravenous Patient-Controlled Analgesia: High Yield for 2011-2012

- PCA provides individualized opioid dosing without extensive nursing intervention.
- PCA allows patients to give themselves pain medication in a highly controlled manner.
- After analgesia has been established with a loading dose of opioid, patients give themselves small doses of opioids to maintain their level of analgesia.
- Reduced contact with the nursing staff and the patient's fear of inadvertently administering an overdose or of addiction to the opioid are potential disadvantages of PCA.
- Advantages of PCA are
  - **Immediate delivery of medication,** ☛☛
  - **Rapid onset of analgesia, and** ☛
  - **Patient control over pain medication.** ☛

- ❒ **Lockout Interval.** This is the period during which the PCA unit is refractory to further demands by the patient. The lockout interval is a needed safeguard to prevent patients from taking a further dose before they appreciate the full effect of the preceding dose.
- ❒ Opioid Selection. The ideal PCA agent would have a rapid onset of action with a medium duration of action. There should not be a ceiling to the analgesic effect, and the agent should not cause nausea, vomiting, or respiratory depression or impair bowel motility.
- ❒ **Morphine is one of the most commonly used analgesics for PCA**
- ❒ Meperidine is the other than morphine that has been approved by the Food and Drug Administration for PCA use.
- ❒ Fentanyl has been used extensively to provide postoperative analgesia. It has a more rapid onset than less lipid-soluble drugs but has extremely variable interpatient requirements. It does not release histamine, has no active metabolites, and has a paucity of other side effects.
- ❒ Other opioids that have been used successfully for PCA include **alfentanil, sufentanil, and hydromorphone.**
- ❒ Complications. The most-feared complication of opioid use is respiratory depression.

➲ Indications of Hypothermia:❋❋❋

- ❒ Neurosurgery☛☛
- ❒ Cardiac surgery☛☛ **PGI 1998**
- ❒ Carotid surgery☛☛
- ❒ ARDS☛
- ❒ Traumatic brain injury☛
- ❒ Malignant hyperthermia☛ **PGI 1998**
- ❒ Prolonged surgeries☛
- ❒ Procedures in which ischemia can occur☛
- ❒ Decreases EEG activity. **AIIMS 2006**

Drugs are associated with Hypothermia are: **AP 2007**

- ➨ Alcohol
- ➨ Amphetamine
- ➨ Chlorpromazine

➲ Neural Destruction: High Yield for 2011-2012

Neurectomy

- ➨ Transection of nerves to relieve pain.
- ➨ Neurectomy is used to treat painful neuromas
- ➨ A number of procedures have therefore been described to prevent this recurrence,
- ✓ **Separating the two nerve ends,**
- ✓ **Burying the nerve in muscle,**
- ✓ **Burying the nerve in bone, or covering the nerve with Silastic**

Rhizotomy

- Refers to **ablation of the sensory root.**
- This can be done either as an open procedure, intradurally or extradurally, or as a percutaneous procedure using radiofrequency coagulation or injection with phenol.
- Patients selected for rhizotomy undergo a **preoperative series of selective root blocks.** Subsequent pain relief does not guarantee equally successful surgical outcome.
- The most common indication is for rhizotomy pain following unsuccessful disk procedures.
- Example: **Retrogasserian Rhizotomy for Trigeminal Neuralgia**

Dorsal Root Entry Zone Lesioning

- Lesioning of the dorsal root entry zone (DREZ)
- Lissauer's tract and the dorsal horn gray matter are coagulated down to the Rexed V lamina, including the second-order neurons in the sensory and pain pathway. Lesions are made in line, close enough together so as to coalesce and produce a continuous zone of obliteration
- The greatest success is achieved for pain secondary to plexus avulsion and spinal cord injury.

Caudalis DREZ Coagulation

- **Nucleus caudalis DREZ coagulation** was introduced as an extension of DREZ lesioning
- The trigeminal nucleus caudalis contains second-order neurons subserving pain, temperature, and crude touch from the fifth, seventh, ninth, and tenth cranial nerves.

Cordotomy

- The goal is to **coagulate the spinothalamic tract in the anterior cord and ventral to the dentate ligament,** which can be visualized myelographically.
- Cordotomy is most useful in patients with cancer who have unilateral pain in the trunk or lower extremity; however, it is possible to treat upper extremity pain. Bilateral procedures should be separated by at least 2 weeks. Immediate pain relief is excellent in 95% of cases.

Myelotomy

- It consists of **splitting the spinal cord in a midline sagittal plane,** usually at and above the level of pain. Myelotomy is of particular value for bilateral and midline pain, especially pain involving the perineum. The resulting pain relief is widespread and often extends beyond the area of analgesia.

Midbrain Tractotomy

- Midbrain tractotomy consists of **stereotactic ablation of the spinothalamic tract at the level of the midbrain, just below the superior colliculus.** At this level, the tracts from the face and body are close to each other, with the face represented more medially. Tractotomy has been performed throughout the brain-stem, including the pons and the medulla.

Thalamotomy

- **Destructive lesions of the thalamus** are probably useful in relieving diffuse pain secondary to cancer or the intermittent neuralgic pain or allodynia and hyperpathia present in some patients with neural injury pain.

Sympathectomy

- **Sympathectomy is a unique form of neuroablation that is indicated for the treatment of causalgia, reflex sympathetic dystrophy, or Raynaud's phenomenon;**
- It is also used to relieve visceral pain, since afferent fibers from the viscera travel in the sympathetic nervous system.

➲ Bispectral Index (BIS): High Yield for 2011-2012

- Is one of several recently developed technologies **which purport to monitor depth of anesthesia.**

AIPGME 2012

- BIS monitors can replace or supplement Guedel's classification system for **determining depth of anesthesia.**
- Titrating anesthetic agents to a specific bispectral index during general anesthesia in adults (and children over 1 year old) **allows the anesthetist to adjust the amount of anesthetic agent to the needs of the patient,** possibly resulting in a more rapid emergence from anesthesia. Use of the **BIS monitor** may reduce the incidence of **intraoperative awareness in high risk procedures** or patients and may also have a role in predicting recovery from severe brain injury.

NOTES